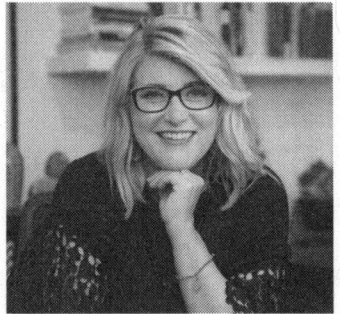

Bec Wilson is one of Australia's most respected authorities on midlife and modern retirement and an expert on modern ageing. She's the bestselling author of How to Have an Epic Retirement, the #1 retirement book in 2023 and 2024, and the founder of the Epic Retirement Institute, a trusted hub for retirement education, insights and tools.

She hosts the *Prime Time* podcast, produced by 9Podcasts, which is the ultimate guide to navigating the potential-filled years leading up to modern retirement, and writes a weekly newsletter at epicretirement.net that brings together an enormous community of pre-retirees and retirees.

Through the Epic Retirement Institute, Bec also runs the hugely popular six-week *How to Have an Epic Retirement* flagship course, and partners with super funds and companies to deliver retirement education that empowers people to plan wisely and live fully.

She writes a widely read syndicated finance column for *The Age, Sydney Morning Herald*, and other Nine newspapers, and manages the vibrant Facebook community, *The Epic Retirement Club*, with a rapidly growing global audience.

Bec is a mother of three teen and adult children, loves to travel and is in her own Prime Time – dreaming of her epic retirement, one day! To get in touch, visit becwilson.net.

becwilson.net
epicretirement.com.au
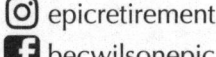 epicretirement
becwilsonepic

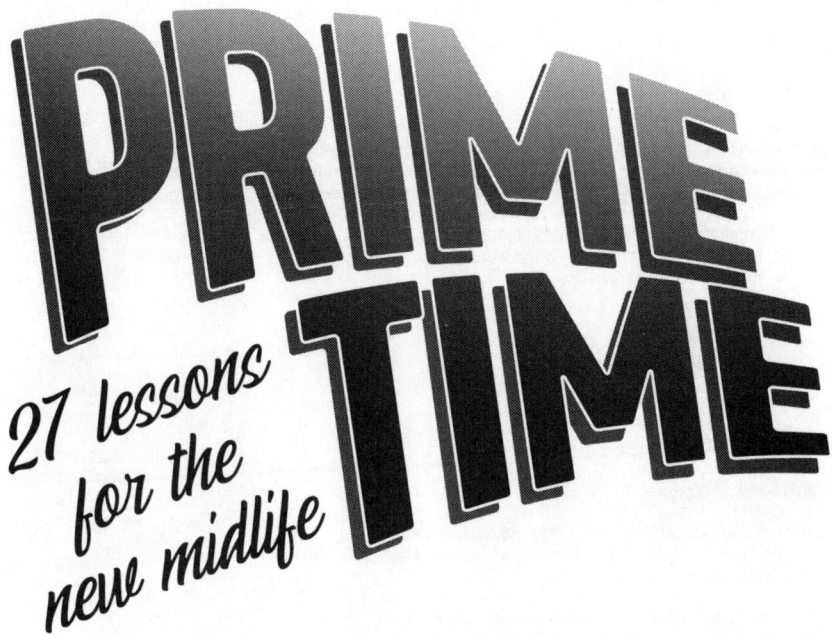

BEC WILSON

BESTSELLING AUTHOR OF
HOW TO HAVE AN EPIC RETIREMENT

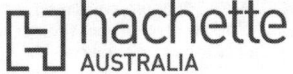

IMPORTANT NOTE TO READERS: Although every effort has been made to ensure that the information in this book is as accurate as possible, it must not be treated as a substitute for professional medical, psychological, psychiatric, financial or legal advice, and may not be appropriate for your particular circumstances. Neither the author nor the publisher should be held responsible for any loss or claim arising out of the use (or misuse) of any of the information in this book, or for any failure to take advice particular to your circumstances.

hachette
AUSTRALIA

Published in Australia and New Zealand in 2025
by Hachette Australia
(an imprint of Hachette Australia Pty Limited)
Gadigal Country, Level 17, 207 Kent Street, Sydney, NSW 2000
www.hachette.com.au

Hachette Australia acknowledges and pays our respects to the past, present and future Traditional Owners and Custodians of Country throughout Australia and recognises the continuation of cultural, spiritual and educational practices of Aboriginal and Torres Strait Islander peoples. Our head office is located on the lands of the Gadigal people of the Eora Nation.

Copyright © Epically Pty Ltd 2025

This book is copyright. Apart from any fair dealing for the purposes of private study, research, criticism or review permitted under the *Copyright Act 1968*, no part may be stored or reproduced by any process without prior written permission. Enquiries should be made to the publisher.

 A catalogue record for this book is available from the National Library of Australia

978 0 7336 5221 9 (paperback)

Cover design by Luke Causby / Blue Cork
Cover illustrations courtesy of Adobe Stock
Author photo by Shae Style Photography
Typeset in Optima by Kirby Jones
Printed and bound in Australia by McPherson's Printing Group

 The paper this book is printed on is certified against the Forest Stewardship Council® Standards. McPherson's Printing Group holds FSC® chain of custody certification SA-COC-005379. FSC® promotes environmentally responsible, socially beneficial and economically viable management of the world's forests.

Contents

Prologue		1
Part 1: Power		**9**
Lesson 1:	The shape of life as we all live it has changed	12
Lesson 2:	Retirement isn't the main goal anymore	20
Lesson 3:	Learn to make active choices that put you back in the centre of your picture	31
Part 2: Money		**35**
Lesson 4:	Stop taking financial shortcuts	38
Lesson 5:	Understand the foundations of financial confidence	45
Lesson 6:	Learn the new lessons of midlife money management: time, income and spending	164
Lesson 7:	Review your big financial picture and your budget	188
Lesson 8:	Work out how much is 'enough'	197
Lesson 9:	Get appropriate financial advice for your situation	208
Lesson 10:	Take a modern, proactive approach to your legacy	221
Bonus lesson: Reconsidering your insurances		239
Part 3: Work, purpose and happiness		**243**
Lesson 11:	Recognise the outdated models of work and retirement: understand your true options	249
Lesson 12:	Choose your path out of the workforce	275
Lesson 13:	Rediscover what brings you joy and fulfilment	282
Lesson 14:	Look beyond work to hobbies, pursuits and communities	288
Lesson 15:	Recognise transitions and embrace the journey they offer	294
Lesson 16:	Remind yourself that curiosity, learning and flexibility are crucial	299
Part 4: Health		**317**
Lesson 17:	Make your health your top priority	319
Lesson 18:	Learn how to age better according to science	338
Bonus lesson: Health insurance – the things no-one tells you		356

Part 5: Family and community — 359
Lesson 19: Prioritise your primary loving relationship — 361
Lesson 20: Revel in your gradually emptying nest — 369
Lesson 21: Give your parents a good last leg — 376

Part 6: Travel and adventure — 387
Lesson 22: Embrace challenge, adventure and active travel: understand your options — 389
Lesson 23: Seek out sabbaticals or 'golden gap years' – several times in your life — 403
Lesson 24: Get better value when you travel — 409
Lesson 25: Don't be afraid to travel solo — 421
Lesson 26: Understand travel money and insurance – and know what to watch out for — 424

Part 7: Taking action — 431
Lesson 27: Make your Prime Time count and prepare for an Epic Retirement — 433
Action and reflection plan — 436

Acknowledgements — 449
Endnotes — 454

Prologue

PUT THE CHANGING SHAPE OF YOUR LIFE INTO PERSPECTIVE

Both life and what we expect from it have changed. We're living longer, and we need to recognise and grab hold of the opportunities that come with that.

We used to think we understood the roadmap of life. You got an education, found a job, left home and started climbing the career ladder. Then, if you followed the map, you met a mate, got married, bought a house and started a family. As your family grew, you moved into a bigger house and progressed in your career, earning more. As a woman, you might have taken time out of the workforce to run the household, then jumped back in once the kids started school or the mortgage became too demanding.

Dutifully and responsibly, you raised your children to the point where they could find their independence, providing for their needs and shielding them from life's brutalities as much as possible.

In the middle of life, just when you thought things were getting good, you might have hit some speedbumps on the stereotypical journey – divorcing a partner, repartnering, or deciding to stay single. Or maybe you just rode out or managed the bumps.

Somewhere in your late 40s to mid 50s, you reached the pinnacle (or peak exhaustion point) of your first career. If you were lucky, you could see the last signs of your mortgage. Your kids got their P-plates and finished school, and you started to see yourself in the mirror again, as you no longer had to spend your days and evenings driving them around, serving their every single need.

Eventually, your kids left home, and you found yourself able to put some money away for your retirement, which still felt a fair way off. Then what? Do you wait? Work? Wonder what happens next? Start counting down? Is full retirement even the ultimate goal anymore?

This is what many of us have been taught by the media, family traditions and stereotypes. But if this is you, and you're a late 40-, 50- or 60-something looking into the years ahead, you might feel there's a blank space in this roadmap.

It feels like we've missed a step. In fact, it feels like we need to add a new section to the rulebook of life, one that comes before retirement. I'm calling it our Prime Time, and it starts when our kids get those P-plates and we start to see ourselves again. Or, if we never had kids, we might be ready to explore a new version of ourselves.

And it's a really interesting stage of life because, for the first time, thanks to the introduction of superannuation 33 years ago, we have a lot more choice about how we live our lives, and at the same time, fewer expectations are placed on us, both personally and societally.

So let's talk about it and shape some new lessons that encourage us to take advantage of it. Let's make our Prime Time count.

UNDERSTANDING THE PILLARS OF YOUR PRIME TIME

This new stage of life calls for a fresh perspective, so I've written a book that takes everything into consideration. It's not a finance book, but it covers your money, and it's not a self-help book, but it teaches you how to help yourself. Ultimately, it's a guidebook that points to the choices you have, explains the new-world ways of looking at them, and inspires *you* to make more active choices. It's like a choose-your-own-adventure book, but it's about real life – your life and the exciting years you have ahead of you.

I've drawn together scientific insights, expert advice, factual information and street-smart lessons from everyday people to make a book that you can hopefully enjoy, learn from and share. I warn you – it's practical. If you read it and do nothing, you'll feel bad. But that's the point. I want you to be inspired and then take action to live the best second half of life possible.

This book is built on six pillars and 27 lessons – essential midlife lessons to make life better than you ever imagined. Each pillar is key to creating a well-rounded, fulfilling life. Let me introduce them.

POWER

You need to recognise the power you have to make the years ahead the best years of your life yet. Recognise the choices you have, understand that your current decision-making templates are broken, and embrace being a little more selfish – in the right ways.

MONEY

There are a lot of financial decisions that, if made well in midlife, can change everything. It's time to learn about them – and to start doing money better.

WORK, PURPOSE AND HAPPINESS

Find what drives you and makes you feel alive in this stage of life. Explore new ways to work, connect with purpose, and find happiness in what you do every day. Midlife is the time to redefine success on your own terms.

HEALTH

Your health is your top priority in midlife. Look after it so your body can keep up with everything your mind and spirit want to do. Use the science of modern ageing and take a preventive approach to stay strong for the years ahead.

FAMILY AND COMMUNITY

Nurture the relationships that matter most. Midlife is a chance to rekindle that spark, support loved ones, create lasting memories and embrace your emptying nest. Family is your foundation in the next phase – invest in it.

TRAVEL AND ADVENTURE

Discover all the ways you can push your boundaries with travel in midlife – and how to get the best value from every dollar you spend on it.

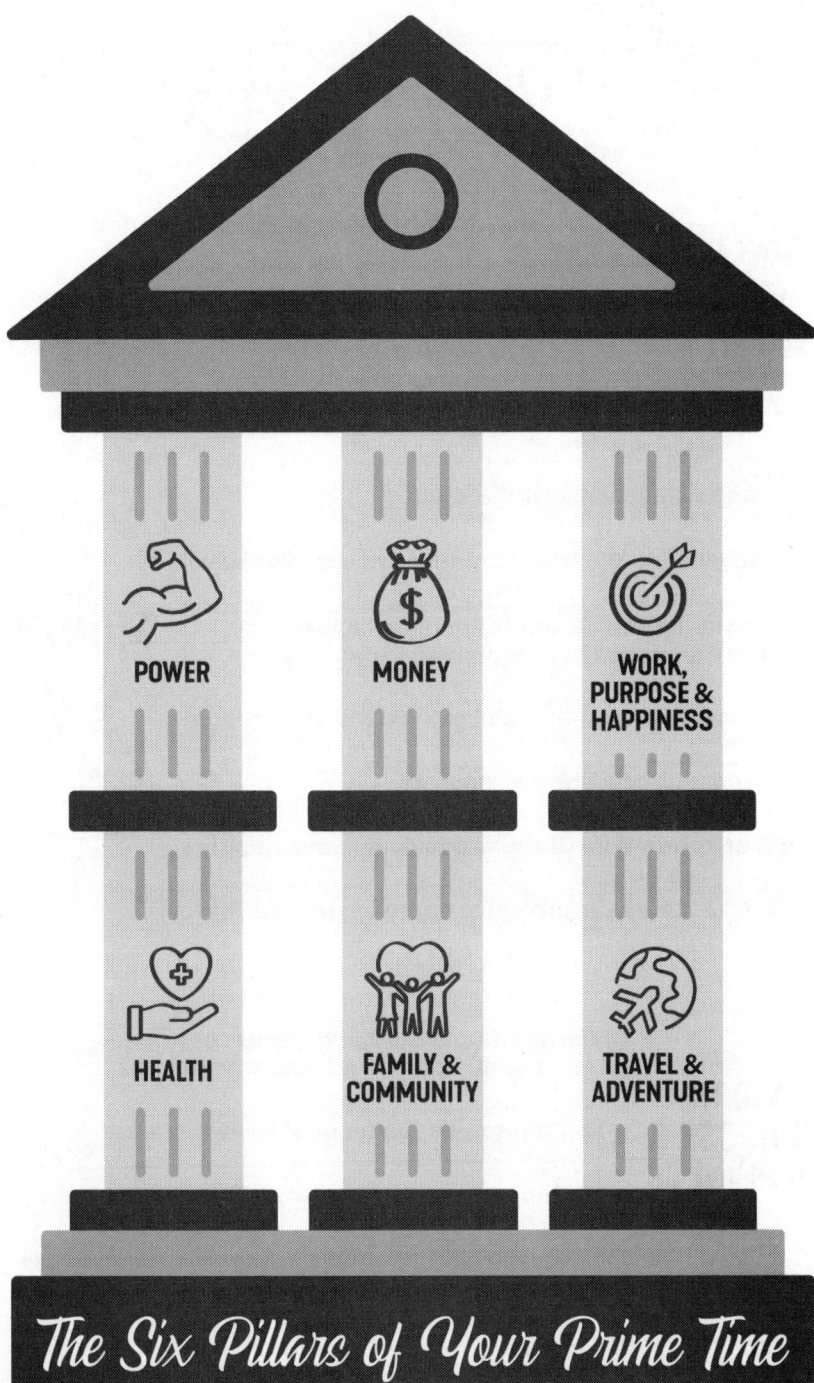

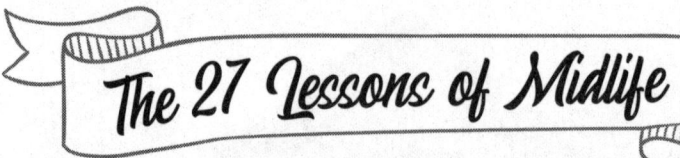

The 27 Lessons of Midlife

ONE: POWER

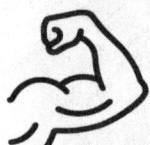

1. The shape of life as we all live it has changed
2. Retirement isn't the main goal anymore
3. Learn to make active choices that put you back in the centre of your picture

TWO: MONEY

4. Stop taking financial shortcuts
5. Understand the foundations of financial confidence
6. Learn the new lessons of midlife money management: time, income and spending
7. Review your big financial picture and your budget
8. Work out how much is 'enough'
9. Get appropriate financial advice for your situation
10. Take a modern, proactive approach to your legacy

Bonus lesson: Reconsidering your insurances

THREE: WORK, PURPOSE & HAPPINESS

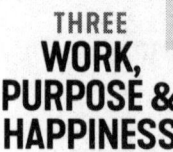

11. Recognise the outdated models of work & retirement: understand your true options
12. Choose your path out of the workforce
13. Rediscover what brings you joy and fulfilment
14. Look beyond work to hobbies, pursuits & communities
15. Recognise transitions & embrace the journey they offer
16. Remind yourself that curiosity, learning & flexibility are crucial

FOUR
HEALTH

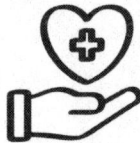

17 Make your health your top priority

18 Learn how to age better according to science

Bonus lesson: Health insurance – the things no-one tells you

FIVE
FAMILY & COMMUNITY

19 Prioritise your primary loving relationship

20 Revel in your gradually emptying nest

21 Give your parents a good last leg

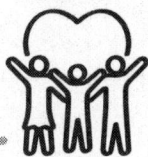

SIX
TRAVEL & ADVENTURE

22 Embrace challenge, adventure & active travel: understand your options

23 Seek out sabbaticals or 'golden gap years' – several times in your life

24 Get better value when you travel

25 Don't be afraid to travel solo

26 Understand travel money & insurance – & know what to watch out for

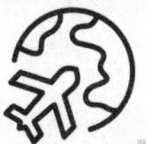

SEVEN
TAKING ACTION

27 Make your Prime Time count & prepare for an Epic Retirement

Part 1
POWER

YOU NEED TO UNDERSTAND WHERE POWER COMES FROM AT THIS STAGE OF LIFE, because it's different now. In your 30s and 40s, power came from hierarchy, achievements and the approval of others. But in your 50s and 60s, power shifts. Real power now comes from within, and you're in the driver's seat.

True power in midlife means understanding the choices you have and actively making them, staying curious, being open to learning, and growing. It's about recognising the impact of the right strategic decisions and knowing what genuinely matters to you – what brings joy and fulfilment, what earns you money, and what makes life meaningful – and then choosing to invest your time, money and energy in those. It's about doing things for the right reasons, not because someone else is expecting it.

This stage of life takes years to reach and it brings a kind of power that's uniquely yours. Now is the time to enjoy that on your terms. When you think about the power you have, but perhaps haven't embraced yet, I want you to think about six types.

THE POWER OF CHOICE

As the kids become more independent, so do you. This new freedom lets you make choices in a way you haven't for a long time, and with a clearer sense of self. Now you can choose how to spend your time, who to spend it with and what to focus on. Every decision reflects your values, rather than obligations or others' expectations.

THE POWER OF KNOWING YOURSELF AND YOUR VALUES

Looking within to explore what you truly value, enjoy and find important can be challenging, but this is the perfect time of life to do it. Knowledge of your strengths, weaknesses and what lights you up is a powerful tool, allowing you to approach life with confidence and purpose. When you understand yourself deeply, you can focus on what brings genuine joy and fulfilment – and you can make better choices.

THE POWER OF STRATEGIC FINANCIAL ACTIONS

In your late 40s, 50s and 60s, you have the chance to make financial moves that can reshape your wealth, even if you're starting with little. Maximising your retirement contributions, leveraging tax benefits, balancing growth with stability, leaning into home ownership and clearing any lingering debts can all have a big impact. It's about making smart choices now to give yourself a wealthier, more flexible Prime Time and an Epic Retirement.

THE POWER OF LETTING GO

Real power comes from knowing what *not* to hold onto. Letting go of old expectations, outdated definitions of success or the need to please others can feel like a superpower. It frees up your energy to focus on things that actually matter to you. Imagine the weight lifted when you're no longer trying to meet others' expectations and standards but are fully focused on what feels right for you and what you want from life.

THE POWER OF PURPOSEFUL ACTION

At this stage, everything you do can carry more intention. You're free to move beyond the busywork of just getting ahead and start taking action that truly aligns with your goals, values and wellbeing, even if you haven't been able to before now. Every choice can be a deliberate, purposeful step toward a life that feels rich and meaningful.

THE POWER OF CONTINUAL GROWTH

Staying curious, open and committed to learning keeps you connected to your power. When you see midlife as a chance to grow rather than settle, you stay energised and engaged. This might mean taking on new challenges, exploring passions or simply learning more about what makes you happy. Growth becomes part of what empowers you to live a better life.

To truly lean into your power in midlife, there are three big lessons to understand:
1. **The shape of life has changed**: The old templates of life don't apply anymore; the journey of midlife is full of new options, directions, and ways to define success.
2. **Retirement isn't the ultimate goal**: Instead of just winding down, think of this time as an opportunity to deepen your experience, find purpose and live fully.
3. **Learn to make active choices**: This is your time to put yourself back in the centre of your picture, making choices that are right for *you*.

Let's dive into each of these.

Lesson 1
The shape of life as we all live it has changed

THE SHAPE OF LIFE HAS CHANGED FUNDAMENTALLY WHILE WE'VE ALL BEEN LIVING IT. Think about it.

Someone born today moves into a childhood that lasts maybe until they're 10–12 years old. That's much shorter than it used to be. In my opinion, childhood ends when you get handed your first iPhone, fully loaded with one or even two social media accounts. At this point, the outside world comes into your life in an uncurated and unrestricted manner that your parents really struggle to control. (And it's doubtful any government age limit will be able to control it for them.) That's when you become a teenager. And your teenage years last a lot longer than they used to!

To me, the teenage years are those years when your parents look after your expenses but you're stepping gradually toward emotional independence. Skyrocketing housing prices in our major cities today mean many children live with their parents, with their expenses subsidised or even fully supported until their mid to late 20s. That's not just impacting the teenager's life but also their parents' lives, limiting their ability to 'cut loose' and launch into their own next stage.

Then the teenager moves into adulthood, working their way through the list of stereotypical steps in young-adult life – building a career, finding a mate, buying a home and paying a mortgage, growing a family, and juggling obligations. Meanwhile, the parents of that child step into this new phase I've coined their Prime Time, where they have quite a bit of financial firepower because the money they have been spending on their kids is now gradually freed up for themselves, and they have less need to meet 'society's expectations' because there are less of them – if any. Many have already achieved the key milestones in their careers, while others are on track for fulfilling roles they can maintain through their 50s and 60s. This is the time when they can start redefining their next set of goals, shaping a future that's focused more on what they want for themselves.

This is not a stage of life that can be defined by age, because your Prime Time can really only kick off when your children become more independent and your financial obligations toward them lessen. If you had children later in life, then your Prime Time will probably begin later in life.

And if you never had children, then you might find you never really 'lost yourself' in the stereotypical parenting roles and lengthy process of supporting teenagers into their 20s. And, alongside this, your level of ongoing financial self-orientation has allowed you to retain the ability to freely choose throughout your life – something many parents can't say they've been able to do. But you may still enjoy a Prime Time priority shift.

No matter how you look at it, though, your entry into Prime Time is marked by an increasing feeling of having more time, adequate financial resources to make more choices, and a desire to seek greater fulfilment in life.

If you embrace it, your Prime Time can be a long window of your life, possibly the longest stage of life you've lived so far. I see it extending from when your adult children get their P-plates, even if they continue to live in your home, all the way through to your active or epic retirement – the time when you give up work completely and forever. These can be the best years of your independent life.

Your Prime Time is a phase of life that has several stages within it.

There are some years when you knuckle down and save hard, taking advantage of your empty nest's lower costs. I call these your *set-up years*. Then there are your *lifestyling years*, when you work passionately, mostly full-time, but start to push more lifestyle into your life. You might take longer holidays or sabbaticals, enjoy a long weekend each month, or adopt a more flexible work structure that fits around your priorities. Then there are your *part-time years*, when you start to step back the volume of work you do and pick up more leisure activities.

Then, as your Prime Time ends, you move into your active or *epic retirement years* when you've stopped working and you fill your life with living. And, if you're healthy, happy and have financial confidence, none of these years are boring.

After your epic retirement come two more life stages you need to be cognisant of, passive retirement and frailty, neither of which are the focus of this book, but you do need to plan for them. The fact is that while we are in our Prime Time, we're often managing our parents through these two stages of life, so that's when we become more familiar with them.

And that's it – seven phases of modern life to think about:
- Childhood
- Teenage years
- Adulthood
- Prime Time (incorporating set-up years, lifestyling years, part-time years)
- Epic Retirement
- Passive retirement, or ageing years
- Frailty.

STOP AND THINK ABOUT HOW LONG LIFE REALLY IS

There's a huge space in the roadmap of life chiefly because one thing has changed – our life expectancies. Over the last 50 years, we've added between 15 and 25 years to modern life expectancies, and, if health advancements progress at the pace of recent decades, we can expect this trend to continue.

Actuaries in Australia expect that today's 50-year-olds, if they make it through to the age of 65, a critical age used in projecting life expectancy, will have a median life expectancy of 90 for men, 92 for women and 95 if they're part of a couple. But men also have a one in four chance of living to 95 and women to 96, and if they're part of a couple, one of them should plan to live to 98.[1]

Life expectancy really does reshape our lives and how we live them.

And I have good news: in recent times, the number of years we spend in poorer health at the end of our lives hasn't really changed that much as a percentage of our lifespan. In the 2022 Australian Burden of Disease Study, the Australian Government said men should expect to spend 88 per cent of their lives in good or full health, while for women the figure was 87 per cent.[2] That puts most people well into their 80s before their health declines and they need to stay closer to regular healthcare services.

The big message I want you to hear is that all those years we've added to our life expectancy are productive, healthy years. We didn't just add 15–25 years to our life expectancy over 50 years. We added those 15–25 years to our Prime Time of life.

TAKE A MOMENT TO UNDERSTAND YOUR OWN LIFE EXPECTANCY

There are a few different ways to approach life expectancy, and I want you to be aware of them all – especially the ones that tend to be underestimated – so you can plan properly for your future.

First, there are the standard Australian Bureau of Statistics (ABS) 'life tables', which are often quoted in the media. According to these, the life expectancy for a 65-year-old today is 85.2 years for men and 88 for women. But let's be honest. These numbers don't account for improvements in health, wealth and living standards, so they can underestimate how long you might live.

A better option is to use the life tables with the 25-year mortality improvement adjustment applied by the Australian Government Actuary. These tell a more realistic story: a 65-year-old today has a

50 per cent chance of living to 88 if they're a man, 91 if they're a woman, and 95 if they're part of a couple. Even more impressively, there's a one in four chance you could live to 94 as a man, 94 as a woman and 97 as a couple.[3]

For the most personalised approach, you could try a life expectancy calculator that takes into account your own health, wealth and happiness. There is one on my website, created by some clever actuaries, which you can try for free – visit becwilson.net/lifeex. It'll give you a much more tailored projection, and all the options if you decide you have a greater than 50 per cent chance of living longer than the median.

Take a moment to lock in the number that feels right for you. This will help you form a clearer vision of your future and make better decisions for the years ahead.

THINK ABOUT THE LIFE YOU HAVE AHEAD OF YOU

Now we're going to get personal. I want you to think about where you are on the roadmap of life. Consider how many years you have ahead of you and contemplate what is really important to you as you move through the different stages of your Prime Time. These are your years of choice, excitement and adventure.

To kick them off, we need to plan for the different phases of our Prime Time:
- Our set-up years
- Our lifestyle years
- Our part-time years.

Then, we plan toward our epic retirement, a crucial phase of the picture we have to build.

THE SET-UP YEARS

The first job you have in midlife, once the kids get their P-plates and you hopefully find yourself with a few more dollars in your budget and more hours in your day, is to get yourself set up. This is a four-part process.

First, you'll want to set yourself up financially, understanding your tipping point – when you will 'have enough' money coming in to relax, meet your obligations, make some healthy savings, and start to enjoy life a little more without sabotaging the finances you'll need to retire.

Second, you'll want to set yourself up purposefully by checking in on your work and career. Ask yourself whether your current job is what you want to be doing for the rest of your life.

Third, you'll want to set yourself up with good health practices, knowing that people who enter their 50s with good health practices age much better than those who do not.

Finally, you'll want to set yourself up socially, making an effort to find and maintain quality relationships with people you have things in common with.

All of these things are essential ingredients for longer, healthier and more satisfying lives. We'll cover each of them in more detail throughout the book, so hold on.

THE LIFESTYLING YEARS

This is the period when you gloriously juggle full-time work or a portfolio of projects that resemble a full-time workload. Alongside that, you have a real sense of purpose and leisure, actively balancing both. You're making enough money to save and compound for retirement and live the lifestyle you want to today. You've knocked over most of the mortgage and can see when you'll get there.

In these years, you find a rhythm that works for you, blending work and play in a way that feels fulfilling. You might pursue hobbies, travel, or invest time in personal projects, all while maintaining a satisfying employed life. This balance allows you to enjoy the present while preparing for a secure future.

THE PART-TIME YEARS

These are the years when you actively decide to start working less and living more. Some people remain in this stage for up to a decade, earning some income from work and supplementing it with a transition to retirement superannuation income stream, or, if they are over 65, a superannuation pension.

It's much easier to adapt to the idea of retiring if you don't have to do it overnight or, even worse, by force – whether through redundancy, being stood down, or health issues. Many people who retire initially find themselves working again, so it's more fitting to describe these years as our 'part-time years' than our retirement.

If you want to convert your superannuation to the retirement phase during this time, you need to meet the conditions of release, having reached the age of 60 and ceased gainful employment – at least long enough to fill out the forms. Because this doesn't stop you from starting work again – in fact, more people than ever are doing this.

YOUR EPIC RETIREMENT YEARS

Eventually, most of us give up working entirely, entering what I refer to as 'full retirement'. This is a time when you no longer engage in paid work of any kind – no Uber driving, no consulting, no Christmas stints as Santa Claus at the local shopping centre. Instead, you live off a combination of your superannuation, investments and quite possibly the age pension.

However, entering active retirement doesn't mean you're stopping. On the contrary, this phase is often filled with important and purposeful projects. You might volunteer, pursue hobbies, travel or engage in community activities. The key difference is that you're not seeking payment for these endeavours anymore; you do them for the sense of meaning and fulfilment they bring.

The epic retirement years are about enjoying the fruits of your labour, maintaining your health and wellbeing, and continuing to find purpose and joy in everyday life.

AFTER THAT

As your health begins to decline, you enter what some might call passive retirement – the first stage of what I consider true ageing, when you start to slip out of the more epic years of retirement. For some, this stage begins in their 70s, while for others it might not occur until their 80s or even early 90s.

Then, as we continue to age and decline in health, we will likely become frail as we head toward the end of life. Unless we die early, these are realities that we can't change, but we can try to delay or reduce their impact by being proactive with our health and social connections during our prime time years.

THERE'VE BEEN NO RULES ... UNTIL NOW

When you stop and think about it, there really are no clear societal rules or expectations for the second half of our lives, except perhaps the outdated perception that we retire and that our health gradually slips away not long after.

That's why I've written a new guidebook for the second half of life – with 27 lessons to help you live well and make your Prime Time count. I've also put together practical activities and how-to tools so you can take those lessons off the page and into your everyday life.

Lesson 2
Retirement isn't the main goal anymore

WHEN I SPEAK TO OTHERS OF MY GENERATION, I FREQUENTLY HEAR QUITE contrasting and contradictory stories.

Sharon, who's 53, says to me, 'Bec, I never want to retire. I just want more flexibility in my life so I don't have to do the stuff I don't enjoy and I'm not that good at.' Sharon loves her job, finds enormous satisfaction in her work, and she's good at it. She's recently restructured her role, asking her company for extra support so she can be more flexible. With their backing, she's starting to really enjoy long weekends and 'working from home' days from her Gold Coast apartment, and three- to four-day weeks in the office. She's embracing her prime time lifestyling phase with long holidays overseas twice a year too.

Geoff, who's 49, says to me, 'Bec, I'm done. I could retire tomorrow and I'd never miss working. And it would probably not miss me.' Geoff works in a declining sector, where he's treated like a number by his employers. He used to enjoy his job when his industry was thriving and his career was on the rise, but now it's turned into a thankless task. He's not even 50 yet and he certainly can't afford to retire. Recently retrenched, he's taken a job he wouldn't have chosen in the same industry for financial security. He doesn't know how to transform his work into something he looks forward to. Geoff could continue like this for some time, or he could face his set-up phase head-on and start looking for new ways to achieve fulfilment, and perhaps seek out a next-phase career. It's not an easy thing to do, but it may well be worth it.

Annie, who's 56, shared with me a different approach. She's not ready to retire, but she's also not chasing promotions or career advancement like she used to. She tells me, 'Bec, I'm focused on finding balance now. I don't want to keep climbing the ladder just because it's expected of me. I'm content with where I am career-wise, but I want to spend more time on my passions and hobbies.' Annie works part-time as a counsellor, having negotiated a flexible arrangement with her company. She dedicates her extra time to gardening, volunteering at a local charity, and travelling with her partner. She's not trying to leave the workforce entirely, but she's transitioned into a phase where she's building a lifestyle she enjoys while still earning a comfortable income. 'I like having something to work on, but I'm glad I don't feel tied to the job anymore,' she explains. Like Sharon, Annie is embracing her Prime Time, but in her own unique way – focusing on life beyond just work.

The fact that Sharon, Geoff and Annie all have different views on retirement highlights the diversity in how people approach this stage of life. Sharon is reshaping her role to enjoy more flexibility while still thriving in her career. Geoff, on the other hand, feels disillusioned with work and is ready to step away entirely, but can't. Meanwhile, Annie is carving out a balance between part-time work and a lifestyle focused on her passions. What stands out to me is that retirement doesn't need to be the ultimate goal for everyone. For many, like Sharon and Annie, it's about creating a fulfilling life now, during their prime time years, rather than waiting for some distant retirement dream. Geoff, however, faces a turning point, needing to decide where to direct his energy and passion next. The reality is that most Australians won't fully retire until their mid 60s, and many will continue working in some capacity even longer. If life at 50 or 60 isn't fulfilling, it's too long to wait for 'the good times'. Wishing away the best years for retirement is a missed opportunity when you can start shaping the life you want today.

So let's aim to make our whole Prime Time count. Learn how to make the most of it today, while still being excited for and planning that Epic Retirement tomorrow. A long, fulfilling, healthy and engaged Prime Time comes before those truly epic retirement years – and it's important to recognise that they *are* different phases. In fact, we should all be excited about these two significant and new phases of life that lie ahead.

But if we want a fulfilling Prime Time that starts long before we retire, we need to build a clearer picture of the years ahead, set some goals, and start creating that life we want to live. Then we need to really enjoy living it.

RETHINKING YOUR VISION

Back in the mid 2000s, a number of scientists led by academic and economist David Blanchflower studied the happiness of more than 500,000 people in the Western world and concluded that our wellbeing or happiness as a population reaches an all-time low somewhere around 47 years of age. This is known as the 'U-shaped curve of happiness', and thousands of scientists have since tried to disprove it, without meaningful success.[4] In fact, Blanchflower revised this data in a much wider study in 2021 to confirm that the low point can now be observed in more than 145 countries in the world, but that because of increases to life expectancies, the low arrives later than originally observed in most western economies.[5] He says that the low in happiness is now being seen at between 50 and 55 years of age.

This low point lines up with the time of life we traditionally associate with the idea of having a midlife crisis, when people might be under greater stress, have become dissatisfied with their lives or are feeling significantly more unhappy. Many don't know why they feel this way; they just know they aren't getting the satisfaction they used to derive from the things they do. The gloss of life has worn off.

If you think about it, there's plenty of logic to why this happens.

We usually progress through our early years with clear, societally set goals, and in the main, people are happy as they achieve them.

There's a great feeling that comes from 'reaching your goals', that's for sure. Our happiness peaks in our early to mid 30s as we achieve milestones in our families and careers. Then, as life becomes more challenging, more tiring and more complex, we often struggle, and for many of us, our happiness declines. In our late 40s to mid 50s, most of us are at the point where life is placing maximum pressure on us, either to achieve more or to make ends meet. Some of us have been successful time and time again and find the excitement just isn't there anymore. Others are tired – really, really tired. We are at the bottom of that U-curve of happiness that many don't even know exists.

Scientists point to three things that fundamentally change for people in this phase of life that sit behind this drop in happiness.

WE ADJUST OUR EXPECTATIONS

We start our lives excited, optimistic and energised about our future. But as life rolls toward midlife, we become increasingly realistic about what we want and expect from our lives and settle into a more down-to-earth set of goals that really might make us happier. We lose our youthful naivety and replace it with pragmatism and sensibleness. It might be because we recognise that the things we've achieved in life haven't actually made us that happy and we can see the need for reprioritisation. Or it might be that we've hit a speed bump and have to change direction. Either way, our expectations of life change and we start to want different things.

WE ADAPT OUR AMBITIONS

As I've mentioned throughout this chapter, by midlife, many of the traditional goals of life have been hit (or not hit) and we've recognised those achievements. Then, we might become jaded about how the constant chasing of professional goals doesn't yield greater satisfaction. And we sensibly start to look beyond workplace success to our values, relationships and sense of meaning, refocusing on personal and community goals that yield a different type of reward – a sense of belonging and purpose.

OUR BRAINS REWIRE THEMSELVES

After midlife, scientists say that our brains start to rewire themselves and become better at managing conflicting emotions. Rather delightfully, they start to react better to positive emotions than negative emotions. This naturally makes us happier and happier as we age, having a huge impact on our self-esteem, confidence and motivation. It's called the positivity effect of ageing.

This is why our 50s are the low point. After these changes to our brain chemistry, our expectations and our ambitions, we usually see an ongoing uptick in our happiness.

Ultimately, what I'm trying to say is that this time of life can be a critical period to reconsider your priorities, if life hasn't already forced you to do so. And you do that by re-exploring your vision of what life looks like in your Prime Time.

THINK ABOUT THESE THINGS

- Who are the people who really matter?
- What do you want to be doing with your time?
- How do you want to be earning money?
- Where will you find fulfilment and belonging in the future?

This is *your* Prime Time, not your boss's or your partner's, and if you aren't prioritising what you want out of it, I can assure you that no-one else will.

It's only after you've stewed on your priorities, and whether they need to change, that you can think about setting goals for yourself in your Prime Time. Let's assume you're ready and go forward.

SETTING YOUR GOALS

Goals really are underrated in midlife. Many of us think we're past the stage of life where having detailed goals matter. But if that's you, then I think you're wrong. Sure, you can 'coast' along if you're happy with where you are in life, but without goals, you're essentially leaving your future up to chance.

Scientifically, a goal is recognised as a desired outcome that wouldn't otherwise happen without some kind of intervention.[6] That is, it's a detour from the path of least resistance in our lives. That makes goals pretty important if we're trying to be actively engaged in what happens in our lives. But when you really dig down, goals are even more important than that.

When we set a goal, we're really saying to ourselves that we want to put the effort in to achieve something that hasn't happened yet and isn't likely to happen on its own. Goals are usually things that we think we will have trouble achieving, so we *need* to define them and work toward them. When we set out to pursue a goal, we usually have to do something differently – create new behaviours, try new activities or foster new knowledge in our lives.

It makes sense, doesn't it. If we want to achieve something, we need to visualise it, set it as a goal, then invest in it, potentially both emotionally and financially, working through the inevitable struggles to strive for the outcome.

It stands to reason that the gap we encounter in midlife and early in the second half of life, where we lack clear goals, can lead to a drop in motivation. And the way out is to set goals, of course. This puts us back in the game of life, striving for things we want to achieve that otherwise would probably not happen to us.

'If you can't see it, you can't be it' is a motivational quote we often hear in workplaces and feminist and racial prejudice conversations. In reality it applies beautifully to midlife too. If we can't see the excitement we want from life, the goals we want to achieve and the sense of fulfilment we aspire to, we can't chase it, strive for it and then enjoy it.

Whether you're 48 or 58 or 68, once you've reconsidered your priorities, put yourself back in the centre of your picture and build a vision of the life ahead of you. The first thing you need to do is set some goals.

Again, I want to remind you that the goals you set are yours. For the first time in your life, they don't have to be socially accepted or hierarchical. You don't need to impress anyone with them except yourself (you don't need to post them on Facebook, LinkedIn or

Instagram). They can't be pulled from any rulebook of life because life has never had a Prime Time before.

So let's get practical and start setting the goals we want to achieve, knowing we might have half our lives ahead of us.

RELATIONSHIP AND COMMUNITY GOALS

Our relationships in the second half of life are important. In fact, science tells us that they are the single most important aspect of life. The Harvard Study of Adult Development, the longest longitudinal study of happiness in the western world,[7] had two key insights: loneliness kills us earlier; and the quality of our social and loving relationships profoundly impacts our health, longevity and happiness.

So I want you to think about the people who are critical to your life's happiness now and in the future. Who are the essential people in your life, the ones who bring you happiness and joy, and what are your goals for those relationships?

- Do you have a partner you share your life with? How do you want this relationship to work in the next phase of your life? Do you want to invest more time, effort or energy in this relationship?
- Do you have a close family that you care for and maintain relationships with purposefully? Do you want to enrich your family connections?
- Do you have friends who are important to you? How do you want to include those friendships in your life?
- Do you feel like you are part of a community or several different communities that you want to prioritise? Set yourself some specific goals around each community and the way you want to involve yourself – or, if there are no communities, in how you might like to build some.
- Or, do you need to do more work on the people part of your life? Again, be specific. If you are single and alone and you don't want to be, don't feel like this leaves you out. Instead, recognise that a life shared with others is often more fulfilling and set some friendship and relationship goals that inspire you.

FINANCIAL GOALS

Later, we'll explore your financial set-up in much greater detail using principles for addressing money in your Prime Time. But for now, I want you to think about the money you have and the way you want to use it in the life ahead of you. Just start to create a realistic vision that you can lean into as we talk about money.

When you think about money, I want you to divide the rest of your life into five phases:

1. **Your set-up years**: These are the years when you lay the foundation for your future, setting financial goals, building good habits and getting on track for the life you want.
2. **Your lifestyle years**: Once your finances are in good shape, you can enjoy more freedom – travel, hobbies and experiences – while still working full-time, rather than deferring everything until later.
3. **Your part-time years**: A transition phase where you slow down work on your terms, reducing hours but staying engaged in meaningful activities.
4. **Your Epic Retirement**: The years when you've fully stepped away from work and are embracing life on your terms – whether that's travel, adventure, learning or just more time for what matters most.
5. **Your passive retirement and, later, your frailty**: As health declines, your focus shifts from lifestyle to managing your wellbeing and financial security, ensuring you have the right support in place.

Then consider:
- What debts do you want to have paid off, and by when?
- How do you want to make money in each phase of your life ahead?
- How much will be made actively, from working?
- How much will be made passively, from investing?
- How affluently or frugally do you want to spend your money in each phase?

- How much income do you need to cover your costs of living in each phase of your life?
- How much do you want to spend on lifestyle and experiences – again, in each phase?
- What is your financial tipping point – so, how much do you need in savings inside and outside superannuation to be able to live the life you want to without ever having to work again? And when do you project you can reach that tipping point?
- What is an ideal amount of money to have invested outside superannuation to support your passive income desires before you retire and/or can access superannuation?
- What is the target amount of money you want to have inside superannuation to support you after you technically retire or reach the age of 65, when you can access your superannuation unconditionally?

I don't expect you to have the answers to these questions yet – you can come back to them later.

HEALTH GOALS

The data on healthy ageing points to the reality that people who come into midlife with good health practices – those who manage their stress, do moderate to vigorous exercise regularly, apply effort to improving their lean muscle mass, eat a healthy and nutritious diet, and have been conscious about posture and movement – tend to live longer than those who don't.[8] Knowing this makes it easier to set some goals for your future health:

- What do you need to work on to build and maintain a healthy body?
- What do you need to work on for better mental health and agility?
- What do you want for your health in the second half of your life and what are you willing to do to achieve that?
- What metrics in your body do you want to monitor to be more aware of the warning signs of chronic disease and what will your approach to prevention be?

CONSIDER YOUR INTERESTS AND YOUR CURIOSITY

Curiosity is such a fundamental part of our lives yet we often overlook it. If you take time to reflect, you might notice that your curiosity isn't as strong as it once was. Curiosity manifests in various ways, such as through an interest in exploration, play, learning, or even a simple hunger for information. It's an intrinsic quality, driven by internal motivation,[9] which becomes especially important to nurture during midlife. So take a moment to consider your goals for your curiosity, and how you can encourage and embrace it.

- What are you curious about or interested in? What do you read? Practise? Expand your knowledge of? Take lessons in?
- What do you want to learn?
- How will you grow your curiosity in your Prime Time rather than let it shrink?

RECONSIDER YOUR PURPOSE

In the early years of our lives, many of us chase goals related to status and money, driven by societal expectations or the ambitions our parents set for us. But by midlife, there can be a hollowness in these, whether we are successful or not, giving us a reason to reflect on what our purpose really could be in the next phase of our lives.

Reflecting on your sense of purpose and fulfilment involves a process in which you actively consider your present and future life, set goals for important areas – social, career and leisure time[10] – and, if required, make concrete plans and undertake actions to align these more closely with your current and future values and wishes.

- Does the work you do give you a sense of purpose and fulfilment?
- How much money do you need to earn from working to meet your prime time and retirement financial goals? Is this realistic and achievable?
- Do you need or want to make changes to your work? What goals do you seek to achieve through these changes?
- What do you do that you are deeply passionate about?

- What do you do for leisure or fun? Is it enough? Are there other things you would like to pursue?

THINK ABOUT YOUR LIFESTYLE AND LEISURE GOALS

When I talk about lifestyle and leisure, I mean the big things you want to plan and look forward to, like holidays, celebrations, experiences and education, *and* the smaller moments and joys in life that you want to prioritise, like your hobbies and pursuits, activities you want to do regularly, and little joys you want to cultivate. All too often we forget how important our day-to-day activities and practices are in driving quality long-term happiness. So let's set some lifestyle and leisure goals:

- Think about the big travel and leisure goals you have for the next one year, three years, five years and ten years of your life. Then look ahead even further. List those big things you're going to plan for and look forward to.
- Now think about the pursuits or hobbies that you want to prioritise, the activities that you want to learn more about and invest yourself in.
- And finally, think about some daily or weekly practices and activities that you want to commit to.

Now that you've put some thought into your goals, and looked at them through many different lenses, you are ready to contemplate the next 25 lessons of the second half of life, knowing you are in the driver's seat.

Lesson 3

Learn to make active choices that put you back in the centre of your picture

WHEN THE KIDS HAVE GOT THOSE P-PLATES AND THE MORTGAGE IS ALMOST PAID off, that for most people is when their Prime Time can start. But for that to happen, you have to take one bold step – you have to choose yourself. You must actively commit to making decisions that prioritise your needs and set the stage for your future goals.

For many people, especially those who've spent years cheering on their kids, partners or friends, prioritising yourself feels strange or even uncomfortable. But if you're reading this, you're already thinking ahead. And that's the first step – you're curious, and you're in the right place. Now it's time to be proactive and take control, because the reality is that this stage of life, while packed with exciting possibilities, can also come with a whole new set of demands.

You're likely familiar with the term 'sandwich generation'. It's that in-between stage when you're caring for both your kids and your ageing parents. And it's not just about physical care but emotional and financial responsibility too. I don't need to tell you that Prime Timers are often the meat in the family sandwich – you know you are. Your late-teen or adult children may still be looking to you for guidance on everything from careers to finances. At the same time, if your parents are still around, you may find yourself becoming their caregiver, helping them navigate medical appointments, finances and other decisions about ageing.

Here's the challenge: this dual responsibility can be mentally and emotionally draining, more so than when your kids were young. Back then, you still had your own parents to lean on. But now? You're the one everyone looks to.

Midlife for many people is also a time of emotional upheaval. There are career pressures, family demands and relationship adjustment challenges. It's a time when things start to go wrong, when life starts to throw curveballs at you that aren't much fun to dodge.

This stage of life also comes with biological changes, from hormonal shifts to declines in muscle mass and cognitive function. These changes can bring about new health challenges, further adding to the emotional and physical load. However, research shows that by making active, informed decisions, you can improve your resilience and adapt to these changes, turning this phase into an opportunity for growth.[11]

It's a time when many of us worry that life isn't turning out the way we planned, or we fear we've chased the wrong goals for too long. Or perhaps we wake up one day and notice that we have lost ourselves almost completely in our long list of obligations. If this is you, you aren't alone. The most important thing you can do as you read this book is acknowledge where you are and start to think about where you want to be.

To make your Prime Time count, you have to take control of the narrative of your life. It's easy to feel overwhelmed by everything going on around you – kids, parents, work, health – but this is also the time to put yourself back at the centre of the picture. By making intentional choices, you can shape how the next 15, 30 or even 40 years will look.

This quote from Jill Tysoe, who did my Epic Retirement Course, says it all:

'Throughout our lives as parents, friends and workers, many of us give our time to others to help them achieve their goals. When we are no longer needed in these situations, we may have lost sight of our own dreams. Where do we even begin to search for our purpose or find and rekindle forgotten dreams?'

That's a conversation for later in the book.

CHOOSE YOUR OWN ADVENTURE

Think of this stage of life as a 'choose-your-own-adventure' novel from the 1980s. Every choice you make will steer your life in a different direction. Just like in those books, where each decision leads to a new outcome, you need to be mindful and intentional about the choices you make. You can't go back once you've turned a page, but you can always peek ahead to see what's coming. So be aware of your options, plan thoughtfully, and navigate your journey using a combination of knowledge and confidence.

SOME PRACTICAL STEPS TO HELP YOU TAKE CONTROL

It's all well and good to tell you that you need to start making active choices. But if you're out of practice at putting yourself first, you might not even know where to start.

SCHEDULE SOME REGULAR TIME FOR SELF-REFLECTION
Set aside time regularly, whether it's a weekend away or a quiet afternoon, to reflect on your current goals, lifestyle and future. Consider what's working, what's not, and what you want to change.

BUILD YOURSELF A SUPPORT NETWORK
Surround yourself with people who lift you up. Whether it's friends, family or a mentor, having the right support can make a huge difference.

STEP UP TO YOUR FINANCIAL PLATE EARLIER

Planning for the rest of your life is hard, but it's enormously rewarding if you start sooner rather than later. Think of all the extra years of compounding – where you'll passively make money while you sleep – that you can enjoy, just because you started now, rather than in your 60s.

START SAYING NO – I MEAN IT

Part of putting yourself first is learning to say no to the things that drain you or don't align with your new priorities. It's not selfish – it's survival. And in place of those things, start to explore and prioritise things that bring you joy or give you a sense of fulfilment.

PRIORITISE YOUR HEALTH

If midlife is showing you some new health challenges, don't ignore them. Prioritise physical and mental wellness, as they really will fuel everything else you want to do.

SET YOURSELF SOME TANGIBLE GOALS

Use the goal-setting strategies from earlier. Break them down into small, achievable steps, and celebrate progress along the way.

EMBRACE MAKING CHANGE IN YOUR LIFE

Whether it's downsizing, switching careers or taking time off, don't be afraid of change. Studies show that embracing life transitions and being curious about where they can lead you, as opposed to resisting them, leads to greater happiness.

Part 2
MONEY

> ### GENERAL ADVICE WARNING
> The information provided in this book, and more particularly this money part, is of a general nature only and does not take into account your individual objectives, financial situation or needs. Before making any financial decisions, you should consider the appropriateness of the information provided in this book, having regard to your own objectives, financial situation and needs, and seek professional advice from a licensed financial adviser.

MOST PEOPLE DON'T START THINKING ABOUT HOW MUCH MONEY THEY'LL NEED for the future until retirement is right in their headlights. But let's be honest, by then it's often too late to make big changes. And here's the thing – not everyone even wants to retire anymore. A lot of people just want to keep working on what they love, but on their own terms, knowing they have the financial flexibility to choose.

That's why I wrote this book, because I believe we need to start thinking about our money and life choices much earlier. When your cash flow begins to free up in midlife is the perfect time to look at how your work, investments, super and home fit into the bigger picture. You then give yourself the power to choose your own adventure through the second half of life.

That power of choice is your greatest superpower in midlife – and I want you to have it. But you have to help yourself to get it.

I want you to think of your Prime Time in stages – the phases of life that are ahead of you. It's not just about coasting along or saving madly for retirement and then stopping work. It's about planning, saving and living fully now, while setting yourself up for what's next. And looking forward to every part of it.

So let's rethink how we approach finances in midlife. It's not just about retirement anymore. Instead, picture this phase of your life – your Prime Time – as three key stages:

- Your set-up years
- Your lifestyling years
- Your part-time years.

Then, if you've planned well, you'll step into your Epic Retirement with confidence. And the best part? You get to decide how you approach each one.

Financially, it's about being ready to shift gears through these stages (or designing your own stages), making sure you're hitting your own goals and chasing your dreams while you've got the health to do it. You need to have enough money, yes, but more importantly you need the confidence to use it to live your life well.

So when I talk about money in Prime Time, I focus on two key things: creating *enough* money, and building the confidence to actually *use* it. Sounds simple, right?

There are seven key lessons in this section that will boost your financial confidence and set you up for success:

1. Stop taking shortcuts.
2. Understand the foundations of financial confidence and put them in place.
3. Learn the new lessons of midlife money management, about income and spending.
4. Understand how your spending will or won't work over time.
5. Work out how much is 'enough'.
6. Get appropriate financial advice for your situation.
7. Take a modern, proactive approach to your legacy.

WHY HAVE MIDLIFE AND RETIREMENT CHANGED?

Midlife and retirement today look completely different compared to how they looked for those currently in their late 70s, 80s and 90s. Previous generations often worked until their mid to late 60s, then relied almost entirely on the age pension to get by in retirement. They lived frugally, preserving their family home as their legacy.

But that's not the path most of us want or need to take anymore. For Australians now in their late 40s, 50s and early 60s, compulsory superannuation has been in place for 33 years, with a solid percentage of salaries being invested – mostly quite wisely – by super funds. Many have built up a healthy nest egg that will continue to grow, compounding well into their later years.

On top of that, we've benefited from a massive housing boom. Most people in this generation bought their homes in the 1990s or 2000s, paid them down steadily, and watched as property values skyrocketed by 300 per cent or more. Even if there's still a mortgage, the equity in these homes is extraordinary.

And here's another game-changer: the way we work has shifted. We're no longer tied to full-time, structured jobs. Work has become more flexible, with plenty of options for part-time or lower-stress roles that simply didn't exist before. This means we don't have to fully stop working when we hit retirement age. In fact, we can keep working in a way that suits us, enjoying the social connections and sense of purpose work can bring, if we choose to.

So, unlike previous generations, many of today's pre-retirees are in a much stronger financial position. While many older retirees still depend on the age pension, the next generation has more options and, crucially, more financial freedom to design their own version of retirement – and really enjoy the prime time years leading up to it too.

Lesson 4
Stop taking financial shortcuts

MIDLIFE CAN BE A CHALLENGING PERIOD, WHEN EVERYTHING SEEMS TO WEIGH heavily on us. Most people in this stage are at the top of their game and under pressure to keep rising. We are or we have been earning the biggest bucks we'll ever earn. But we're also likely saddled with the tail end of the largest mortgage and the most financial responsibilities we'll ever carry. And on top of that, we may be quite bored or frustrated with our jobs and afraid of our future employability. We may still have teenagers or young adults in our homes, or ageing parents looking for support, or a partner we barely find time for, and a career we have to keep looking invested in while we work out how to juggle all these things. And we feel the pressure of planning for retirement too. That's a lot of pressure for one person.

To put some light in the tunnel, while running on that wheel, many midlifers take financial shortcuts, looking for ways to avoid having to do the hard work required to be financially successful into the next stage of life. And there are lots of shortcuts to try. They take on risky investments, hoping for high returns without really understanding the market. They operate without a budget and spend on 'whatever they need', racking up the credit card debt to cover shortfalls in income, and ending up with piles of debt. And my favourite, putting off saving for retirement or paying down the mortgage faster to free up cash flow in the short term. But these quick grabs rarely lead to financial stability. And they certainly don't help you set proper foundations for the future.

Instead of ignoring the shortcuts, let's crack them open and then focus on what truly works for a healthier, wealthier and wiser second half of life.

SHORTCUT #1: I DON'T HAVE TIME TO FOCUS ON MY MONEY

Most people in midlife face a common challenge: they don't prioritise time to focus on their finances. This lack of attention costs them. They miss opportunities to understand how financial systems work, set goals for their future and consistently practise the right things to build their wealth. Yet the changes we need to make at this time of our lives can make us truly wealthy, even if we have no wealth today to speak of. What should you prioritise learning about? Superannuation is the big one – as you get closer to wanting to use it, you need to know how it works. Investing is also important to understand, and so is managing your cash flow sensibly, with a set of financial and lifestyle goals firmly in focus.

SHORTCUT #2: I DON'T NEED A BUDGET – I UNDERSTAND HOW MONEY WORKS AND SPEND AS I NEED AND WANT TO

Many people in midlife spend as they need and want to, often covering any shortfall with credit cards or by dipping into the redraw account on their mortgage. In today's challenging economy, this has become more common than we might admit, leading many to find their finances spiralling out of control.

I hate to break it to you, but if you want to plan for the future, you need a budget. Your budget is the framework that tells you the truth about your spending habits: how much you spend on your cost of living, how much you spend on discretionary items, and how much you spend on your lifestyle.

Understanding your spending gives you power – the power to save, the power to compound, the power to make decisions more easily, and the power to live a better quality life.

SHORTCUT #3: EVERYONE HAS A NEW CAR AND DRINKS FANCY WINE – I SHOULD TOO

If you live in the suburbs of a big city, it might feel like everyone around you has a new car, a selection of stunning posh-brand jeans and a passion for fancy wine. I have one message for you: buying into this is a trap that can delay your Prime Time and your retirement, not to mention cause you massive anxiety.

It's a hard trap to avoid, and you need good friends to be able to do it. A few years ago, my friends and I got together and agreed on four principles so we could prioritise seeing each other *and* paying off our mortgages:

1. When we dined together, we'd stick to 'at home' events during our saving years.
2. No-one was to bring wine costing over $25.
3. There was no need to dress fancy or buy new stuff, just be who we were and use the opportunity to put our existing going-out clothes on and feel good about ourselves.
4. We would always, always bring a plate to each other's house, so there was no pressure on anyone to supply all the food when they hosted.

We all wanted to pay off our mortgages and grow our wealth, not our egos. And none of us wanted to stop having fun as we did so. I think these simple principles have stood the test of our younger years and are still relevant in midlife. In fact, they are probably more relevant now because we have less time to save and more things to do with our money that we'll get to really enjoy in our Prime Time – if we achieve those savings goals.

SHORTCUT #4: I NEED A BIGGER HOUSE IN A FANCY NEIGHBOURHOOD

Many people make the mistake of upsizing one last time in their late 40s, 50s or even 60s, just as their cash flow starts to free up (when the kid-related expenses drop). Some are trying to shake off midlife stagnation with a fresh start in a fancier home, while others decide that the logical 'next step' is a bigger, better house in a more prestigious suburb.

There comes a point in life, though, when we don't need a bigger house. Somewhere in midlife, we move from needing a big house to hold all of our family in separate rooms, to the next phase of life where we need a powerful pool of income-generating assets to drive our compound growth and power our future passive income streams. What we need is strong financial foundations, and while your principal place of residence is a valuable growth asset, it will probably never generate you any income. So having too much tied up in your home can be a frustration in the second half of life, unless it is a conscious strategy to shield assets from the age pension later in life.

SHORTCUT #5: I DON'T NEED TO SAVE FOR RETIREMENT NOW – I'LL START SAVING LATER AND EVERYTHING WILL BE FINE

If your life expectancy extends into your 90s and you plan to retire at the average age of 65, you'll need to save enough money to support yourself for 25–35 years. While you might qualify for an age pension, which is currently up to about $30,000 per year for singles and $45,000 per year for couples (in 2025), depending on your assets and other income, it probably won't provide the quality of life you aspire to.

There's a crucial secret about saving for retirement that we don't discuss enough in our 40s and 50s: compound investment over the long term is the easiest way to do the hard work. Sounds boring, right? Stay with me. It is, but it's also incredibly powerful. And if you get it right it can change your life.

It involves investing in high-quality, long-term growth assets that typically increase in value each year and provide a steady income stream that can be reinvested. For instance, starting at 50 with a $100,000 investment in assets averaging 7–10 per cent annual returns (typical for Australian equities over the past decade), you really could double your money every 7–10 years through compound returns alone. Adding $10,000 annually to these investments could grow your initial $100,000 to about $334,880 at 7 per cent or $418,740 at 10 per cent return over 10 years. Remarkably, you'd have contributed only $200,000 from your own savings efforts during that period. Plus, if you used superannuation tax concessions and saved this money within your superannuation fund, you could potentially save 15–30 per cent in tax on each dollar invested. That's free money! Why don't we talk about this some more, later on.

SHORTCUT #6: I CAN TRADE (OR BET!) MY WAY OUT OF TROUBLE

This one really gets under my skin, and I've seen it far too often. People, easily swayed by others, dive headfirst into stock trading, currency trading, or worse, cryptocurrencies, without fully understanding the complexities of short-term trading – all to fix their financial problems or clear a credit card bill. Even worse is when they turn to gambling, betting on horse racing or other sports to try to fill that financial hole.

You might have heard someone brag about taking $5000 or $10,000 for a punt and thinking they'll strike gold. But that same money could've been invested in something stable, allowing it to compound and grow over time. And here's the thing – people only ever tell you how much they've made, never how much they've lost along the way. The real danger is when someone gets lucky the first time, and they start believing they're invincible and go all in.

Short- and medium-term investing requires highly developed skills, and let's be real – most of us don't have those just sitting in our back pocket. And when it comes to gambling, the odds are always stacked in favour of the house. As I'll show you, focusing on long-term investments can lead to solid returns, so why take a gamble?

Now, I'm not saying you need to play it *too* safe in midlife. If you've got a decade or a good few years until you can access your super, there's still plenty of time to ride out economic swings if investing in growth assets. But be smart about it – take calculated risks, not reckless ones.

SHORTCUT #7: I NEED A HIGHER-PAYING JOB TO FUND MY MIDLIFE EXPENSES AND SAVE FOR RETIREMENT

Don't get me wrong. Big incomes are an incredible way to build retirement savings, so if you have one, don't fail to appreciate it – *if* you like your job. But one of the biggest lessons people often learn in midlife, if they haven't already, is that while having a big income is exciting, managing how you spend that income is even more crucial.

You'd be surprised by how many middle-aged doctors with sky-high incomes live pay cheque to pay cheque because they don't manage their finances well. Budgeting, saving and investing wisely are the real keys to financial security. You can achieve financial stability by living within your means, prioritising savings and making smart investment decisions, regardless of your income level. Truly!

SHORTCUT #8: I'LL JUST WORK LONGER IF I DON'T SAVE ENOUGH FOR RETIREMENT

In midlife, when you want to spend every dollar, it's easy to tell yourself, 'I don't need to save. I'll just work a year or two longer to fund my retirement.' But the reality is that this plan is far from foolproof.

Counting on being able to extend your working years can be risky. Only 31 per cent of Australians who retired in 2022–23 did so by choice, timing their retirement to fit their lifestyle and savings goals.[12] The rest retired because they were retrenched, hit with health issues, or they became frustrated with their job but couldn't find another suitable role. Or they faced head-on the need to care for a loved one.

Employers also point out, discreetly, that there is a sensible point in everyone's working life where they should choose to move into the next phase, so they don't have to be forced into it by a mind or an attitude that doesn't want to keep up. And everyone should prepare themselves for this, so they have the power to choose.

It's far smarter to recognise that retirement as we know it has changed. We don't have to aim anymore for a window in our mid to late 60s where we get laid off or give up work and finally get to step back from life.

Instead, most people want to reach a point somewhere between 50 and 67 when they become financially independent, and know they can afford to live off the income generated by their investments, superannuation, assets and pension (if they're eligible) for the rest of their lives. Then, if they want, they can choose to step back from working full-time and start to do work on *their* terms.

My aim for you is that you work out how much is enough, then reach that point with your financial plans securely in place and your non-financial plans ready alongside them.

Now that we've seen the damage taking shortcuts can do, let's learn about how to do it the smarter way.

Lesson 5
Understand the foundations of financial confidence

I BELIEVE THERE ARE NINE BIG FINANCIAL FOUNDATIONS THAT EVERYONE NEEDS TO understand and take more active control of as they hit their midlife, if not before. The earlier you grasp them, the wealthier you have the opportunity to become. I'm not kidding! This is a big section, so hang in there because you need to understand all these things, in order, in your Prime Time.

1. Make time for managing your money.
2. Create a detailed household budget and your big financial picture.
3. Understand how much you need to live comfortably.
4. Understand the power of compound investing.
5. Develop a solid understanding of tax, tax deductions and tax concessions.
6. Pay off a home that's within your means.
7. Get the most out of superannuation.
8. Explore your investment options.
9. Consider your future eligibility for the age pension.

We'll go through each of these in detail, examining how they work in midlife. These foundations are key to managing your finances effectively as things change. There will be some new-age lessons in the next chapter that develop these foundations.

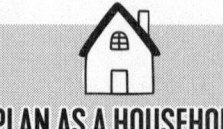

PLAN AS A HOUSEHOLD

One important thing to keep in mind as you go through this section is that, if you're in a couple and expect to stay together in the years ahead, it's crucial to plan as a household. Not only does this help you align your decisions on cost of living, housing, investments and superannuation, but there are also significant tax benefits. By planning together, you can take advantage of strategies like income splitting, spousal super contributions and tax offsets that can reduce your overall tax burden and maximise your combined wealth.

If you're a single person, you still need to plan as a household – meaning you should factor in how your cost of living will likely be higher on your own. Without the ability to split costs or pool resources, it's important to be realistic about expenses such as housing, bills and retirement savings. You may need to build a stronger buffer to cover these higher living costs or explore ways to reduce expenses, like downsizing or taking advantage of concessions available to single-income households. Planning carefully as a single person ensures you're well prepared to meet your financial needs independently.

1. MAKE TIME FOR MANAGING YOUR MONEY

Understanding your financial situation and setting goals and strategies, then committing to working toward them, can be one of the most important steps you take in life.

Superfunds and financial advisers often point out to me that there are three different types of people. See which one you are:

- **The proactive**: who know where they want to go and make the effort to learn about how to get themselves there
- **The reactive**: who only take action when prompted or when something goes wrong, and will otherwise tend to ignore their financial management

- **The inactive:** who don't really want to know about their budget, their superannuation or their big financial picture; perhaps they feel like they'll never be able to improve their situation.

If you're currently in the reactive or inactive category, it's time to get proactive. And if you're already proactive, then giddy up – let's go learn!

EMBRACE BECOMING FINANCIALLY PROACTIVE

This week, I want you to schedule a quiet, intentional dinner at home, with your partner if you have one or your best friend of a similar age if you don't. Get a nice bottle of wine out of the cupboard, cook one of those special 'going out but staying in' dinner recipes you haven't made time to do in a few years, and sit down. Tonight is all about discussing your midlife money expectations, possibly for the first time.

If you're a part of a couple, there are two reasons why you have this conversation *after* you've set your individual goals and before you learn all the deeper lessons about money in your midlife. Firstly, it's so you can open up the conversation and start to learn together, bring your dreams together and plan. It's also so you can hold onto your individuality, recognising the importance of your own identity in the next stage of life – especially when many will be feeling they lost it along the way.

If you're single, you might ask why I suggest that you do it with your best friend. Well, chances are you're both at a similar crossroads in life, each with individual goals, and when shared, you can learn from each other and put in place the mutual bonds that will help you cheer each other on, help each other achieve those goals, and celebrate the big milestones.

If you're really alone, with no-one to share your time with, then remember you're doing it with me – I'll help you with ways to find new connections for your Prime Time later in the book.

'So what's on the menu for our dinner discussion?', I hear you asking. Well, tonight I want you to look the other person in the eyes and talk about what you think you want in the next phase of your life.

1. Talk about how it feels to be entering or in the next stage of your life, and what you want it to mean for you.
2. Talk through the way you see life panning out in stages, and the goals you set for yourself when you worked through lesson #2.
3. Talk about how much money you have, in which assets, and how much debt you have. Also talk about what your main expenses and income sources are, how that has changed over the last five years, and how you think it might change in the future.
4. Talk about how long you have been working for, how much you enjoy your work, how long you think you want to keep working for, and how work might change for you.
5. And finally, talk about the things you want to do with the second half of your life other than work.

Share this early picture with the other person in an open, honest and curious way. Listen to their picture and, if you're a couple, see how it feels to start exploring what it might look like together. And then, let it rest. There will be plenty of time to shape these initial visions into real-life plans. You don't need to rush it.

2. CREATE A DETAILED HOUSEHOLD BUDGET AND YOUR BIG FINANCIAL PICTURE

Budgeting and keeping track of your household balance sheet are two of the most important financial skills you'll ever use. It still amazes me that this isn't taught in schools. You need to understand your true cost of living today, and know how to adjust it when your income or goals change – it's crucial. Smart budgeting and saving give you the ability to allocate funds for paying down debts and investing for your future.

These two processes together form what I call your *big financial picture*. It's best to lay this out in a simple spreadsheet that you can update at least once a year, because you will use this information all the way through your life. Once you have this big picture, you can figure out your next steps, or even take it to a financial adviser for help.

Building this big financial picture is your springboard for other activities later in the book:

- Spotting savings you can make in your everyday living costs
- Setting realistic savings goals and tracking them year after year
- Mapping out your spending and income streams in phases, so you can see how your money will work for you over time
- Deciding how much is really *enough*.

So let's build it together. There are five simple steps I want you to work through, gathering all the information you need about your current financial position.

> Download the Prime Time 'Big Financial Picture' spreadsheet to build your own big financial picture using the instructions below – visit becwilson.net/primetime_resources

Step 1: Understand your assets. Start by listing *all* your assets: the things you own that have a legitimate saleable value. This includes your home, superannuation balance, financial investments, rental properties and other income-generating assets. Don't forget to include lifestyle assets like furniture, cars, boats and caravans – even though they don't contribute to growing your wealth, they could be considered for age pension eligibility later on.

For most people, this is a straightforward process. You can use the prime time budgeting spreadsheet, which has a dedicated tab for this purpose. Start by listing each asset and its current market value. In a separate section, note the value of your lifestyle assets, at a price you could realistically sell them for in the second-hand market today.

Assets	Current market value	Income generated per month
Principal place of residence (PPOR)	$900,000	Nil
Equities investments (outside super)	$200,000	$900
Rental property	$650,000	$3033
Car 1	$20,000	Nil
Car 2	$30,000	Nil
Boat	$10,000	Nil
Furniture	$20,000	Nil
Cash at bank	$20,000	Nil
Gross assets outside super	**$1,850,000**	
Superannuation (Nivek)	$300,000	
Superannuation (Bob)	$470,000	
Total household superannuation	**$770,000**	

Note: This is an example built with commonly held assets. Please build your own with your assets.

Step 2: List your liabilities. To get a full picture of your financial situation, continue by listing your liabilities: everything you owe. Include the total value of each debt, interest rate, the terms of each loan, and the monthly payments you need to make. This includes your home loan, car loans or leases, personal or investment loans, and any credit card balances you carry. Don't forget to add any buy now, pay later accounts you maintain, especially if you're not paying them off monthly.

Once you have all of this mapped out, then along with your assets, you'll have a much clearer understanding of where you stand financially. This will allow you to start making informed decisions about how to save, invest, and reduce your debt, setting you up for a better financial future.

Liabilities	Value	Interest rate	Terms	Payments	Payment frequency
PPR loan	$275,000	6%	12 years remaining	$2684	Monthly
Investment loan on equities	$100,000	7%	10 years remaining Interest only	$583	Monthly
Rental property loan	$400,000	7%	10 years remaining Interest only	$2333	Monthly
Credit card	$800	19%	Pay down monthly in full	$800	Monthly
Gross liabilities	**$775,800**		**Total debt outgoings**	**$6400**	

It's easy to get overwhelmed about the big numbers in these tables. But we need to look at our assets net of the debt we are holding on them. So now let's calculate your net assets.

I also want to point out that we list superannuation separately. It receives a particularly attractive tax treatment both in the accumulation phase and the retirement phase. So it's worth isolating it, as we may decide to focus on growing the money *inside* super, particularly as we get closer to retirement, when we can access it.

Gross assets outside super	$1,850,000
Less gross liabilities	$775,800
Total (net) assets	$1,074,200
Total household superannuation	$770,000

Step 3: Estimate your income. Estimate your current annual income by listing all your sources of cash flow. Start with your take-home pay. Use a calculator to figure out how much you earn *after* tax and what you receive in superannuation. The Australian Taxation Office (ATO) income tax calculator is a helpful tool for this: see moneysmart.gov.au/work-and-tax/income-tax-calculator

Now add any other income, such as income from small businesses, trusts, investments outside of superannuation, rental properties or side hustles. Be sure to itemise each source as a separate line item.

As you write down each income stream in the spreadsheet, note how often each one is paid and when you expect to receive it. This helps keep everything organised and provides a clearer picture of your cash flow.

	Super (paid on top of salary)	Net income per year	Payment notes
Salary 1 – Bob (gross $140,000)	$16,800	$105,883	Paid monthly on the 15th of the month
Salary 2 – Nivek (gross $100,000)	$12,000	$76,408	Paid fortnightly on Fridays
Estimated investment income (outside super)		$6300	Drawn once per year after 30 June

	Super (paid on top of salary)	Net income per year	Payment notes
Nivek's side hustle (gross $10,000)		$6800	Drawn quarterly at quarter-end
Total	**$28,800**	**$195,391**	

Step 4: Itemise your current expenses. It's time to get real about your spending by itemising your expenses, by category. This should include everything you spend money on throughout the year: food, clothing, utilities, rent or mortgage payments, insurance, entertainment, health care, memberships, subscriptions, even life's little luxuries. Be honest with yourself, as this is the only way to get a true picture of your finances.

You can make this process easier by using your banking app to summarise these things, if that function is offered, or consider a budgeting app that can aggregate your spending by reviewing payments from your bank accounts. Otherwise, get hands-on. Grab your transactional account and credit card statements, open up my 'Big Financial Picture' Excel spreadsheet template, and manually work through each expense, categorising it.

When building your version of the spreadsheet, I recommend separating your everyday living expenses from lifestyle or discretionary spending, and one-off expenses that don't recur. This helps you distinguish between your needs and wants, making it easier to make active choices about your future spending and saving.

If you've been flying by the seat of your pants financially, just spending what you have without really tracking it, this process might feel painful the first time you do it. But trust me – it's incredibly empowering. And if you're already on top of your money, you'll find this process simple and even more valuable.

The prime time big financial picture spreadsheet includes a budgeting tab with sections for all the categories listed below. This structure allows you to benchmark your spending against the average Australian household at retirement. It lines up with the Association of Superannuation Funds of Australia's budget benchmarks, helping you check yours and make it a more realistic and effective budget.

Here's a table that sets out the categories and line items for your budget. We'll build a current budget now, then later in the book we'll build a prime time budget that's future focused. Let's go!

Housing expenses	
Building and contents insurance	$–
Council rates	$–
Water charges	$–
Home improvements	$–
Repairs and maintenance	$–
Electricity and gas bills	$–
Body corp fees (or similar)	$–
Rent (deducting rent assistance)	$–
Fresh food expenses	
Supermarket	$–
Butcher/fruit shop	$–
Other	$–
Internet and mobile phones	
Internet and mobile phone bundle (or)	$–
Internet	$–
Mobile phone	$–
Household goods and services	
Household cleaning	$–
Cosmetics and personal care items	$–
Hairdresser and barber costs	$–
Digital media	$–
Computer, printer and software	$–
Household appliances, air conditioners and smartphones	$–
Other household expenses	$–
Clothing and footwear	
Clothing	$–
Footwear	$–

Car, transport and running costs	
Car registration	$–
Car insurance	$–
Fuel and other operating costs	$–
Servicing and maintenance	$–
Public transport costs	$–
Tolls	$–
Personal health	
Health insurance	$–
Chemist	$–
Doctor's co-payment and out-of-pocket expenses	$–
Vitamins and over-the-counter medicines	$–
Exercise and fitness	$–
Entertainment and leisure	
Membership to clubs	$–
TV	$–
Streaming services	$–
Alcohol consumed	$–
Charity or church donations	$–
Cinema, theatre, sports and day trips	$–
Meals out	$–
Domestic vacations	$–
International vacations	$–
Takeaway foods, coffees and so on	$–
Other insurance	
Life insurance (not held in super)	$–
Total and permanent disablement (TPD) insurance (not held in super)	$–
Trauma insurance (not held in super)	$–
Pet insurance	$–
Work-related expenses	
Professional memberships and other subscriptions	$–
Other work-related expenses	$–

Family and friends	
Gifts (Christmas and birthdays)	$–
Other family expenses	$–
Travel and experiences	
Domestic travel per year	$–
International travel per year	$–
Debt repayments	
Credit card payments	$–
Loan payments	$–
TOTAL EXPENSES	$–

Step 5: Build a subscriptions list. Creating a subscriptions and direct debits list is a savvy way to monitor your recurring expenses. This list can be a powerful tool for identifying opportunities to reduce discretionary spending and improve your financial health. By tracking your subscriptions, you can easily see where your money is going and make decisions about which ones to keep or cancel.

	Monthly, or annual payments	Monthly amount	Annual amount	Contract term	Date paid monthly/ annually
Netflix	Monthly	$18.99	$227.88	None	18th of each month
Optus mobile	Monthly	$45.00	$540	12 months	3rd of each month
Microsoft	Monthly	$9.95	$119.40	None	30th of each month
Apple iCloud	Monthly	$4.49	$53.88	None	30th of each month
Spotify	Monthly	$15.99	$191.88	None	5th of each month
Sydney Morning Herald	Weekly	$5	$260	None	10th of each month
Gym	Monthly	$60	$3120	None	10th of each month

Use this subscription list as a living document – add new subscriptions as you sign up, update amounts when companies raise their fees and remove any cancellations. It helps you track where your money is going and stay mindful of its value.

BRINGING IT ALL TOGETHER

It's now time to finish your big financial picture, establishing one of your critical foundations. You now have a solid understanding of each of your important numbers:

How much your family home is worth: It's important to stand this one alone, and see if it represents a good amount to have tied up in a non-income-producing asset as you move forward.

How much you hold in assets excluding super and your family home: Knowing the value of your investments, properties and other assets outside super gives you a clear picture of your wealth.

How much you have in superannuation: Ultimately in your retirement years, you can draw income from your superannuation tax-free so this amount is important.

How much you have in liabilities: Understanding your debts, including mortgages, loans and credit card balances, helps you prioritise your repayments.

How much you spend on your cost of living per year today: Including both essential and discretionary spending, so you can track your cost of living accurately and adapt it if you have the opportunity.

How much you generate in income (ideally an estimated after-tax amount): Knowing your income sources and amounts, whether from work, investments or pensions, is crucial for financial planning.

UNDERSTAND YOUR CURRENT SURPLUS (OR DEFICIT)

Now I want you to isolate the surplus amount in your spending each month and each year. This is the difference between your after-tax income and your expenses.

Just observe that picture, and see how it feels to better understand your whole financial situation as it currently stands.

Your big financial picture really is one of the fundamental inputs into the decisions you will need to make in your coming years. So keep it handy. You'll use it later, after we understand the other foundations.

3. UNDERSTAND HOW MUCH YOU NEED TO LIVE COMFORTABLY

'How much do I need to be able to live comfortably in my Prime Time and then, later, to have an Epic Retirement?'

This is the biggest question most people ask themselves as they approach the time of life when they might want to change things up. But it's a bit like asking, 'How long is a piece of string?', because everyone's situation is different. Your standard of living, everyday expenses, expectations of working and lifestyle goals will vary depending on where you live, how much you earn and the kind of life you want to lead.

The best way to figure out how much you'll need is to *build your own* prime time cost of living and lifestyle budget, like we've just done, and extrapolate how that might change over time. From there, you can tailor your financial plans to fit your own needs.

But alongside this, it can be helpful to explore how much others are really spending. So here's a look at some benchmarks to help you compare your cost-of-living budget with other people's budgets and see how you stack up. Always remember: there's no right answer, only *your* answer.

PRE-RETIREMENT SPENDING BENCHMARKS

It's tough to find reliable 'average' figures for what everyday people spend on their costs of living during their Prime Time, especially before retirement, as much of the data is closely guarded by the banks who commercialise it. The reality is that spending varies widely depending on where you live and the standard of living you can afford.

To give you a clearer picture of this diversity, here's a snapshot of basic household expenses for a 60-year-old living in the Sydney metro area across three different income levels, compared to someone living in regional Queensland on the same income bands. These averages are based on publicly published credit card data from one of the major banks and provide insights into the varying costs of living in different parts of the country.[13]

Similar data isn't publicly available for 50-year-olds, and there's no ability to adjust the data for couples, so you'll have to use your imagination to spin it up.

Average spending of someone aged 60–64, living in a NSW metropolitan area.

Average spending	Aged 60–64, income of $1001–$2000 per month NSW metro area	Aged 60–64, income of $2001–$3000 per month NSW metro area	Aged 60–64, income of $3000+ per month NSW metro area
Groceries and food	$265	$335	$473
Housing expense (incl. insurance)	$200	$274	$395
Health	$123	$204	$327
Utilities and finance	$144	$172	$215
Clothing and appliances	$106	$164	$296
Eating and drinking out	$78	$139	$307
Travel	$56	$135	$319
Transportation	$101	$127	$187
Total cash spending	$147	$114	$112
Other	$68	$111	$226
Leisure and entertainment	$44	$80	$173
Total spend – NSW metro area	$1461 per fortnight	$1855 per fortnight	$3028 per fortnight
	$37,986 per year	$48,230 per year	$78,728 per year

Average spending of someone aged 60–64, living in a Queensland regional area.

Average spending	Aged 60–64, income of $1001–$2000 per month Qld regional area	Aged 60–64, income of $2001–$3000 per month Qld regional area	Aged 60–64, income of $3000+ per month Qld regional area
Groceries and food	$322	$372	$465
Housing expense (incl. insurance)	$242	$274	$456
Health	$125	$204	$362
Utilities and finance	$99	$172	$140
Clothing and appliances	$124	$164	$303
Eating and drinking out	$85	$139	$231
Travel	$73	$135	$362
Transportation	$137	$127	$218

LESSON 5: UNDERSTAND THE FOUNDATIONS OF FINANCIAL CONFIDENCE

Average spending	Aged 60–64, income of $1001–$2000 per month Qld regional area	Aged 60–64, income of $2001–$3000 per month Qld regional area	Aged 60–64, income of $3000+ per month Qld regional area
Total cash spending	$115	$114	$91
Other	$91	$111	$206
Leisure and entertainment	$49	$80	$142
Total spend – Qld regional area	$1463 per fortnight	$1855 per fortnight	$2901 per fortnight
	$38,038 per year	$48,230 per year	$75,426 per year

It's not surprising to observe that as our income rises, so does our standard of living and our expenditure on almost everything – both non-discretionary and discretionary.

POST-RETIREMENT SPENDING BENCHMARKS

The other benchmarks that can be helpful when trying to figure out how much you need are post-retirement benchmarks.

The Association of Superannuation Funds of Australia (ASFA) provides estimates of the annual cost of living for retirees. These estimates are updated every quarter in a report called *The Retirement Standard*.[14] The report gives clear guidelines for two different lifestyles for people aged 65–84: a comfortable retirement and a modest retirement. This can help you figure out if your retirement budget is on track.

ASFA Retirement Standard – annual budget (March quarter, 2025)

	Single	Couple
Comfortable lifestyle	$52,383	$73,875
Modest lifestyle	$33,386	$48,184

A comfortable lifestyle allows for a good standard of living, including things like household goods, private health insurance, a decent car, and the ability to take an interstate holiday once a year.

A modest lifestyle is better than relying solely on the age pension, but it only covers the basics.

How much super do you need to afford this? ASFA also estimates that if you retire at 67, and expect to live until 87 if a man or 90 if a woman, you'll need to have saved a significant amount to maintain this level of income throughout retirement.

	Single	Couple
Comfortable lifestyle	$595,000	$690,000
Modest lifestyle	$100,000	$100,000

(Figures current at January 2025, subject to change)

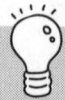

TAX-FREE SUPER MAKES YOUR MONEY GO FURTHER

One really important thing we often forget when comparing pre- and post-retirement income is that superannuation income in the retirement phase is tax-free. This means that once you're retired, your super provides up to double the real value of your cash flow compared to pre-retirement, after-tax income. That tax-free status makes a huge difference, significantly boosting the value of the cash you have available to live on once you stop working and can draw on superannuation income.

The Retirement Standard assumes that you own your own home outright when you reach retirement, are eligible for a part or full aged pension, and do not pay rent.[15] It does not factor in body corporate costs. It's important to point out that the budgets do not allow much for travel, even in the comfortable budget, which accounts for a low-cost international trip every seven years and an interstate trip each year. If you plan to travel more frequently or take more expensive trips, you would need to account for that extra spending on top of the standard budget.

If you plan to retire before the age of 67, or live longer than 87 as a man or 90 as a woman, you'll want to consider how much more to factor in to support you during those years.

ASFA benchmarks are based on real, regularly revised cost-of-living budgets that you can download from the ASFA website, with all the line items available for you to review (visit superannuation.asn.au/consumers/retirement-standard).

BUILD YOUR OWN NUMBER

Finally, to determine how much you need each year, you should take three simple steps:
- Build your cost-of-living budget: this provides you with a true baseline, using the standard you live at today.
- Assess how much you want to add to your budget for one-off spending and epic experiences.
- Estimate an annual budget to build your plan with.

We'll work through this process later in the book.

4. UNDERSTAND THE POWER OF COMPOUND INVESTING

This next lesson should be a fun one. Understanding compound investing and how it drives the growth of your wealth is truly one of the most important financial principles you'll ever learn. It's crucial that you understand it as you plan for the second half of your life. And the earlier in life you embrace it, the more money you'll have, sooner. Have I got your attention now?

Compound investing happens when you invest money and you generate income. At this point you have a choice: you can either withdraw that income or you can reinvest it. If you reinvest the income you receive, your total investment 'compounds', which means it grows by the amount you earned in income that year. Then, in the second year, you earn interest on this larger amount. If you continue reinvesting your earnings each year, your investment keeps growing, and that growth becomes more significant over time.

It really is an amazing concept. There are two fundamental components you need to understand to grasp how compound investing works: the *value of time* and the *rate of return*.

The value of time refers to the number of years over which you invest and compound your money. This is crucial because compound investing generates the best returns over the long term.

The rate of return from your investments is equally vital. It determines the income you receive each year, which is added to your principal investment, thereby boosting your returns in subsequent years.

Here are some simple examples.

Sam has $150,000 in his superannuation at age 48, and he's getting an average return of 8 per cent, but those returns vary year to year. Sam wants to understand how this $150,000 could compound over the years ahead if it retains the same long-term rate of growth and he makes no more contributions – ever. (For simplicity, this example does not demonstrate the impact of taxes, tax concessions or fees.)

Year	Age	Opening balance of principal – compounding	Returns in year	Annual earnings	Yearly investment	Closing balance at year end
1	48	$150,000	8%	$12,000	$0	$162,000
2	49	$162,000	13%	$21,060	$0	$183,060
3	50	$183,060	6%	$10,984	$0	$194,044
4	51	$194,044	15%	$29,107	$0	$223,150
5	52	$223,150	4%	$8,926	$0	$232,076
6	53	$232,076	10%	$23,208	$0	$255,284
7	54	$255,284	8%	$20,423	$0	$275,706
8	55	$275,706	–3%	–$8,271	$0	$267,435
9	56	$267,435	12%	$32,092	$0	$299,527
10	57	$299,527	7%	$20,967	$0	$320,494
11	58	$320,494	10%	$32,049	$0	$352,544
12	59	$352,544	5%	$17,627	$0	$370,171
13	60	$370,171	11%	$40,719	$0	$410,890
14	61	$410,890	10%	$41,089	$0	$451,979
15	62	$451,979	6%	$27,119	$0	$479,098
16	63	$479,098	8%	$38,328	$0	$517,425
17	64	$517,425	4%	$20,697	$0	$538,122
18	65	$538,122	12%	$64,575	$0	$602,697
19	66	$602,697	8%	$48,216	$0	$650,913
20	67	$650,913	6%	$39,055	$0	$689,968
21	68	$689,968	8%	$55,197	$0	$745,165

Year	Age	Opening balance of principal – compounding	Returns in year	Annual earnings	Yearly investment	Closing balance at year end
22	69	$745,165	12%	$89,420	$0	$834,585
23	70	$834,585	4%	$33,383	$0	$867,968
		Average return	8%			

THE RULE OF 72

There's a handy rule called 'the rule of 72' that vividly illustrates the power of compounding. It estimates the number of years it takes for your invested funds to double at a given annual rate of return. It's quite simple: divide 72 by the annual rate of return on your investments. This will tell you how long it will take for the money invested to double through the power of compound investing.

6% return – 72/6 = 12 years
7% return – 72/7 = 10.2 years
8% return – 72/8 = 9 years
9% return – 72/9 = 8 years
10% return – 72/10 = 7.2 years

Now let's look at what would happen if Sam invested $10,000 per year over his working life until he finally retires at 70. He's still getting an average 10-year return of 8 per cent. (Again, this example does not demonstrate the impact of taxes, tax concessions or fees.)

Year	Age	Opening balance of principal	Returns in year	Annual earnings	Additional contributions	Closing balance at year end
1	48	$150,000	8%	$12,000	$10,000	$172,000
2	49	$172,000	13%	$22,360	$10,000	$204,360
3	50	$204,360	6%	$12,262	$10,000	$226,622
4	51	$226,622	15%	$33,993	$10,000	$270,615
5	52	$270,615	4%	$10,825	$10,000	$291,439
6	53	$291,439	10%	$29,144	$10,000	$330,583
7	54	$330,583	8%	$26,447	$10,000	$367,030

Year	Age	Opening balance of principal	Returns in year	Annual earnings	Additional contributions	Closing balance at year end
8	55	$367,030	–3%	–$11,011	$10,000	$366,019
9	56	$366,019	12%	$43,922	$10,000	$419,941
10	57	$419,941	7%	$29,396	$10,000	$459,337
11	58	$459,337	10%	$45,934	$10,000	$515,271
12	59	$515,271	5%	$25,764	$10,000	$551,035
13	60	$551,035	11%	$60,614	$10,000	$621,648
14	61	$621,648	10%	$62,165	$10,000	$693,813
15	62	$693,813	6%	$41,629	$10,000	$745,442
16	63	$745,442	8%	$59,635	$10,000	$815,077
17	64	$815,077	4%	$32,603	$10,000	$857,681
18	65	$857,681	12%	$102,922	$10,000	$970,602
19	66	$970,602	8%	$77,648	$10,000	$1,058,250
20	67	$1,058,250	6%	$63,495	$10,000	$1,131,745
21	68	$1,131,745	8%	$90,540	$10,000	$1,232,285
22	69	$1,232,285	12%	$147,874	$10,000	$1,390,159
23	70	$1,390,159	4%	$55,606	$10,000	$1,455,766
		Average return	8%			

Next let's do two examples that show how the two variables of compounding work. First, let's look at the rate of return.

Let's see how Sam's situation might change if he invests in higher-growth assets and gets a long-term return of 10 per cent, compounding, and he continues to save $10,000 per year too.

Year	Age	Opening balance of principal	Returns in year	Annual earnings	Additional contributions	Closing balance at year end
1	48	$150,000	9%	$13,500	$10,000	$173,500
2	49	$173,500	13%	$22,555	$10,000	$206,055
3	50	$206,055	8%	$16,484	$10,000	$232,539
4	51	$232,539	15%	$34,881	$10,000	$277,420
5	52	$277,420	6%	$16,645	$10,000	$304,066
6	53	$304,066	14%	$42,569	$10,000	$356,635
7	54	$356,635	13%	$46,363	$10,000	$412,997
8	55	$412,997	2%	$8,260	$10,000	$431,257

LESSON 5: UNDERSTAND THE FOUNDATIONS OF FINANCIAL CONFIDENCE

Year	Age	Opening balance of principal	Returns in year	Annual earnings	Additional contributions	Closing balance at year end
9	56	$431,257	12%	$51,751	$10,000	$493,008
10	57	$493,008	9%	$44,371	$10,000	$547,379
11	58	$547,379	11%	$60,212	$10,000	$617,590
12	59	$617,590	7%	$43,231	$10,000	$670,822
13	60	$670,822	12%	$80,499	$10,000	$761,320
14	61	$761,320	10%	$76,132	$10,000	$847,452
15	62	$847,452	12%	$101,694	$10,000	$959,147
16	63	$959,147	8%	$76,732	$10,000	$1,045,878
17	64	$1,045,878	4%	$41,835	$10,000	$1,097,714
18	65	$1,097,714	12%	$131,726	$10,000	$1,239,439
19	66	$1,239,439	14%	$173,521	$10,000	$1,422,961
20	67	$1,422,961	9%	$128,066	$10,000	$1,561,027
21	68	$1,561,027	8%	$124,882	$10,000	$1,695,909
22	69	$1,695,909	13%	$220,468	$10,000	$1,926,377
23	70	$1,926,377	9%	$173,374	$10,000	$2,109,751
		Average return	10%			

Now let's look at the power of time.

What if Sam was to kick off this more aggressive growth strategy eight years earlier, at the age of 40, with a $150,000 super balance when he started? How would he benefit from those extra eight years when he reached his Prime Time, and what could he do with that extra income?

Year	Age	Opening balance of principal	Returns in year	Annual earnings at 8%	Additional contributions	Closing balance at year end
1	40	$150,000	9%	$13,500	$10,000	$173,500
2	41	$173,500	13%	$22,555	$10,000	$206,055
3	42	$206,055	8%	$16,484	$10,000	$232,539
4	43	$232,539	15%	$34,881	$10,000	$277,420
5	44	$277,420	6%	$16,645	$10,000	$304,066
6	45	$304,066	14%	$42,569	$10,000	$356,635
7	46	$356,635	13%	$46,363	$10,000	$412,997
8	47	$412,997	2%	$8,260	$10,000	$431,257

Year	Age	Opening balance of principal	Returns in year	Annual earnings at 8%	Additional contributions	Closing balance at year end
9	48	$431,257	12%	$51,751	$10,000	$493,008
10	49	$493,008	9%	$44,371	$10,000	$547,379
11	50	$547,379	11%	$60,212	$10,000	$617,590
12	51	$617,590	7%	$43,231	$10,000	$670,822
13	52	$670,822	12%	$80,499	$10,000	$761,320
14	53	$761,320	10%	$76,132	$10,000	$847,452
15	54	$847,452	12%	$101,694	$10,000	$959,147
16	55	$959,147	8%	$76,732	$10,000	$1,045,878
17	56	$1,045,878	4%	$41,835	$10,000	$1,097,714
18	57	$1,097,714	12%	$131,726	$10,000	$1,239,439
19	58	$1,239,439	14%	$173,521	$10,000	$1,422,961
20	59	$1,422,961	9%	$128,066	$10,000	$1,561,027
21	60	$1,561,027	8%	$124,882	$10,000	$1,695,909
22	61	$1,695,909	13%	$220,468	$10,000	$1,926,377
23	62	$1,926,377	9%	$173,374	$10,000	$2,109,751
24	63	$2,109,751	7%	$147,683	$10,000	$2,267,434
25	64	$2,267,434	12%	$272,092	$10,000	$2,549,526
26	65	$2,549,526	6%	$152,972	$10,000	$2,712,498
27	66	$2,712,498	14%	$379,750	$10,000	$3,102,247
28	67	$3,102,247	13%	$403,292	$10,000	$3,515,539
29	68	$3,515,539	10%	$351,554	$10,000	$3,877,093
30	69	$3,877,093	6%	$232,626	$10,000	$4,119,719
31	70	$4,119,719	12%	$494,366	$10,000	$4,624,085
		Average return	10%			

Why is this important? Well, if you begin investing actively in growth assets in your late 40s or 50s, you have the potential to double your money every 7–10 years at the average rates of return we are seeing from growth investments at Australian superannuation funds today. This strategy can be a game-changer for building wealth. By holding compounding investments inside super for your post-access years and outside super for the pre-access years, you can ensure your assets are working for you – generating passive income when needed and growing tax-efficiently over time.

SUPER IS DESIGNED TO GROW YOUR MONEY THROUGH COMPOUNDING

Superannuation is all about harnessing the power of compound investing. In Australia, the system is set up so that 12 per cent of your salary goes straight into a super 'accumulation' account – this happens automatically from 1 July 2025. Plus, the government gives you a big incentive to boost that amount, allowing you to contribute up to $30,000 a year from your income at a concessional tax rate of 15 per cent up until you're 75. On top of that, you can throw in another $120,000 per year in after-tax dollars, if you have more to invest. And there's a $300,000 one-off tax-free downsizer concession too.

Your super fund then invests that money across different options – stocks, bonds, property, you name it – and the returns from these investments are reinvested, compounding over time. This snowball effect, with fees kept relatively low, helps your super grow faster than if you were just saving the cash on your own.

Most Australians start putting money into super from the time they're 16–18 and can't touch it until they're 60–65. That means you could have up to 49 years of compounding returns working in your favour, giving your retirement savings a huge boost by the time you're ready to kick back and enjoy them.

Compound investing is at the heart of building a solid financial foundation. It drives the growth of your superannuation, increases the value of your home over time, and powers any long-term investment strategy. As we continue, keep this simple concept in mind and think about how you can harness compounding to grow your wealth steadily and effortlessly.

5. DEVELOP A SOLID UNDERSTANDING OF TAX, TAX DEDUCTIONS AND TAX CONCESSIONS

One of the most effective ways to grow your wealth is by understanding and taking advantage of the tax system, including the tax concessions on offer. Stay with me here – I know tax can be heavy stuff! In simple terms, this means finding smart strategies to pay less tax and keep more of the income and capital gains you earn.

With the right approach, you can minimise what you pay in taxes, legally, and invest those savings to supercharge your financial growth. Whether you're saving for your Prime Time and Epic Retirement using superannuation, or investing outside super, making the most of the tax benefits you're eligible for should be one of your big financial priorities.

But where do you start? First, it's important to understand the two primary taxes that affect your financial life: income tax and capital gains tax (CGT). Once you grasp how these work, you can start exploring juicy tax concessions and the clever strategies that can help reduce your tax burden and maximise your wealth.

Let's dive into the basics of these two types of taxes.

INCOME TAX

We all pay tax on the money we earn in any financial year. This type of tax is called income tax and it's the most well understood (and disliked) of the taxes.

There are three different ways to earn an income and pay income tax:

1. By doing work and earning a salary or wage, you pay income tax through your employer in what's called pay as you go (PAYG).
2. By running a business and drawing a combination of wages and a dividend, both of which you pay income tax on.
3. By investing money, and generating income from the investments – all the money you earn from these investments is taxable as income.

Ultimately, we pay income tax at our 'marginal tax rate' on all of these. The most recent Australian tax rates are detailed below.

AUSTRALIAN TAX RATES 2025	
Taxable income	Tax on this income
0 – $18,200	Nil
$18,201 – $45,000	16c* for each $1 over $18,200
$45,001 – $135,000	$4,288 plus 30c for each $1 over $45,000
$135,001 – $190,000	$31,288 plus 37c for each $1 over $135,000
$190,001 and over	$51,638 plus 45c for each $1 over $190,000

* Note: The Australian Government will cut the lowest tax bracket from 16c to 15c from 1 July 2026, and to 14c from 1 July 2027.

INCOME TAX DEDUCTIONS: LEARN HOW TO PAY LESS INCOME TAX

We all want to legally pay less income tax, and most people can achieve this by claiming tax deductions. These deductions, which you claim once a year when submitting your tax return, reduce your taxable income, meaning you pay less tax overall. Keep in mind that the ATO is increasingly automating returns for people with simple finances, and they're using AI to check things, so being proactive and honest is key.

The ATO has a long list of allowable tax deductions on its website. The most common deductions include:

- Protective clothing for work, if your job requires it
- Sun-safe clothing and sunscreen if you work outdoors
- Job-related training courses
- Running costs of your car for work (not commuting), which can be claimed at standard rates
- Home office expenses if you work from home, like energy, stationery and office equipment.

One of the most sizeable deductions available is there to help you invest. If you earn income from investments, you can claim the interest paid on money borrowed to invest. This is a very popular deduction, used by many people to turbocharge their investing with leverage.

By understanding and claiming these deductions, you can reduce your tax bill or get a nice tax refund at the end of the year. It's nothing new for most people, but it's a key part of managing your money smartly.

Another way to lower your tax is through superannuation, a tax-friendly way to invest for the long term, which I'll dive into later.

DEDUCTIBLE DEBT AND NON-DEDUCTIBLE DEBT

You need to understand the difference between the two types of debt – deductible and non-deductible – to make smarter financial decisions.

Deductible debt is when you borrow money to invest in income-generating assets, like rental properties, shares or managed funds. This is often considered 'good debt' because the interest is tax-deductible, meaning you can reduce your taxable income. For example, with an investment property, if your costs (like loan interest) are higher than the income, you can use that loss to reduce the tax you pay over a year – and get a sizeable refund at year end (negative gearing).

Non-deductible debt is when you borrow for things that don't generate income, like your home, car or personal loans. This is generally seen as less favourable since you can't claim the interest as a tax deduction. While borrowing for a home isn't bad as such, it doesn't offer the tax perks that deductible debt does. Remember that any gains made on your principal place of residence are capital gains tax-free – making it a potentially valuable long-term asset.

A common strategy for building wealth is to focus on paying off non-deductible debt (such as your home loan) early and then using the equity in the home to borrow for investments that grow over time. Knowing how to manage each type of debt is essential. A financial adviser can help you make the best choices.

CAPITAL GAINS TAX (CGT)

CGT is the tax you pay on the profit made when selling assets. It doesn't get as much attention as income tax, but trust me, it's just as important, especially if you're aiming to grow your financial resources.

When you sell an asset for more than what you paid for it, the difference is called a capital gain, and that's where CGT comes into play. Here's how it works:

Selling investments: If you sell shares, property or other investments for a profit, CGT applies. To figure out your gain, subtract what you originally paid (including purchase costs like stamp duty and legal fees) from the sale price. The difference is your capital gain and you may owe tax on that.

Selling a business: If you sell your business (or part of it) and make a profit, CGT kicks in here too. Whether it's the whole business or just a portion, the ATO will want a cut of the profit you made.

Transferring assets: Giving assets away doesn't let you dodge CGT. The market value at the time of the transfer is treated like a sale, even if you didn't get any cash. For instance, if you transfer your rental property to your daughter, you'll still have to pay CGT on the profit you've accumulated over the years if the property has gone up in value.

Calculating capital gains tax

Capital gains are added to your assessable income and taxed at your marginal tax rate. Here's a simplified example:
- Purchase price of asset: $100,000
- Selling price of asset: $150,000
- Capital gain: $50,000

So you would then add $50,000 to your taxable income and pay tax on it at the overall levels.

There is an incentive to invest for the long haul. If you hold onto the asset for more than 12 months, you could be eligible for a 50 per cent discount on the capital gain (if you're an individual or a trust). This reduces the amount that's taxed. So in this case, it would look like this:

- Purchase price of asset: $100,000
- Selling price of asset: $150,000
- Capital gain: $50,000
- 50 per cent discount on long-term capital gain: $25,000
- Amount added to your taxable income: $25,000.

Reducing capital gains tax

There are a few smart moves you can make to reduce the CGT you pay when selling assets:

Hold assets for longer: Hang onto your assets for more than 12 months and you could score a 50 per cent discount on the capital gain.

Offset gains with losses: If you've had a rough year and made a capital loss, you can use it to offset any gains. And if your losses outweigh your gains, you can carry them forward to reduce future tax.

Leverage superannuation: Investing through your super fund can offer some handy tax perks and may reduce CGT on assets sold within the fund.

Use trusts and companies: Holding assets in structures like family trusts or companies can help manage CGT, but it's not straightforward. This strategy requires careful planning, as trusts and companies come with different tax rules. To make sure you're doing it right – and to avoid any unwanted tax surprises – it's essential to seek professional advice from an accountant, financial adviser or both.

By understanding these strategies and managing your capital gains wisely, you can legally reduce the amount of tax you pay.

CGT concessions

Now we need to talk strategy. It's important to understand how you can minimise the CGT you pay when selling assets. The following tips can help you make smarter decisions about when to buy, sell or hold onto your assets.

Main residence exemption

This one is important to understand. In Australia, the family home is exempt from CGT, meaning that when you sell your primary residence, any profit you make is not subject to capital gains tax. This is why owning a home has been such a huge wealth builder in this country. And it's one of the reasons why a home bought early in life is so much more valuable than any other asset, which might only be eligible for a 50 per cent discount on CGT if held longer than a year.

50 per cent CGT discount

As mentioned, if you hold onto an asset for more than 12 months, individuals and some trusts can claim a 50 per cent discount on the capital gain. This cuts the taxable portion in half and can be a big win for long-term investors. It's a solid incentive to hold assets longer and reduce the tax bite on your profits.

Small business CGT concessions

Small business owners in Australia can tap into a range of CGT concessions when they sell their small business. These are especially useful for those in their Prime Time. There are three you should become familiar with:
 1. **The 15-year exemption**: wipes out CGT entirely if you've owned the business asset for at least 15 years and are over 55
 2. **The retirement exemption**: gives up to $500,000 in CGT relief when you retire or wind up the business, and if you're under 55, the amount needs to go into super
 3. **The CGT rollover option**: lets you defer CGT if you're reinvesting in new business assets, helping you grow or transition the business.

Knowing these concessions can make a huge difference when planning your business exit or retirement in your prime time years, to maximise your gains. If you're considering this, seek advice about your own circumstances. Your tax accountant is best placed to help you.

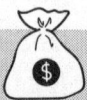

SUPERANNUATION AS A TAX STRUCTURE

Superannuation is a tax structure designed to help you save for retirement in a tax-efficient way. Concessional contributions to your super are taxed at just 15%, which is much lower than most income tax rates, making it a powerful way to reduce tax and build your retirement savings. The earnings on your investments inside super are also taxed at 15% while you're in the accumulation phase. And when you retire and start drawing down your super, those withdrawals can be tax-free if you're over 60 and cease working or 65 unconditionally. So, while super itself isn't a tax, it is a smart tax structure that offers significant concessions to help your money grow.

FRANKING CREDITS AND COMPANY TAX

When it comes to investing, understanding how company tax and franking credits work can give you a major advantage.

In Australia, companies pay tax on their profits at a flat rate of 30 per cent (or 25 per cent for eligible small businesses, known as base rate entities). When a company distributes its profits as dividends to shareholders, it has already paid tax on those profits. To avoid double taxation, companies attach franking credits to the dividends.

Franking credits essentially say, 'We've already paid some tax on this, so you don't have to.' When you file your tax return, these credits reduce the income tax you owe on that dividend, and if you're in a lower tax bracket, you might even get a refund on the credits. This system makes investing in Australian companies more tax-efficient, which is why dividend-paying shares are so attractive to investors.

How it works for individuals

Let's say you own shares in an Australian company that's taxed at 30 per cent, and the company pays you a $700 dividend. They'll attach $300 in franking credits (because they've already paid 30 per cent tax on the dividend). Here's what happens:
- Gross dividend received: $700
- Franking credit: $300
- Assessable income: $1000 (the total of your dividend and the franking credit).

Now, let's say your marginal tax rate is 30 per cent (which is the current rate for income between $45,001 and $135,000):
- Tax owed on assessable income ($1000): $300
- Franking credit applied: $300
- Additional tax to pay: $0.

So you would have no additional tax to pay.

If your marginal tax rate is lower (say 19 per cent, which applies to income between $18,201 and $45,000):
- Tax owed on assessable income ($1000): $190
- Franking credit applied: $300
- Tax refund: $110.

In this case, because your tax owed is less than the franking credit, you'd receive a refund of $110.

How it works for superannuation

Franking credits can also provide great tax efficiency within your superannuation, whether it's in the accumulation phase (taxed at 15 per cent) or the retirement phase (tax-free if below the transfer balance cap).

Super in the accumulation phase

If your super is still in the accumulation phase, your super fund pays 15 per cent tax on earnings, including dividends. Here's an example of how franking credits would work in this case:

- Dividend received: $700
- Franking credit attached: $300 (company has already paid 30 per cent tax on the dividend)
- Assessable income: $1000 (the dividend + franking credit)
- Tax owed at 15 per cent on assessable income ($1000): $150
- Franking credit applied: $300.

In this scenario, the franking credit of $300 is greater than the $150 tax owed by your super fund. The super fund would receive a refund of $150, boosting the overall return on that investment.

Super in the retirement phase

When your super is in the retirement phase, it's even better – there's *no tax* on earnings. Here's how franking credits work:

- Dividend received: $700
- Franking credit attached: $300
- Assessable income: $1000
- Tax owed at 0 per cent: $0.

In this case, because your super fund owes no tax, the full $300 franking credit is refunded to the fund. This refund directly boosts the return on your investment.

GOODS AND SERVICES TAX

While the goods and services tax (GST) doesn't really offer any special perks or deductions for people in midlife, it's good to know how it works, especially if you're running a business or working for yourself. GST is the 10 per cent tax that's added to most goods and services in Australia, and if your business turnover hits $75,000 or more a year, you need to register to charge it.

For most of us, GST is just baked into the price of the stuff we buy, but if you're running a business, remember to claim back the GST you pay on business expenses (called input tax credits). This can help reduce your costs and keep more money in your pocket.

And if you hold investments within a GST-registered entity, you may also be entitled to a GST refund on brokerage fees, transaction costs and other charges related to managing those investments.

TAX CONCESSIONS YOU SHOULD BE AWARE OF

Tax concessions are basically the taxman's way of giving you a break – legal ways to pay less tax and keep more of what you earn. These are special opportunities designed to help you make smarter investments, save for the future and reduce your overall tax bill.

There's a range of tax concessions out there, especially for those in midlife and beyond, that can help you trim down how much tax you fork over each year.

The downsizer concession

If you're over 55 and ready to sell the family home you've lived in for at least 10 years, the downsizer concession is your friend. This one-off deal lets you throw up to $300,000 per person (or $600,000 per couple) into your super without paying tax on that contribution. There are a few conditions to watch out for, but it's a fantastic way to boost your super with the sale of your home, giving your retirement fund a nice bump without giving a chunk to the ATO.

Senior Australians and pensioners tax offset (SAPTO)

SAPTO is a fairly limited perk for senior Australians and pensioners. If you're of pension age (but you don't have to be receiving the age pension) and have an income within the qualifying thresholds, this offset can help reduce your tax bill. In fact, if your income is within the qualifying range, it could knock your tax down to zero. It's a great way to ease the tax burden and keep more of your hard-earned money as you enjoy your retirement.

Private health insurance rebate

The private health insurance rebate is designed to make private health cover more affordable by reducing the cost of premiums. It's income-tested, meaning the lower your income, the higher the rebate you receive. The federal government offers this rebate as either a direct discount on your premiums (applied by your insurer) or as a tax offset when you lodge your tax return. For singles earning under $97,000 and families earning under $194,000, the rebate is at its highest, but it gradually reduces for higher earners and phases out completely at $151,000 for singles and $302,000 for families. This means many Australians can keep their hospital and extras cover more affordable without taking a big hit to their budget.

However there are extra costs if you don't take out private hospital cover at the right time. If you delay getting hospital cover past the age of 31, you may have to pay Lifetime Health Cover (LHC) loading, which adds an extra 2 per cent to your premiums for every year you wait, up to a maximum of 70 per cent. This stays on your policy for 10 years, making late entry into private health insurance much more expensive.

There's also the Medicare Levy Surcharge (MLS) – if you earn over $97,000 (singles) or $194,000 (families) and don't have private hospital cover, you'll have to pay an extra tax of up to 1.5 per cent of your income on top of the 2 per cent Medicare Levy that everyone pays.

So while private health insurance isn't compulsory, there are financial penalties for higher-income earners and those who delay taking out cover, making it something worth considering before costs start adding up.

NOW LET'S GET STRATEGIC

Now that you've got a better handle on the tax system, it's time to start thinking about how to use it to grow your wealth. Let's break down the major strategies.

Adding a concessional contribution

Consider salary sacrificing extra funds into your superannuation. You can contribute up to $30,000 a year in total (this amount is indexed with rising wages and includes your employer contributions) and pay just 15 per cent tax on it instead of your regular income tax rate. The best way to take advantage of this is by asking your employer to contribute more than the standard 12 per cent super guarantee from 1 July 2025, salary-sacrificing those funds before you see them, allowing you to benefit from the lower tax rate. Alternatively, you can make personal contributions and claim a tax deduction when you file your tax return.

If you've already hit your concessional contributions cap, you can still make non-concessional contributions (after-tax contributions) of up to $120,000 per year in the 2025/26 financial year (this amount is also indexed). While non-concessional contributions won't give you an immediate tax break, the money grows at just 15 per cent income tax and 10 per cent capital gains tax in your super, and there's currently no tax on the earnings once you're in retirement, unless you are over the transfer balance cap.

Example (2025/26 financial year): Jake earns $150,000 and adds a concessional contribution via salary sacrifice. Jake's employer contributes the 12 per cent super guarantee, which totals $18,000. Wanting to grow his super faster, Jake decides to salary sacrifice an additional $12,000, bringing his total contributions up to the $30,000 concessional cap.

Normally, if Jake took that extra $12,000 as part of his salary, he'd be taxed at 37 per cent (his marginal tax rate), leaving him with just $7560 after tax. However, by salary sacrificing the amount into his super, he only pays 15 per cent tax on that $12,000, meaning $10,200 ends up in his super account, giving him an extra $2640 compared to taking it as regular income.

Over time, the tax savings, combined with the compounded returns on that extra money inside super, can significantly boost Jake's retirement savings.

Adding a non-concessional contribution

Now let's say Jake has additional savings and wants to invest even more into his super after hitting his concessional cap. He can make a non-concessional contribution.

Example: Jake adds $10,000 as a non-concessional contribution. Because Jake has already paid income tax on this $10,000, he can contribute it to his super tax-free as a non-concessional contribution.

By investing this $10,000 in his super instead of a regular investment account, Jake benefits from the tax-free growth inside super when he retires, compared to being taxed on earnings outside of super.

Over time, this additional non-concessional contribution will compound alongside his concessional contributions, helping Jake build a larger retirement nest egg.

Leveraging your family home to invest and receive a tax deduction

Gearing to invest lets you use borrowed money to invest in income-generating assets like shares, managed funds or rental properties. The goal is two-fold: to pay off your non-deductible home loan, and to grow your wealth using borrowed funds (often secured against your home) while taking advantage of the tax-deductibility on investment loans.

Here's how it works. After paying down your home loan, you can borrow against the equity in your home to invest. Since this new loan is tied to income-producing investments (like dividends from shares or rental income), the interest is tax-deductible. As your investments grow and generate returns, those returns can help cover the interest costs, allowing you to invest more over time.

While this strategy offers potential benefits, there are two key things to consider. First, you need to ensure you can service the debt, which means having enough income to cover repayments even if your investments don't perform as expected. And second, you'll need to be in a position where the tax deductions actually benefit you. If your income isn't high enough to make the most of the deductions, this strategy may not be a smart one.

Example 1: Anita, earning $100,000. Anita earns $100,000 per year and has recently paid off a big chunk of her home loan. Feeling financially comfortable, she decides to borrow $100,000 using an interest-only loan at 6 per cent to invest in Australian shares. She plans to hold the investment for at least five years. Her investment is expected to deliver:

- 4 per cent cash dividend yield, fully franked – that's $4000 per year in cash
- Capital growth of 4 per cent per year.

Each year:
- Interest paid: $6000
- Tax benefit from interest deduction: $1800 (30 per cent of $6000)
- Net interest cost: $4200
- Cash dividends received: $4000
- Franking credits: $1714
- Gross dividend: $5714
- Tax on dividend: $1714, fully offset by franking credits
- Net tax on dividend: $0.

Net cashflow shortfall per year = $4200 − $4000 = $200

Over five years:
- Total cash dividends: $20,000
- Total franking credits: $8571
- Total out-of-pocket funding: $1000
- Investment grows to: $121,665
- Capital gain: $21,665
- CGT (after 50 per cent discount): $3250
- Net capital gain after tax: $18,415.

Final outcome after five years	
Item	Amount
Net after-tax capital gain	$18,415
Total cash dividends received	$20,000
Less total cashflow shortfall	−$1000
Total net benefit after five years	**$37,415**

In short: By borrowing to invest in fully franked Australian shares with a 4 per cent cash yield and 4 per cent growth, Anita ends up around $37,415 ahead after five years – after covering all her loan costs and yearly top-ups.

> **IMPORTANT POINTS TO CONSIDER**
>
> **The timing difference:** While Anita gets a tax deduction, the benefit only comes when she files her tax return. Until then, she covers the full interest payments.
> **The lumpy income:** Dividends are not paid monthly, so she needs to plan for cash flow gaps between her monthly interest payments and when the dividends arrive.
> **The tax savings come a year later:** While the tax deduction reduces her overall interest cost, she still needs to cover those interest payments during the year.
> **The market risks:** Borrowing to invest works well for her in rising markets, but in falling markets it could cause her financial stress as she would still have to meet loan repayments even if her investments drop in value. If companies reduce or stop paying dividends – something that can happen in tough economic conditions – and Anita was relying on those payments to cover loan interest, so she could face serious financial pressure.

Example 2: Nikos, earning $250,000. Nikos earns $250,000 a year, putting him in the top marginal tax bracket – 47 per cent including the Medicare levy. Confident in his income and borrowing power, he takes out a $100,000 interest-only loan at 6 per cent and invests it in Australian shares. He plans to hold the investment for at least five years. His investment is expected to deliver:
- 4 per cent cash dividend yield, fully franked – that's $4000 per year in cash
- Capital growth of 4 per cent per year.

Each year:
- Interest paid: $6000
- Cash dividends received: $4000
- Franking credits: $1714
- His total taxable dividend income is $5714 (gross)
- Tax on that income at 47 per cent = $2686
- After applying the franking credit of $1714, he still owes $971 in tax
- He also deducts the $6000 interest expense. The tax saving from the deduction = 47 per cent of $6000 = $2820.

Nikos's cashflow each year:
- Interest paid: $6000
- Tax benefit from interest deduction: $2820
- Extra tax on dividends after franking credit: $971
- Cash dividends received: $4000.

Net out-of-pocket cashflow shortfall = $6000 (interest) − $2820 (benefit) + $971 (dividend tax) − $4000 (dividends) = $151 per year

He needs to top up about $151 each year from salary or savings to keep the strategy going.

Over five years:
- Total cashflow shortfall: $757 ($151 × 5)
- Total cash dividends received: $20,000
- Total tax on dividends: $4857
- Net dividends after tax: $15,143
- Total franking credits received: $8571
- Total tax savings from loan interest: $14,100.

Meanwhile, his $100,000 investment grows at 4 per cent annually. After five years, it's worth about $121,665.

Capital gains tax:
- Capital gain = $121,665 − $100,000 = $21,665
- After 50 per cent CGT discount: $10,833 taxable

- Tax at 47 per cent = $5091
- Net capital gain after tax = $16,574.

Final outcome after five years	
Item	Amount
Net after-tax capital gain	$16,574
Total cash dividends received	$15,143
Less total cashflow shortfall	−$757
Total net benefit after five years	**$30,960**

In short: By borrowing $100,000 to invest in fully franked Australian shares with a 4 per cent cash yield and 4 per cent capital growth, Nikos comes out $30,960 ahead after five years – even after covering loan costs, tax, and out-of-pocket top-ups.

> ### BORROWING TO INVEST: KEY TAKEAWAYS
>
> Borrowing to invest isn't a set-and-forget strategy. It requires careful planning, strong cash flow and the ability to handle market downturns. If you're not prepared for the risks, it might not be the right approach. If you're considering this approach, here are some important lessons to keep in mind:
>
> - **Tax benefits don't come straight away**: Yes, you can claim interest as a tax deduction, but that doesn't mean the cost disappears. You still have to cover the interest payments every month and the tax break only kicks in when you do your tax return.
> - **Dividends aren't a safety net**: They provide income, but they aren't guaranteed, they're taxable and they don't always arrive when you need them. Franking credits help with tax, but they don't magically make an investment profitable.
> - **Capital gains tax still takes a chunk**: Holding an investment for more than a year gives you a 50 per cent CGT discount, but of course you still pay tax on half the gain. Selling when the market is strong helps, but timing is everything.

- **Cash flow really is key**: Interest is charged monthly, but dividends are usually paid quarterly or annually. You need a plan to cover expenses while waiting for income.
- **Markets don't always cooperate**: Leverage works both ways – when markets rise, borrowing can accelerate gains. But if markets fall, you're still on the hook for loan repayments even if your investments drop in value.

Two reasons why people use leverage:
1. **The pursuit of capital gains**: The main reason people use leverage is to increase their potential capital growth. While you can claim a tax deduction on the interest paid, the real goal is to grow your wealth over time by holding appreciating assets.
2. **Leverage to build wealth faster**: Borrowing to invest allows you to leverage your existing equity to grow your wealth faster than if you were just using your own savings. It's about using other people's money (the bank's) to make money for yourself, faster – but please make sure it fits within your risk tolerance and financial strategy.

Negative gearing your investments

At first, the idea of losing money on an investment might sound like a bad strategy, right? But negative gearing is actually a popular strategy in Australia, used chiefly by property investors because it offers short-term tax benefits and the potential for long-term capital gains.

Negative gearing happens when the costs of owning an investment property – like mortgage interest, maintenance, and property management fees – are higher than the rental income. In other words, the property is costing you more than it's earning, so you're making a loss. Now while this might sound counterproductive, here's the clever part: you can use that loss to reduce your overall taxable income, meaning you'll pay less tax in the short term.

Here's a basic example:
- **Income**: Say you're earning $20,000 a year in rent from your investment property.
- **Expenses**: The costs of owning the property – loan interest, maintenance, insurance and other fees – total $30,000 a year.
- **Net loss**: You're making a $10,000 loss on the property ($30,000 in expenses minus $20,000 in rent).

Because of negative gearing, you can take that $10,000 loss and offset it against your other taxable income, like your salary. So if you earn $100,000 a year from your job, the loss reduces your taxable income to $90,000. As a result, you pay less tax, which helps you manage the ongoing costs of the property.

But you might be thinking, why would anyone choose to make a loss on purpose just to pay less tax?

The goal of negative gearing is long-term capital growth. Sure, you might be out of pocket in the first years, but the idea is that the property's value will increase over time, and that when you sell it you will more than cover those early losses. Many people use this strategy in areas where property prices are expected to rise, with the hope that property will be a key part of building their long-term wealth.

Embracing franking credits

As we learned earlier in the section, franking credits can offer a powerful additional line of income, particularly for people who are living on a tax-free or low-tax income, as you might be during your part-time and retirement years.

Franking credits are a tax benefit that can boost your investment returns if you hold shares in Australian companies. Since the company has already paid tax on its profits, you get a credit for that tax. If your personal tax rate is lower than the company tax rate (30 per cent), you can use the credits to reduce your own tax or even get a refund. It's a smart way to avoid double taxation and maximise your income from dividends.

6. PAY OFF A HOME THAT'S WITHIN YOUR MEANS

This is a big, important lesson.

I hope you own your own home. And I hope one of your big financial goals is to pay it off (or at the very least pay it down to the last $10 and keep the loan open and the redraw account full). There's simply no better way to build wealth and give yourself financial freedom and security later in life than by owning your own home.

Home ownership in Australia is very attractive. When you buy a house and pay it off over your working years, you get to use a mortgage to access leverage that isn't available at that scale on other asset types. If you rent during those years, you miss out on that leverage. You also miss out on the CGT exemption offered on your principal place of residence. That adds up over a lifetime.

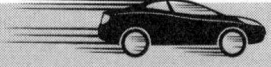

BUYING A HOUSE GETS YOUR FINANCIAL ENGINE STARTED

Here's why buying a house fires up your financial engine:
- It kickstarts compound investing through home ownership.
- You can use borrowed money (your mortgage) to amplify your growth. Banks will lend more against a home than they will against shares or rental properties.
- It allows you to benefit from CGT incentives, making your investment more efficient.
- It acts as a compulsory savings system, where you're essentially forced to invest by making regular mortgage payments.
- And when you own your own home, you no longer have to pay rent to a landlord!

What we don't often talk about is that houses don't generate income like some other investments do. Instead, they provide an 'implied yield' by saving you from paying rent. While home

> ownership offers potential capital growth and the security of a roof over your head, it can also tie up a large portion of your wealth. As you move into the second half of life and income generation becomes increasingly important, it's worth considering how much of your wealth is locked in your home – as this can limit your ability to access funds to invest for income.

But let's put it in real life terms. Think about how home ownership has played out for many Prime Timers. You bought your first home, allowing you to get on the housing ladder. As your family and career grew, you probably upgraded your home to a larger one, often in a better suburb (because you could), taking a larger mortgage and hopefully increasing the pace of your compound growth. And then you lived in it, using the mortgage payments as a compulsory savings scheme, and over many years your capital grew – on paper.

If you managed to avoid divorce, you might be entering your Prime Time with more than four-times returns on your housing investment, potentially even more. Statistically over the past 30 years, Australian housing has grown by 382 per cent. In annual compounding terms, this translates to an average house price rise of 5.4 per cent per year since July 1992.[16] This significant growth has made many Prime Timers in Australia property-rich. In fact, for many, their family home is their biggest asset.

If you didn't manage to avoid divorce – and let's be real: with around 33 per cent of marriages ending in divorce, you're definitely not alone – it can be a harder road to navigate. Divorce can take a significant financial toll, often meaning you have to work a lot harder to get back on the property ladder, especially if you're doing it on your own. Still, many Prime Timers manage to rebound financially by making strategic choices about property, investments and lifestyle. For others, it might mean navigating the complexities of re-partnering and figuring out how to blend families and assets in new ways.

In fact, post-divorce, this phase can be an opportunity to rethink your long-term housing and lifestyle goals with more clarity, particularly if you're free of earlier life obligations. The key is recognising that even with life's twists and turns, there's still room for your prime time goals.

Do yourself a favour, though. Try to find a way to own your own home before you stop working for good. It will give you so much more financial freedom and security as you move into the later stages of your Prime Time, and then your Epic Retirement, helping you live the life you envision without the stress of rent, landlords or mortgage payments hanging over your head.

THE ULTIMATE GOAL

The goal for most Australians looking to maximise their Prime Time is to pay off their home, whatever its size, by their mid-50s, ideally earlier. Once you reach this point, you gain a financial advantage you may not have seen coming:

- When you no longer have mortgage payments, you can use that money to save more aggressively for your Prime Time and Epic Retirement.
- You end up with a mortgage-free asset that can provide a secure roof over your head for the rest of your life.
- You may find your home is larger than needed or located in a more expensive suburb, which allows you the option to sell, release equity, and reallocate funds into superannuation or income-generating investments for your second half of life.

Future generations approaching their Prime Time may find it harder to fully own a valuable home by retirement. However, for today's boomers and generation X, property remains their number-one financial asset, and I believe it will continue to be in the future. Governments just haven't learned how to make that happen yet. But rest assured, in other countries they're working out how to get younger generations on the property ladder despite its challenging affordability – so in time it's likely that we will too.

SHOULD YOU REALLY PAY OFF YOUR MORTGAGE IN FULL?

We've always been told that the ultimate financial goal is to pay off our home loan and finally receive those mortgage papers from the bank. But is that really the smartest strategy? Many people now opt to pay their mortgage down to the last $10 while keeping a healthy sum in an offset account. This reduces the payments on the loan to almost nothing but allows access to the money if needed, rather than completely closing off the loan.

The reasoning behind this is simple: as you get older, it becomes much harder to secure a new loan. If you're property-rich but cash-poor, having access to funds through a redraw or offset account could be a lifesaver, giving you financial flexibility without needing to go through the hassle of applying for a new loan.

That said, it's worth considering the costs. Some banks might charge fees for keeping the loan open, while others allow you to keep it running for the full 25 or 30 years without penalty. Weigh it all up to decide what's right for you.

WHEN DO MOST PEOPLE PAY OFF THEIR HOMES?

It's interesting to contemplate when average Prime Timers are paying off their homes today in Australia. The latest Housing Occupancy and Costs survey by the ABS shows that 43 per cent of Australians aged 55–65 own their own homes with some sort of mortgage, and 36 per cent have no mortgage. The ratio changes dramatically between 65 and 75, with 13 per cent holding a mortgage and 68 per cent owning their home outright. About 18.2 per cent of those aged between 55 and 65 rent in Australia – 4.3 per cent of these people live rent-free in government accommodation, while the other 13.9 per cent pay private landlords. The percentage of people renting falls dramatically when you talk about those over 65. Around 9.5 per cent of those between the ages of 65 and 75 rent from a private landlord, and 3.8 per cent live in government accommodation.[17] It will be interesting to see if these trends change – or if ultimately most people strive to pay their home off or downsize just as they retire.

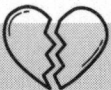

REALITY CHECK: LATER LIFE DIVORCE MESSES UP HOME OWNERSHIP GOALS

Here's a hard truth: divorce rates later in life are rising. When divorce happens, it often forces people to sell assets and divide wealth just when financial stability is most crucial. For many, this means halving assets, making it difficult to re-enter the housing market or take on a mortgage alone. Rebuilding on a single income, especially in your 50s or 60s, can feel overwhelming.

If this is your situation, it's important to recognise that securing a home loan as you age becomes a greater challenge. Lenders are often more cautious about offering mortgages to older borrowers, particularly if retirement is less than 20 years away. This can make it harder to get back into the property market after a late-life divorce, as banks worry about your ability to repay over a shorter timeframe.

But don't lose hope. Owning a smaller, more affordable home with a manageable mortgage still provides you with significant leverage, potential for growth, and long-term security – advantages that renting simply doesn't offer. If home ownership isn't immediately feasible, consider rent-vesting – buying an investment property and renting it out. While it doesn't give you the CGT exemption of a principal residence, lenders can be more flexible because investment properties generate income.

As you approach retirement, if you've paid down a significant portion of the loan on your investment property, you could convert it into your primary residence. While you won't receive the tax benefits for the years it was rented, you'll still enjoy living mortgage-free. Banks may not love this, but there's little they can do once you've significantly reduced the mortgage.

If you don't own another property, you may be able to treat your investment property as your main residence for tax purposes for up to six years – as long as you live in it for at least three

> months first. It's called the six-year rule, and it can soften the CGT blow if you switch it to your home later on.
>
> If neither home ownership nor rent-vesting works for your situation, renting may be your only option. In that case, explore support programs like Commonwealth Rent Assistance to see if you're eligible. Also focus on building up investments that can provide a reliable income in retirement, whether they are shares, superannuation, lifetime annuities or other financial products.
>
> No matter which path you choose, the key is to live within your means and make financially sound decisions that reflect your current situation while still supporting your long-term goals. Rebuilding after divorce is tough, but with the right plan, it's absolutely possible.

Let me tell you the story of Mark and Lisa. Both 58, they have four kids ranging from 17 to 27 in age. They got into the Sydney property market in the late 1990s, buying their first home just before the big boom of the early 2000s. In their 30s, they upgraded to a larger home, and in their mid 50s, as they neared paying that off, they made a bold leap, upgrading to a flashy waterfront suburb with an equally flashy mortgage. Now, looking back, they say it's a move they deeply regret.

At the time, it was all about lifestyle, ego, and the belief that they could afford it. They wanted a large, beautiful home to show off their success. But life had other plans. About a year later, Mark's corporate job was suddenly cut, and his generous salary vanished almost overnight. Around the same time, one of their kids moved overseas and another moved out. Suddenly, their bustling six-person household shrank to four, and their income took a serious hit.

That flashy waterfront house no longer seemed like such a good idea. After six months of job hunting with no success, Mark and Lisa made the tough decision to sell the property and downsize to a more practical home in the suburbs again, one very similar to the home they left. The move ended up costing them around $200,000 in stamp duty, real estate commissions and fees. Worse still, the experience shattered their financial confidence.

To top it off, they sold their long-time family home and upgraded when they were both 54. So they've now missed the window in which they would have been eligible for the downsizer contribution scheme, which starts at 55 (if they hadn't been upgrading, that is). If they'd waited and downsized later, that could have allowed them to put a one-off $600,000 into super, tax-free. Sure, they can hang around for another 10 years in the house they're in, but they're unlikely to want to, they say.

In reality, Mark and Lisa were acting ego-centrically. They hadn't even thought about where they wanted to live after their kids left home or whether they should start reallocating funds from their home to their superannuation, leaving them in a state of uncertainty about whether they'd done the right thing at all. Neither of them have a large super balance, but until now, that never seemed important.

You might be thinking, 'Rich people's problems', but the truth is that many ordinary people face the same dilemma in their Prime Time. Rather than upscaling, top of mind in their 50s and 60s should have been right-sizing or rethinking how to reallocate the capital tied up in a larger-than-necessary family home. Timing it right could save you tens or even hundreds of thousands of dollars.

THE ROLE OF YOUR HOME CHANGES IN THE SECOND HALF OF LIFE

For many people in their 50s and 60s, a big chunk of wealth is tied up in property. And why not? Watching your home's value climb can feel pretty satisfying. It's more than just bricks and mortar; it's a symbol of status and stability.

But as you move through the second half of your life, how you view your home as an asset might shift. Sure, it provides shelter and costs less than renting, but it's often the only part of your portfolio that doesn't generate income to support your lifestyle. In fact, a large, valuable home can end up being under-utilised. That's where the idea of 'right-sizing' comes in – finding a place that better suits your financial goals *and* your living needs.

A lot of people choose to downsize at least once in their later years, moving from the big family home to something smaller and easier to manage, or to a home that offers more in terms of 'lifestyle'. It's not just about cutting down on upkeep but also about freeing up equity that can be invested (inside or outside super) to help fund your retirement lifestyle.

As you approach midlife and start thinking about downsizing, remember: it's not just about cashing in. You need to think about your entire housing journey. You deserve to live in a home you love, but it's equally important to make sure your money, lifestyle and confidence are all considered in a long-term plan.

Previous generations of retirees have been reluctant to leave their big family homes, preferring to age in them, but often unable to manage the maintenance and upkeep in their later years. Today's generations of Prime Timers and Epic Retirees have been incentivised to consider downsizing by the federal government, as explained in the box opposite and on the following pages.

THINK ABOUT HOW MANY TIMES YOU'LL MOVE

Most people in their midlife think about their moves one at a time, but as you prepare for your Prime Time, you need to look further ahead. Reflect on how many moves you've got left in your lifetime, including how many you can afford without burning savings you've spent a lifetime building up. Real estate commissions, stamp duty and moving and renovation costs can really eat into your wealth.

Understand the types of housing suitable in different phases of your life

A lifestyle home might be perfect now, but later on you might need something smaller, lower maintenance, more accessible, or closer to services or family. Start thinking about it and discussing it with your partner and your family early on so you can avoid rushed or ill-considered decisions later. It becomes much harder to move in your 70s and 80s than it is in your 50s and 60s.

Think about where you'll age

The government has made it clear that it wants you to age in your own home if you can. To that end, we're seeing the systems of ageing change to drive this outcome; for example, aged care is becoming more expensive and scarcer, and home care is receiving more government investment. Retirement villages are growing in popularity too, as they provide supported living without the 'care home' vibe. Whatever your path, finding a home you can age in gracefully before you hit a health crisis is important, as is preserving enough money to fund your lifestyle and care needs. And don't forget – many will end up single later in life and should be prepared for that.

Think about how you'll fund aged care

Aged-care costs are increasingly being self-funded, especially for those not relying on the age pension. Most Prime Timers should expect to contribute to their care, so preserving some wealth for that is a must. Many people who own their own homes outright consider this a valuable safety net for their later care needs.

AUSTRALIA'S UNIQUE HOUSING RULES: STRATEGIC OPPORTUNITIES FOR PRIME TIMERS

Australia has some unique property rules that offer significant opportunities if you know how to use them. Here are a few to consider.

1. The downsizer concession

Under the downsizer concession, people aged 55 and over who have owned their family home for at least 10 years can contribute up to $300,000 per person (or $600,000 per couple) into superannuation, tax-free, from the proceeds of selling their home. This is a powerful, one-off chance to significantly boost your super.

2. The age pension assets test exemption

Your principal place of residence is exempt from the age pension assets test, meaning its value won't be counted when determining your eligibility for the pension. Even if your home is worth millions, you could still qualify for a full or partial age pension if your other assets and income fall within the limits. This exemption allows retirees to maintain a valuable asset while still accessing government support.

3. The CGT exemption on your primary residence

Another key benefit of owning a home is the CGT exemption on your principal place of residence. If you sell your home, you don't have to pay tax on the capital gains as long as it's been your primary residence throughout your ownership. This makes it easier to sell and downsize without worrying about losing a chunk of your profits to taxes – a significant advantage for retirees freeing up equity.

4. The six-year CGT rule (great for rent-vesters)

If you rent out a property you've lived in and you don't own another principal residence, you may be able to treat it as your main residence for CGT purposes for up to six years. This rule can work in your favour if you've used a rent-vesting strategy, living in the property first, then renting it out while you live elsewhere. If you sell within that six-year window, you may avoid CGT entirely.

5. The Home Equity Access Scheme (HEAS)

If you're of pension age (67+) and want to access your home's equity without selling, the government's Home Equity Access Scheme can provide a solution. It's essentially a reverse mortgage that allows you to borrow against your home and receive regular payments to supplement your income. This scheme is open to both pensioners and self-funded retirees. The interest rate is extraordinarily low compared to commercial reverse mortgages, at 3.95 per cent. Still, remember that a reverse mortgage uses compounding in reverse, so the longer you borrow the funds for, the more interest you'll pay over your lifetime.

6. The First Home Super Saver Scheme (FHSS)

While primarily aimed at younger Australians, the First Home Super Saver Scheme could benefit you if you're looking to help younger family members get into the housing market. The scheme allows first-time buyers to save for a deposit through superannuation, taking advantage of super's lower tax rates. Supporting your children or grandchildren with FHSS contributions into their superannuation can help them get ahead in the housing market while maximising tax efficiency.

7. Rent assistance for retirees

If you're forced to or choose to live in a rental property, you might be eligible for Commonwealth Rent Assistance as you become eligible for the age pension. It's a program designed to help retirees cover up to 75 cents in the dollar of their rent costs, up to a cap. While it's income-tested, this assistance can potentially reduce the financial impact of renting if you're navigating later life without home ownership.

These programs are of course subject to change – so do your homework and check the latest thresholds, eligibility and rates.

PAYING DOWN YOUR MORTGAGE: AN IMPORTANT PRIORITY

As you move into your Prime Time, that exciting phase where life opens up and your choices expand, you might still have a mortgage weighing you down. The sooner you ditch that non-deductible debt, the sooner you can unlock the financial freedom this stage of life offers.

Remember: every dollar you free up from your mortgage in midlife can go toward lifestyle choices or boosting your super, making it well worth tackling head-on. And while your mortgage may feel like a noose, most people have more options than they think to demolish that debt. It might involve some tough decisions, but brave people do hard things. Here are eight ways to demolish your mortgage debt sooner.

1. Keep working (full-time or part-time)

For some, extending their working years – either full-time or part-time – makes sense. Keeping a steady income allows you to continue paying down the mortgage while slowly transitioning into retirement. If you're earning a higher salary in your final years of work, you can use that extra income to speed up mortgage repayments while still building up your super balance.

2. Downsize your home
Downsizing is another popular option, especially if your current home is larger than you need for your prime time and retirement years. Selling your home and moving to something smaller and more affordable can help you pay off the remaining mortgage. Plus, a smaller home generally comes with lower ongoing costs, like maintenance and utilities, making it easier to manage.

3. Use your superannuation to pay off the mortgage
Once you're over 60 and meet the conditions to access your super, you could use a lump sum to wipe out the rest of your mortgage. While this reduces your super balance, it can give you peace of mind knowing you're debt-free as you enter retirement. Alternatively, using a transition to retirement (TTR) strategy can allow you to supplement your income while directing more of your salary toward paying down the mortgage.

4. Refinance or extend your mortgage term early
If you haven't refinanced recently, now could be a good time to secure a better interest rate or improve your mortgage terms. Extending your mortgage term can also lower your monthly payments, though it might mean paying more interest over time. Still, this could give you some breathing room as you ease into your Prime Time.

5. Rent out part of your home
If you're not ready to downsize but need extra income, renting out a room or granny flat could help. This can provide additional cash flow to pay down the mortgage while letting you stay in your home.

6. Look harder at your budget
Let's be real – creating a prime time budget early on, with a focus on paying down the mortgage, can be a game-changer. By trimming

non-essential expenses in the set-up phase, you'll free up more cash to tackle your debt now. The pay-off? More freedom during your lifestyling and part-timing years, when the money you're currently throwing at the mortgage can be redirected toward super savings or lifestyle upgrades.

7. Restructure some investments

You might want to think about restructuring your investments, such as selling off assets like shares or investment properties, if it means making your right-sized home all yours before you stop working. But make sure to weigh up the potential capital gains and taxes you'll face when selling, as well as the long-term value of those investments, before making any big moves.

8. Seek good financial advice

Finally, don't underestimate the value of financial advice. A good adviser can help you balance your mortgage, super and lifestyle goals, ensuring you make the most of your options as you move into retirement.

THE REALITY OF RENTING IN YOUR PRIME TIME

People often stop me and say, 'But what about me? I rent! Don't leave me out!'

In Australia, owning a home has traditionally been seen as the foundation of financial security, especially in retirement, and I can't see that changing anytime soon. But with rising housing costs, nearly 20 per cent of households approaching retirement are renting. For many, renting isn't a choice but a necessity, while for others it's part of a financial strategy. Whatever the reason, renting comes with its own unique challenges, trade-offs and lessons, particularly for those nearing retirement. Let's look at the big ones:

1. Renting has no finish line – and it's exhausting!

One of the most significant downsides of renting is the uncertainty. While owning a home gives you the security of a finish line – a point where you no longer have to pay for housing – renting is an endless cycle. Every year or two, when your lease is up, you face the possibility of a rent increase or even eviction if the landlord decides to sell. And you often don't think about how hard it might be later in life until it's too late to buy.

This uncertainty becomes more difficult as you age. Take Susan, who's 70 and living on Melbourne's northern fringe. She's widowed, broke and relying on the single age pension after her husband's business went under during COVID and he died of a heart attack not long after. She had to sell everything they owned. She moved out of the city, away from her friends and community, in order to find an affordable place to rent. She pays $370 per week, which she can afford thanks to rent assistance.

It took her a year of lining up at rental inspections and submitting applications to find a place because landlords took one look at her application as a single woman on the full age pension and offered the home to someone younger or more affluent. She lives in constant fear that her lease won't be renewed.

If you have the chance to avoid this by being more strategic earlier in life, please do so!

2. Home ownership remains the best way to build wealth

Despite the challenges of today's housing market, owning your principal place of residence is still the most effective way to build wealth in Australia. Here's why: capital gains on your principal residence are tax-free, and home loans offer greater leverage compared to other investments. As your property grows in value, so does your wealth.

If you rent, you could miss out on this valuable opportunity. But if you're still a couple of decades away from full retirement and haven't yet climbed onto the property ladder, there's still time.

Take Sarah and Mike, both in their late 40s with one child. They've been renting in Sydney for years, and with a combined household income of $200,000, they're paying $50,000 in rent annually. They've grown accustomed to the inner-city lifestyle and would love to own a home close to where they've spent their entire adult lives.

But with property prices skyrocketing, the mortgage payments for even a modest apartment would be close to $70,000 per year, plus additional costs like body corporate fees. They worry about whether they can handle that level of financial commitment at this stage of life, but they know there's no other way to achieve the safety and security that comes from owning your own home when you retire.

While they feel discouraged about not having bought earlier, Sarah and Mike still have options. They could save longer for a deposit for the apartment in their dream area, or they could rethink their dream of living in the inner city and consider moving to a more affordable suburb, or even a more affordable city.

3. Renting can be a financial and lifestyle choice

Not all renters are forced into it. Some, like Greg, who is 65, recently divorced and renting on Sydney's northern beaches, chooses to rent for flexibility and financial reasons. After selling his $2.5 million family home and dividing the proceeds with his ex-wife, Greg has $1.25 million in investments generating a 6–7 per cent return – enough to comfortably cover his $700-per-week rent. By renting, Greg keeps his capital working for him in the markets rather than tying it all up in property.

If Greg were to shell out for an apartment like the one he is living in, he says it would cost him well over $1 million and leave him living on a much lower passive income and drawing on the age pension. And he wouldn't be able to draw down money for holidays or help his child get on the property ladder.

His numbers add up if he can manage two things: avoid nibbling away at his capital over time, leaving himself with a much smaller pool of assets that in a bad-investment year won't cover the bills; and his biggest risk, which he can't see yet – that of ageing without a home and having to live in fear of moving more regularly.

For some, especially those with significant assets or defined-benefit pensions, renting can be a strategic choice. It offers the flexibility to live in desirable locations without the financial commitment of home ownership, and it allows capital to be invested elsewhere.

4. The clock is ticking on your mortgage window

When you reach the topside of fifty, no-one tells you that time is running out to get a home mortgage – and then, one day, you can't. Banks are restricted from lending to older people who don't have enough earning years left to pay back their mortgage before they turn 67. The door silently closes on buying a principal place of residence somewhere in your early 50s, because you realistically need 20–30 years to pay down a decent-sized mortgage. Then you're left with only one choice: to buy an investment property and later kick the tenants out, just as that property is to be assessed for the age pension assets test, because if you live in it, it's exempt.

Grant, 50 and divorced, rents in Brisbane and prioritises paying for his children's private education over buying a home. While that's a noble decision, by the time his children finish school he'll be 54 and may find it difficult to enter the property market. Time isn't always on your side when it comes to mortgages and leaving it too late can mean missing out on property ownership altogether.

5. Renting offers flexibility, but there are trade-offs

Renting certainly provides flexibility that home ownership doesn't. If you're not ready to settle down, are thinking about moving to a new place, or anticipate changes in your lifestyle and aren't sure what's right for you yet, renting can be a very appealing option. It allows you to live in areas that might be unaffordable to buy into and helps you avoid the added costs of home ownership, such as maintenance, repairs and council rates.

But that flexibility comes with trade-offs. Renters face ongoing uncertainty about their housing situation. And while that might not concern you today, it's something to consider as you move through your Prime Time. Rising rents, lease renewals and the risk of being evicted can cause a lot of stress, especially in a high-inflation and tight housing market.

Take Karen and Peter. They're in their mid-50s and rent a beautiful house in Sydney's eastern suburbs. It's the perfect spot, close to the beach, cafes and the community they've been part of for decades.

They're paying $1200 per week in rent, which seemed manageable when they both had solid incomes. But Peter recently shifted to part-time work, and Karen is considering early retirement. The couple is starting to feel the pinch. Last year, their landlord increased the rent by 5 per cent, and there's always the looming worry that the property could be sold. They love the flexibility of renting, but they're also starting to realise that, as their incomes change in their prime time years, managing these rising costs will become much harder and they may perhaps want to buy a townhouse in a lower-cost area.

The flexibility of renting is great in your younger years, but as you get older, particularly when living on a fixed income, those rising rents can quickly become overwhelming. It's essential to have a plan for how you'll manage these trade-offs, and to think about long-term housing security as part of your prime time strategy.

6. The hidden costs of renting

While renting frees you from the expenses of home ownership, it comes with its own hidden costs. Constantly moving due to rising rents or other circumstances can be expensive. Bond payments, moving costs and the potential loss of community add up with every relocation. For older renters, the stress and cost of frequent moves can become burdensome. You may not see that now, but later you'll feel it.

Additionally, renters don't benefit from the capital gains that homeowners enjoy. While property owners see their wealth grow as housing prices rise, renters are subject to increasing costs without the long-term financial pay-off of ownership.

7. Home ownership provides security in old age

And finally, one of the greatest advantages of home ownership is the security it offers in your Prime Time, Epic Retirement and ageing years. When you own your home outright, you no longer need to worry about rent increases or the possibility of being evicted. You have a stable, predictable living situation. Additionally, if you're relying on the age pension, your home is exempt from the assets test, meaning its value won't reduce your pension entitlements.

For renters, the risk of rent increases and potential eviction becomes more concerning as they age. Without a stable housing situation, managing these risks on a fixed income can be difficult.

STRATEGIC OPTIONS FOR RENTERS IN RETIREMENT

If you find yourself renting later in life, here are some strategies to consider:

Build a stable income stream

If home ownership isn't possible, focus on building a robust investment portfolio that generates reliable income to cover your rent and living expenses throughout retirement.

Understand Commonwealth Rent Assistance

If you expect to be eligible for the age pension, explore rent assistance from the government. It's a means-tested payment that can ease the burden of rent payments for eligible retirees. You have to reach pension age to become eligible.

Consider co-housing or shared living

Think like the Golden Girls – 50 years later! Co-housing with other retirees can reduce rent costs and offer a sense of community, making it easier to manage living expenses while enjoying social benefits.

Plan for future rent increases

If there's one thing that's certain in today's tight property market, it's that your rent will rise. Make sure you've built a financial buffer so rent hikes don't take you by surprise. This gives you some security against the inevitable inflationary pressure on your housing costs.

7. GET THE MOST OUT OF SUPERANNUATION

No matter your age or how far off retirement may seem, the best time to start understanding your super is as early in life as possible. Your goal should be to build up the desired amount of super to fund your retirement as soon as you can, and to understand how it works, so you have the confidence to spend it on living comfortably.

Prime Timers in their late 40s, 50s and even their early 60s really are at the pivotal age for taking advantage of superannuation. So do yourself a favour – learn about it and embrace it.

As discussed earlier, superannuation is a tax structure designed to force you to save for your retirement over many years. It requires employers to deduct 12 per cent of your salary and put it into a dedicated superannuation fund that you can't withdraw from until you reach the age of 60 and retire or turn 65. You pay just 15 per cent tax on the amount you contribute up to $30,000 per year, a percentage that is usually a lot lower than the rate you pay on the rest of your income.

Then you choose how those funds are invested, with the goal of driving powerful compound investment returns over many years. While the amount is growing, you pay just 15 per cent tax on the money it earns within the fund, allowing the compounding to work better for you inside super than outside.

When we consider the power of compound investing, which is the fundamental basis for superannuation, we know that super invested in balanced growth or growth assets and getting a 7–10 per cent return can double every 7–10 years, or faster when you account for your contributions consistently flowing in. So the earlier you start contributing, the more passive compound growth you'll enjoy.

When you reach the age of 60 and retire from work, or the age of 65 when you can access your super without needing to retire, you can take the money held in your superannuation fund as either an income stream or a lump sum. In the retirement phase, both the income from your superannuation and any capital gains are tax-free, unless your balance is over $3 million, for which the government has proposed the new Division 296 tax.

Concessional contributions to superannuation are one of the most powerful ways in which you can both save for retirement and, later, generate an income in retirement. The earlier you understand how your superannuation works, the better you can leverage the power of it.

THE TWO PHASES OF SUPERANNUATION

Superannuation has two key phases: the accumulation phase and the retirement phase. There's also a transitional phase in-between that's worth a closer look.

1. The accumulation phase

The accumulation phase of super is where you are contributing funds while you work. In this phase, your employer makes contributions into your super fund that are 12 per cent of your salary. You can also contribute additional funds from your pre-tax income, called concessional contributions, and from your post-tax income, called non-concessional contributions.

In the accumulation phase, it's crucial to understand how your superannuation is invested. Your superannuation fund offers various investment options with different risk levels.

Your goal should be to contribute as much as you can to your superannuation before retirement and choose investments with strong growth potential that match your risk tolerance. This will help grow your super faster, giving you a larger retirement fund when you're ready to retire.

I touched on this in the tax section, but now we need to dive deeper. There are four core ways to get money into superannuation:

1. Concessional contributions
2. Non-concessional contributions
3. The downsizer contribution
4. Small business CGT concessions.

Concessional contributions

Concessional contributions are the contributions you make to superannuation from pre-tax dollars, which are taxed at just 15 per cent, which is usually lower than your marginal tax rate. You can contribute up to $30,000 per year in concessional contributions, which are made by employers but also through voluntary contributions. They are one of the most powerful ways to get money into super incrementally.

If you make concessional contributions that amount to less than the cap, you can accrue these unused amounts and carry them forward for up to five years before they expire, so long as your superannuation fund balance is below $500,000 at the prior financial year end. It's called a 'catch-up concessional contribution'. And you can carry forward unused cap amounts from up to five previous financial years, including when you were not a member of a super fund.

Non-concessional contributions

Non-concessional contributions are your after-tax contributions. You have already paid tax on this money, so it goes into your super tax-free. You can contribute up to $120,000 per year in non-concessional contributions. This is a good option if you've got extra savings or a windfall and want to bump up your super without affecting your concessional cap. You can make non-concessional contributions up to the age of 75. If you're under 67, you can bring forward up to two years of the non-concessional contributions caps, allowing you to contribute $360,000 over three financial years. It is important to note that you can't make non-concessional contributions once your superannuation fund balance exceeds the transfer balance cap of $2 million or if you're 75 or over, because you can't make non-concessional contributions after 28 days past the month you turn 75. The bring-forward rule only works if you're under 75 at the *start* of the financial year and still have enough years left to use the cap you trigger.

The downsizer contribution

If you're 55 or older and sell your principal place of residence, having owned it for at least 10 years, you can put up to $300,000 per person or $600,000 per couple tax-free from the sale of your home into your super. This is a once-in-a-lifetime opportunity to turn some of your home equity into retirement savings and, later, retirement income, especially if your super balance needs a boost in the years leading up to and during retirement.

There are some important conditions:

- You must have owned the home for at least 10 years.
- You must put the money into superannuation within 90 days of the settlement of the sale – exemptions are available under certain conditions but you will need to apply proactively.
- You must have lived in the home for a portion of the 10 years, making it exempt or partially exempt from CGT.

Small business CGT concessions

If you sell a small business, there are some special rules allowing you to put part of the sale proceeds into your super without it counting toward your contribution caps. This is a really powerful and fair way for small business owners to convert their hard-earned business success into a comfy retirement fund. There's more information in the section on small business tax concessions (see page 73).

2. The retirement phase

This phase of superannuation is triggered when you open a retirement phase superannuation account and start to draw down on your superannuation funds. The money you move over into the retirement phase is completely tax-free; that is, you don't pay income tax on the money earned, and you don't pay CGT on the growth in value. This is a great reason to take superannuation seriously.

To open a retirement phase account and move your money across from the accumulation phase, you need to meet the 'conditions of release'. You can move up to $2 million, which is the 'transfer balance cap', into superannuation in your lifetime. The rest must be kept in the accumulation phase, where it continues to be taxed.

Let's have a closer look at the retirement phase of superannuation.

Conditions of release

To access your superannuation and enter the retirement phase, you need to meet two key eligibility criteria, known as the conditions of release:

1. You've reached the age of 60, your preservation age.

2. You cease a gainful employment arrangement on or after the age of 60, with no intention of working more than 10 hours a week. This part is simple: you just declare your retirement from work on your super fund's retirement account application form.

Alternatively, if you wait until you're 65, you can keep working and still transfer your super into the retirement phase, with no conditions attached.

A question I often get asked is, 'How does this actually work in practice?' The reality is that at the time you apply to your super fund, you need to have genuinely stopped working. You don't have to be done forever, but you need to cease employment with no plans to work over 10 hours a week. You declare that intent, and once that's done, you're free to transfer your super into the retirement phase.

But here's the flexibility: if, after you've made the switch, you decide to get back into work – whether that's full-time, part-time, or even starting a small business – you absolutely can. The only catch is that you'll need to open a new accumulation account for your new contributions. Your existing retirement account will keep ticking along with non-preserved, tax-free income, and you'll need to make the required minimum drawdowns.

If for any reason you breach these provisions, the ATO might step in and reclassify your retirement pension as a transition to retirement pension. This means you wouldn't be able to make lump sum withdrawals and things might become more restricted.

It's all about timing and intent – and staying within the guidelines when making that switch from the accumulation phase to the retirement phase.

Here are some common scenarios.

You must genuinely cease employment, but you can change your mind later. Carlos, 63, a full-time employee at an engineering firm, ceased his full-time employment and was paid out his leave entitlements, ending his relationship with the firm. At the time, he had no intention of rejoining the workforce for more than 10 hours a week, so he decided to convert his superannuation into a retirement phase account. Three months after he retired, he reached out to his former employer for a role identical to his previous one, but as a part-time employee. There was a clear break in employment, so Carlos has satisfied the definition of retirement.

You can't just switch or downshift roles for the one employer. Catherine, 61, a nurse in a large regional hospital, gives her employer notice that she will cease her full-time nursing unit manager role. During the notice period, Catherine and her employer agree that she will be employed as a home-help nurse in a casual capacity. While Catherine's employment contract has been terminated, there has been no break in the employment relationship, so it is unlikely that Catherine will have satisfied the retirement conditions of release even though her role has substantially changed, meaning she'll be unable to open a tax-free retirement phase account yet.

In small business, you need to create evidence of the cessation. Jenny is a small business owner running a bookkeeping enterprise. To access her superannuation at 60 she would need to genuinely cease employment. And to demonstrate that her employment had ceased, she might be expected to provide evidence of the cancellation of her ABN or the cessation of her business income.

Using the window of opportunity. Robyn quit her job in teaching to care for her ageing mother at 58. Upon turning 60, Robyn declared permanent retirement to her superannuation fund and commenced an account-based pension. At age 62, with her mother having passed a year prior, she accepted a full-time role as a teacher. If Robyn had no intention of returning to the workforce full-time when she made her retirement declaration, all her superannuation benefits at the time of making that declaration would become unrestricted (they enter the retirement phase and can be drawn out without limitations). The fact that Robyn decided to return to work does not invalidate her earlier declaration and she can continue to receive her account-based pension, tax-free.

The transfer balance cap

The government has set a limit on the amount any one person can transfer from the accumulation phase into the tax-free retirement phase of superannuation in their lifetime. It is called the transfer balance cap, and it is currently set at $2 million and the government reviews and indexes it every financial year. Your total balance in the retirement phase can grow beyond the $2 million with investment returns – you just can't transfer any more into your account than the cap over your lifetime.

If you have more than $2 million in superannuation, you will need to keep the remaining amount in an accumulation phase account and continue to pay 15 per cent tax on earnings. If your total super balance exceeds $3 million, it may become eligible for the proposed new Division 296 tax.

Accessing your money

Once you're in the retirement phase, there are three different ways to access your superannuation.

An account-based pension. This is the most common type of account inside superannuation. It is used to invest your superannuation and pay you a regular income stream. The investments held in an account-based pension are exposed to market fluctuations, so you need to think carefully about your asset allocation to ensure maximum resilience in times when the market is down. When you move your money into an account-based pension, there is a mandatory drawdown of a percentage of the balance each year, calculated on your age.

Annuities and lifetime income streams. These are financial products that provide a guaranteed income for either a pre-agreed period of time or, in the case of lifetime annuities, for life, no matter how long you live. These products are often used by retirees to secure a steady income stream that offers financial confidence and stability. Most people who buy them choose to invest just a portion (ie 10–50 per cent) of their retirement savings in annuities, rather than their entire nest egg, to maintain some flexibility while guaranteeing part of their income.

Lifetime annuities, also known as lifetime income streams, are an evolving product category in Australia. They'll likely become hotter as super funds gradually start to offer them within their mix of solutions – the wheels of the industry are certainly in motion for this product. One key benefit is that many provide a guaranteed income stream for life, ensuring you never run out of money no matter how long you live. Some also offer market-linked bonuses, adding potential upside to your payments. This allows people to spend on their cost of living and lifestyle with greater confidence. Another benefit is that they may offer assets test discounts for the age pension. These discounts can make lifetime annuities an attractive option for retirees seeking to maximise their pension entitlements. For eligible products, 40 per cent of the funds invested are exempt from the assets test between the ages of 60 and 84, and this exemption increases to 70 per cent after the age of 84.

Lump sum drawdown. Many people choose to make lump sum drawdowns from their superannuation fund, which they can do once they meet the conditions of release, whether it is in the accumulation phase or the retirement phase. But remember – once it's gone, it's gone! It can't compound and it won't generate you an ongoing income.

Investing your superannuation

Once your money is in the retirement phase, there are some important investing considerations that are different to pre-retirement considerations, namely:
- How much to hold in low-risk assets that can fund your next 1–3 years of income needs
- How much to hold in balanced and/or growth assets to drive longer-term asset growth
- How you are going to manage your portfolio to ensure you shift assets in between when markets are outperforming. This is commonly referred to as a 'bucket strategy'.

Most people don't realise that superannuation makes up to around 50 per cent of the earnings you will see in your lifetime *during* the retirement phase, depending on how you have it invested. Many people entering retirement today have more than 25–30 years of life ahead of them, so moving all your money to conservative investments can see you miss out on a significant financial upside.

> ## THE 10/30/60 RULE: SUPERANNUATION DOES ITS BEST WORK 'PASSIVELY'
>
> The United States has what's known as the 10/30/60 rule, which says that over your lifetime, your retirement income is saved and grown chiefly through passive investment. It says that if you start saving for retirement early, at around 25 years of age, then you'll save 10 per cent of your retirement income during your working years from contributions; you'll grow 30 per cent of your retirement savings from the compound investment returns that you achieve before you retire; and you'll grow 60 per cent of your returns from the investment returns achieved during your retirement.
>
> In Australia, actuaries have calculated the ratio to be closer to 15/35/50. Of course, it all relies on you being proactive about investing.

Drawing down your superannuation

Once your super moves into the retirement phase, you're required to start drawing it down at a rate based on your age, something the government calls a 'mandatory drawdown'. While this might feel like a structured process, it's a reminder that super was designed to be spent – to fund your best years, not just sit as a tax-effective vehicle for passing on wealth.

In fact, most retirees should be drawing down more than the minimum to make the most of their early retirement years. The government wants you to use your super for living well, not hoard it for future generations.

It's also worth noting that mandatory drawdowns only apply to your account-based pension – not your entire super balance – and must remain within the $2 million transfer balance cap. So, the real question isn't just about how much you have, but how you'll use it to live the retirement you've worked for.

Age	Default minimum superannuation drawdown rates from 1 July 2023
Under 65	4%
65–74	5%
75–79	6%
80–84	7%
85–89	9%
90–94	11%
95+	14%

Transition to retirement (TTR)

Many people are gradually moving into retirement by stepping back from full-time to part-time work and then transitioning to casual or consulting roles before fully retiring. As you reduce the amount of time you spend at work, you usually reduce your income from work too, so many people look for ways to fund this lifestyle shift.

To support this gradual transition, superannuation funds offer a transition to retirement (TTR) account. This account allows you to draw an income stream from your super before you retire, supplementing your income from working.

You can apply for a TTR account once you reach the preservation age, which is currently 60. Here's how it works and why it can be beneficial:

Accessing your super

Through a TTR account, you can access up to 10 per cent of your superannuation balance as an income stream per year. This flexibility allows you to supplement your part-time or reduced income without having to dip into other savings or investments. For example, if you have $300,000 in your super, you could draw up to $30,000 per year through your TTR account, tax-free.

Tax efficiency

The money you receive from your TTR account is not subject to income tax, making it a highly tax-efficient way to manage your finances during your transition to retirement.

While drawing from your TTR account, you can continue to make concessional (pre-tax) contributions to your superannuation. These contributions up to the concessional contribution cap of $30,000 are taxed at only 15 per cent, which is typically much lower than your marginal tax rate. This can be particularly beneficial if you have a high income, as it allows you to reduce your taxable income and grow your super at a lower tax rate. For example, if you earn $100,000 a year and salary-sacrifice $18,000 into your super, you'll only pay 15 per cent tax on that $18,000 instead of your higher marginal rate.

Here's an example. Debbie is 60 years old, works 4 days a week and earns $100,000 per year. She has $400,000 in her superannuation fund. Debbie sets up a TTR account and starts drawing $30,000 per year tax-free from her super. This additional income can help cover living expenses or allow her to reduce her working hours further without compromising her lifestyle. Debbie's employer contributes 12 per cent of her salary to super, which is $12,000. She salary-sacrifices an additional $18,000 to bring her total concessional contributions to the $30,000 cap. Without salary sacrifice, Debbie's marginal tax on $18,000 would be $6210 (34.5 per cent, including Medicare levy). By-salary sacrificing into super, she pays just $2700 in concessional tax (15 per cent of $18,000), saving $3510 in tax. Every dollar counts when you're saving for the future.

THE REAL VALUE OF A TRANSITION TO RETIREMENT ACCOUNT

The real value of a TTR account is the flexibility it gives you in your Prime Time to choose how much work you want to do. It allows you to access some of your superannuation before you retire fully, to supplement your income if you choose to do less work. Or you might simply want to step up your lifestyle with some additional income without retiring.

GETTING A RETIREMENT BONUS FROM YOUR SUPER FUND

The concept of receiving a retirement bonus from your superannuation fund might sound appealing – a lump sum payment when you transition from the accumulation phase to the retirement phase. But what exactly is a retirement bonus, and how does it work?

In Australia, a retirement bonus is a one-off payment that some super funds offer when their members move from an accumulation account or a TTR account into a retirement income stream. This bonus comes from tax provisions that were set aside during your working years, while your super was in the accumulation phase. These provisions are no longer needed once your money shifts into the retirement phase, where no tax is payable on earnings or capital gains.

The idea is that as you stop contributing to your super and start drawing from it, the tax provisions your fund has built up are returned to you as a bonus. However, not all funds offer retirement bonuses, and those that do use different methods to calculate them.

When you shift from the accumulation phase (where your super is taxed at 15 per cent) into the retirement phase (where you pay no tax on income or capital gains), your super fund no longer needs to put money aside for tax. This is called 'provisioning', and some funds build up a decent reserve of these tax provisions.

Now, when you retire, your fund can either absorb this money back into the pool for everyone's benefit or hand it back to you as a retirement bonus. About 50 per cent of funds are currently paying it back, while the others are keeping it in the pool to boost overall fund performance.

The marketing behind these bonuses is clever, with some funds calling them 'retirement boosters' or 'rewards'. It sounds great, but here's the catch: just because you're getting a bonus doesn't mean your fund is the best performer. Let's unpack the two ways in which these bonuses are calculated.

Type 1: Pooled provisions. Some funds, like Australian Retirement Trust, MLC and Brighter Super, pool all the tax provisions from members retiring that year and divvy it up as a percentage of their balance. This is simple and easy to promote because everyone gets the same percentage. For example, in 2023/24, MLC offered 1.25 per cent, Brighter Super gave out 0.8 per cent and ART handed out 0.5 per cent.

But it's not technically fair. Members in high-growth investments have more tax provisioned than those in safer assets like bonds or cash, yet they all get the same bonus percentage. Some funds try to balance this by only offering bonuses to those who have invested in growth assets.

Type 2: Individual provisions. Other funds, like HESTA and AustralianSuper, calculate retirement bonuses based on each person's unique situation – what investments you've been in, how long you've been with the fund, and how much you're transferring into your retirement account. To work out how much you might be eligible for, you'll likely have to call your fund and get them to run the calculation. This approach tends to reward members who have been in growth assets longer and had more tax provisioned for them.

In both cases, the bonus is paid automatically when you move into the retirement phase. But there are a few caveats. If the fund has had a bad year and no taxes are provisioned, don't expect a bonus. Also, you generally need to be with the fund for a set period, usually 12 months, and have money in growth assets to qualify. There's usually a clawback period if you leave the fund soon after receiving it, too.

What if your fund doesn't offer a bonus?

Don't panic. That money goes back into the investment pool, which should boost overall performance. If your fund is performing well and has low fees, you could be better off in the long run. Look at the bigger picture: consistently strong returns and low fees can often outweigh a one-off bonus.

The real consideration

For context, the average super balance for Aussies aged 65–69 in 2023/24 was around $453,075. A 1.25 per cent bonus from MLC would give you $5663, while Australian Retirement Trust's 0.5 per cent would give you $2265. These are decent amounts, but if your fund has consistently outperformed by even 0.25 per cent annually or has lower fees, you might end up better off without a bonus in the long term.

Remember, if your fund is offering strong growth, low fees and a bonus, that's the ultimate win.

HOW DO YOU KNOW IF YOUR SUPER FUND IS PERFORMING?

Funds are really only starting to grasp this new era, when people who have built up their super now want to start drawing it down. Most of them have not refined their services and product offerings to the extent that they will over the years ahead. It will be up to you to push them, moving away from funds who don't offer good products and services more appropriate for this phase of life.

There are at least 14 things I think super funds should be offering members in their Prime Time:

1. Good long-term investment performance

Super funds have become some of the most powerful investment houses in the world. They have teams of experts scouting the globe for top-notch investments, and long-term performance is their bread and butter. You need your super to perform consistently to feel financially secure. Don't be swayed by flashy one-year returns – dig deeper and check out their 10-year numbers. That's where the real magic happens. Remember compounding?

Here's the average superannuation fund performance in 2023/24 in the accumulation phase – accumulation performance is net of investment fees and tax.[18]

	One-year returns (%)	Ten-year returns (% pa)
Balanced (41–60% growth assets)	7.3	5.7
Growth (61–80% growth assets)	9.1	7.2

And here's the average superannuation fund performance in 2023/24 in the retirement (pension) phase – pension performance is net of investment fees.

	One-year returns (%)	Ten-year returns (% pa)
Balanced (41–60% growth assets)	8.0	6.4
Growth (61–80% growth assets)	10.0	7.9

2. Investments specific to the pension phase of retirement

Many funds invest in the same way regardless of whether you're still in accumulation or drawing down in retirement. That's mainly because retirement phase investing is relatively new for most funds. But things are changing. Some funds are starting to offer tailored options specifically designed for retirees. These investments focus on balancing long-term growth with reduced sequencing risk, which I explain later in this chapter. This is definitely a space to watch.

3. Administration fees under the average

Fees can quietly chip away at your returns without you even noticing, so pay close attention to the administration fees on your statement (investment fees matter less if your returns are strong and quoted net of fees). Administration fees come straight off your balance, so aim to have them as low as possible to keep compounding working in your favour, but make sure your fund isn't skimping on providing you adequate services to cut their fees.

4. Lifetime income stream products and trustworthy insights into how to use them

The government wants super funds to offer lifetime income streams – products that provide an income for life, no matter how long you live.

While not all funds have embraced this yet, these products could be a game-changer for ordinary Australians, offering greater confidence in retirement spending. Many retirees say they would gladly invest a portion of their super in a product that guarantees certainty and security in later life. Yet, most consumers aren't aware these options exist. If your fund doesn't offer lifetime income streams (and most don't yet), it's worth asking them why not and when they might. And watch this space – more super funds are likely to start offering solutions in this category as the demand and the conversation grows.

5. Drawdown strategies

When you hit retirement, mandatory drawdowns kick in. Some funds make it easy to choose something other than the minimum, while others leave you to figure it out on your own or just take out the minimum. Keep an eye out for funds that help you navigate how much you can sustainably draw down to help you live the best retirement life you can.

6. Advice that's helpful for the average person

Some funds offer advice that actually helps, others not so much. Whether they charge you for every call or only offer advice once a year, not all funds are equally helpful. Look for funds that include practical, personalised advice as part of their service, especially leading up to and at the point of retirement. With new financial advice laws expected in 2025, funds should be doing more to offer affordable, useful advice – especially as you approach retirement.

7. Intra-fund advice

Your super fund should provide free advice via call centres on managing your investments, risk profile and insurances within your super fund. This is called 'intra-fund advice' and it's a must-have service. Make sure you use it.

8. Ways to seek more comprehensive advice

If you're looking for more comprehensive advice, your super fund should be able to guide you to financial advisers who know how their funds work and can work with you to build a more comprehensive financial plan.

9. Great calculators and tools

Funds have been investing in tools to help you plan for retirement. There are investment and drawdown calculators that can help you visualise how different strategies will work for you, robo-advice that will guide you on the best decisions to make, and retirement planning advice that brings all your decisions together. Every fund does it differently. It's worth looking at what your fund provides and playing around with it. Their tools should help you build your confidence and make important decisions.

10. Transparency of your retirement bonus

When you shift from the accumulation phase to the retirement phase, many funds hand back the tax provisions that were set aside during your working years as a lump sum 'retirement bonus'. But not all funds do so, and those that do use different methods to calculate them. It's important to be able to understand the details of how your fund treats retirement bonuses and look at them alongside long-term returns.

11. Retirement education

Your super fund should be helping you learn about your money and, more importantly, your superannuation and how you can grow it, especially as you approach retirement. Look for structured educational programs and/or webinars from your fund that break down the systems and strategies you'll need for the years ahead. Whether they're offered online or in person, retirement education programs are a great way to receive bite-sized info. Not all education is created equal, though. Look for the offerings that are engaging and offer practical next steps.

12. Nudges

Do you get friendly reminders from your fund to review your super? These 'nudges' help keep you engaged and on top of things. If your fund isn't nudging you, they might prefer you don't look too closely at their fees or returns. A good fund will keep you informed.

13. Soft defaults

Some funds offer soft defaults in retirement that act like recommendations based on what they know about you – settings that make it easy for people who aren't super-savvy about investing to still get decent outcomes. If you're the 'set and forget' type, this can be a big help.

14. A reasonable standard of service provision
We've seen serious issues where super funds delay paying out death benefits, and where poor adoption of multi-factor authentication has left members vulnerable to hacking. Service standards are one of the first places funds cut corners to keep fees low – but what's the real cost of that? A fund with tech failures, poor security or slow insurance payouts can cause real harm at the worst possible time. Watch the media and refer to our Epic Retirement Tick (see pages 123–24) to learn how your fund stacks up on service, not just fees.

Activity: REVIEW YOUR SUPERANNUATION
Grab your phone and open your super fund's app or pull out your latest super statement. Let's go through it step by step and see what actions you might need to take to get your super working smarter for you. You should be checking these things every three years at a minimum! Ideally you will look at them once a year – for good practice.

Check your balance. First things first. What's your current super balance? Keep it handy because we're going to put it to work.

See how your fund is investing for you. Find out where your money's invested. What types of assets is your super fund investing in on your behalf? Your statement or app should explain what you're invested in, including the percentage of growth assets and defensive assets. And you really should know 'why' you're invested in this way. If you don't, book an appointment with your fund's financial planner and discuss it.

Look at your returns. Now dig a little deeper. What are your fund's one-year and 10-year average investment returns? These numbers will give you a snapshot of how well your investments are performing over time. Are they above or below the averages?

Understand your fees. Are your fees quoted excluding investment fees? They should be. Add up all the other fees on your statement and calculate what they add up to as a percentage of your total balance. How much are you really paying?

Why do we exclude investment fees? Funds report their earnings after deducting investment fees, so the net performance you see already accounts for these costs. This means that for a fund achieving high performance, charging higher fees isn't necessarily a downside. It could even reflect the fund's resources and expertise in delivering stronger returns.

Compare the numbers. Now take a moment to compare your returns and fees with those of the top performers in your asset class. Are you getting a good deal or is it time to explore other options?

REVIEW YOUR INSURANCES

Many people don't realise they have life insurance – and sometimes income protection and total and permanent disablement (TPD) insurance – sitting inside their superannuation fund. If you haven't reviewed it in a while, it may not reflect the life you're living today.

Insurance through super can be an affordable way to stay covered, but it can also quietly eat away at your balance if you no longer need it. If you've paid off your mortgage and the kids are financially independent, the original reason for holding that insurance may no longer apply. It's worth checking whether your cover still serves a purpose – or if it's time to adjust or cancel it.

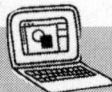

WHERE DO YOU GO TO COMPARE SUPER FUNDS WHEN RETIREMENT'S AROUND THE CORNER?

Epic Retirement and one of Australia's most trusted names in super fund research, Chant West, have joined forces to create the Epic Retirement Tick, a certification program that recognises super funds delivering on the things that matter most in midlife and as you head into retirement. This classification, underpinned by research from one of Australia's most respected fund assessment providers, offers a clear and transparent view of the criteria outlined in the previous pages – and more.

The government offers benchmarking for default accumulation funds through the ATO's YourSuper comparison tool (visit ato.gov.au), but this is far from comprehensive, focused only on the accumulation phase and only on default superannuation funds, and it doesn't assess how funds perform in the retirement phase.

That's why we created the Epic Tick, and why, at the end of each financial year, I share updated fund ratings and service level insights at epicretirement.com.au/epictick.

8. EXPLORE YOUR INVESTMENT OPTIONS

Investing is something every Australian needs to understand if they want to enjoy a great Prime Time and an Epic Retirement. The level of complexity of your investment strategy is entirely up to you, and fortunately, today's superannuation and investment funds have made it easier than ever to access world-class investments at a very low cost.

Here, I want to help you understand the basics: how risk and investing work, the different ways in which you can invest, and the workings of the various investment products you hear about. With this foundation, you'll have the knowledge and confidence to engage with financial advisers and your super fund, and make informed decisions about the investment strategies that suit your goals and lifestyle. Hopefully this will help you ask the right questions!

UNDERSTANDING YOUR RISK APPETITE

Before we talk about investments and the ways in which you can hold them, we need to discuss your risk appetite, or how much risk you are prepared to take to achieve your goals. Most people don't understand their risk profile until they've been through a challenging time where they've lost money in the markets. Thinking sensibly about your profile is very important, because you use it to guide the level of risk you are prepared to take on investments, and you will adjust it at different stages of your life.

Technically, your risk profile measures your tolerance for making investment losses while you are seeking investment gains. But to me it's much more than that. I believe your risk profile is a carefully balanced consideration of time, money and safety.

In the event of a market crash, for example, you must consider:
- How much time you can afford to wait for your portfolio to recover
- How much of a financial loss you can withstand
- And how much security you need for financial peace of mind.

There are five elements that typically underpin your risk profile:

Your time horizon
The length of time you intend to hold an investment before needing to access the funds. If you have a long time horizon, you can usually afford to take more of a risk, as there is greater opportunity to recover from market downturns.

Your financial goals
These play a crucial role in determining your risk profile. For many people, their goals may include saving for retirement, paying off their home, taking a pre-retirement sabbatical or a grey-nomad year of travel, or affording themselves a pre-retirement phase with part-time work only. All these objectives can impact how much risk you're prepared to take.

Your financial situation
Your big financial picture, including your income, savings, debts and assets, all impact your ability to take on risk. People who have a stable income and significant savings tucked away usually have a higher risk tolerance than someone with very limited resources.

Your knowledge and experience

Your knowledge of financial markets and investment products, as well as your past investing experience, will likely heavily influence your risk profile. Experienced investors will be more comfortable with certain types of risks compared to novice investors.

Your risk capacity

This is your financial capacity to withstand potential losses without jeopardising your financial stability or long-term goals. Your capacity to take risks usually takes into account things like your net worth, need to access liquidity, and the other financial obligations you are weighed down by.

Most people who are investing in midlife will take into consideration the time horizon for their investment, seeking longer-term compound growth over many years. But it really will depend on what you're investing for.

Some may be investing for the period before retirement, when they will want to access money outside superannuation to fund dialling back their work and stepping up their lifestyle choices. And everyone will be investing inside superannuation for the period after retirement, which may still be some time away. Different time horizons usually mean different risk profiles because of a thing called sequencing risk.

> **WHAT IS SEQUENCING RISK?**
>
> Sequencing risk comes into play when you start drawing on your funds. It refers to the risk of a market downturn occurring early in your withdrawal phase, requiring you to take money out of your portfolio without allowing your assets time to recover. This can hurt your portfolio because you're selling assets at a low point, making it harder for your savings to bounce back. It's a concern for anyone relying on their investments, not just retirees. To manage this risk, diversify your investments, keep a cash reserve for tough times, and adjust withdrawals based on market performance. This way, you can protect your savings from the bad luck of a poorly timed market dip.

Once you've considered your time horizon, you can focus on your financial goals and determine whether taking more risk for higher returns is your priority, or if it's more important to protect your savings with a lower-risk approach. Wealthier people often have a higher capacity for risk because losses won't threaten their entire financial stability. Likewise, experienced investors are generally more comfortable taking calculated risks in areas they understand well.

Increasingly, super funds are encouraging people to keep a portion of their investments in balanced or even growth options. This reflects the reality that, with retirement potentially lasting over 30 years, achieving strong returns is essential to ensure savings last throughout that period.

So think about your overall risk capacity, and consider leaning into risk strategically when it fits your profile.

For example, after the 2008 financial crisis, the S&P 500 took about six years to recover and nearly a decade to achieve substantial gains. Investors heavily exposed to equities before the crash faced tough choices: sell at a loss, or hold on through extreme volatility? Those who held on eventually recovered, while those who had cash on the sidelines and embraced the risk of buying at lower prices recovered faster and saw bigger gains. It's often in times of adversity that real wealth is built.

BUCKET STRATEGIES

You'll hear the term 'bucket strategy' tossed around a lot as you approach Prime Time and start looking at what to do with your super in the retirement phase. It's one of those ideas that people either love or hate. For some, it's a simple way to understand retirement income planning, while to others, it feels like a gimmick that distracts from real risk-based asset allocation tailored for you by a financial adviser. So what's it really about?

At its core, a bucket strategy is just a way to divide your super between cash and growth assets, giving you a short-term reserve for immediate expenses and a long-term growth pool to keep your super working for you. By structuring your super in this way, you're balancing cash reserves for near-term needs with higher-growth investments for the future.

Here's how a two- or three-bucket strategy might look:

1. **Short-term bucket**: This is your 'safe cash' for the next couple of years, which you set aside in low-risk investments like cash or term deposits. This bucket covers your everyday needs while avoiding worry over market swings. You decide how many years you want to have at call.
2. **Long-term bucket**: This is your 'growth pot', invested in things like shares and property that you *don't* need to touch right away. The key here is to leave this bucket alone in a market downturn so it has time to recover and grow. You don't want to be forced to sell shares or property at a low point just to pay your bills. This bucket gives you the freedom to wait for better market conditions.

If you want even more flexibility, you can add a middle bucket with moderate-risk investments, giving you another way to refill your short-term bucket as needed.

In reality, the bucket strategy is less about complicated finance and more about balancing cash for today and investments for tomorrow. By keeping a clear boundary between what you need now and what you're growing for later, it can help you feel more secure about your retirement income without overcomplicating things.

UNDERSTANDING RISK PROFILES AND COMMON INVESTMENT CATEGORIES

In Australia, superannuation funds commonly categorise their investment options based on risk profiles, which help members choose strategies that align with their goals and risk tolerance. Here's a breakdown of the four common risk profiles, with the percentage of growth assets typically allocated in each.

Conservative investor (low risk)

Conservative investors focus on capital preservation and stability over high returns. They prefer low-volatility investments like bonds and cash. The goal is to protect their principal while generating modest returns.

Super fund equivalent: Often called 'conservative' or 'capital stable'.

Asset allocation: Funds typically allocate 20–35 per cent of the money to growth assets (shares, property) and the rest to defensive assets (bonds, cash).

Balanced investor (medium risk)

Balanced investors seek a mix of growth and stability. They are comfortable with moderate market fluctuations for potentially higher returns over time, with a diversified portfolio.

Super fund equivalent: Usually referred to as 'balanced' or 'moderate'.

Asset allocation: Balanced super options generally invest 50–70 per cent of the money in growth assets, with the rest in defensive assets.

Growth investor (high risk)

Growth investors focus on long-term capital growth and are willing to accept higher volatility. A significant portion of their portfolio typically consists of stocks and equity funds.

Super fund equivalent: Commonly labelled as 'growth' or sometimes badged 'high growth' when they're not quite.

Asset allocation: These funds typically hold 60–85 per cent in growth assets, making them suitable for those with a long-term investment horizon.

Aggressive investor (very high risk)

Aggressive investors aim for maximum capital gains and are willing to take on high levels of risk, investing in speculative or volatile assets. They prioritise returns over security.

Super fund equivalent: Often called 'aggressive' or 'high growth'.

Asset allocation: Aggressive options in super funds typically have 85–100 per cent in growth assets, offering higher return potential but with increased volatility.

These risk profiles, and their associated asset allocations, help investors and superannuation fund members understand how their money is invested and the level of risk they are comfortable with. The percentage of growth assets reflects the potential for returns, but also the volatility, making it crucial to align the investment strategy with your life stage and goals.

> **WATCH OUT FOR TERMINOLOGY**
>
> Superannuation funds often use risk-profile terms in their branding and marketing, but they don't always apply them consistently.
>
> While the general asset allocations mentioned earlier are common, individual super funds may adjust their definitions and asset mixes. For example, one fund's 'balanced' option could include 60 per cent growth assets, while another's could have 70 per cent, making it more growth-focused than you might expect. This inconsistency means you can't always compare apples with apples. In fact, it can make a fund appear to perform better if you're unknowingly comparing it to others with less aggressive asset mixes – which is exactly why some funds do it.
>
> To avoid surprises, always check the specific asset allocation of any investment option to ensure it aligns with your risk tolerance and goals. Don't rely on the label alone – dig deeper to understand what you're really investing in.

TYPES OF INVESTMENTS COMMONLY OFFERED BY SUPER FUNDS

The most common way in which Prime Timers invest is simply by selecting an investment option offered by one of the major superannuation funds. Super funds generally provide a range of investment options catering to different risk profiles, financial goals and time horizons. Understanding the types of investments available in your super fund can help you tailor your strategy to suit your needs.

Growth assets

Growth assets, like shares (equities) and property, are designed to deliver higher returns over the long term but they come with more risk and price fluctuations. These investments tend to make up the majority of growth or high-growth options within a super fund. Within a growth portfolio you'll often find:

Shares (equities): Investments in Australian and international companies offering long-term capital growth and dividends.

Property: Direct investment in commercial or residential property or through property trusts, providing a combination of rental income and capital growth.

Infrastructure: Assets like airports, roads and energy grids, offering steady income from essential services with long-term growth potential.

Private equity: Investments in privately held companies, providing access to new growth opportunities not listed on public exchanges, though they carry higher risk.

Commodities and natural resources: Exposure to assets like metals, oil and agricultural goods, which can hedge against inflation and offer portfolio diversification.

Hedge funds: These have growth strategies that aim to capture returns uncorrelated to broader markets, but come with higher fees and complexity.

Defensive assets

Defensive assets are lower-risk investments aimed at providing income stability and capital protection. These assets are commonly found in conservative or balanced investment options within super funds, adding stability when growth assets fluctuate.

Bonds (fixed interest): Loans to governments or corporations that pay regular interest over a set period, offering more stability than shares.

Super funds may invest in a mix of Australian and international bonds to provide steady income and cushion against equity market volatility.

Cash and term deposits: Offer capital preservation and low but stable returns. While not high-yielding, cash is the safest option and forms a solid foundation in conservative strategies, helping preserve value while providing immediate liquidity.

Balanced or diversified investment options

If you're looking for a blend of growth and stability, many super funds offer balanced or diversified options. These portfolios mix growth assets like shares and property with defensive assets like bonds and cash. A balanced option might contain 60–70 per cent growth assets and 30–40 per cent defensive assets, aiming to deliver moderate returns while managing risk. Every fund mixes their balanced funds differently, so it's worth taking a close look at the detailed levels of exposure to different asset classes that they are offering with their investment mix, and comparing their returns with other funds with a similar mix.

Ethical and socially responsible investments

For investors who want their super to align with their personal values, many funds now offer ethical or socially responsible investment (SRI) options. These portfolios focus on companies and industries that meet environmental, social and governance (ESG) criteria. Typically, they avoid investing in industries like tobacco, gambling and fossil fuels while focusing on companies with sustainable business practices. While returns from SRI funds have sometimes lagged behind broader market benchmarks in the past, recent years have seen many ethical funds delivering competitive, even superior returns. As always, it's important to do your homework to ensure the fund aligns with both your values and financial goals.

Lifecycle investment options (sometimes called target-date funds)

Lifecycle investment options are a growing trend in many superannuation funds, offering an evolving investment strategy that adjusts as you move through your working life toward retirement. The idea behind these options is to match your changing financial needs and risk tolerance as you age. Early on, your investments focus on growth, but as retirement nears, the strategy gradually shifts toward preserving your capital by increasing the proportion of defensive assets.

In the early stages of your career, typically when you're in your 20s and 30s, the focus is on maximising growth. With decades ahead before you access your super, your portfolio is heavily weighted toward growth assets like shares, property and infrastructure. These investments come with higher risk, but with time on your side, the potential for long-term capital growth outweighs short-term volatility.

As you move into the mid-career period, generally in your 40s and 50s, the mix begins to shift. While growth assets still dominate, defensive assets like bonds and fixed-interest products begin to make up a larger portion of the portfolio. This stage is designed to continue building your super balance while introducing some stability, reducing the risk associated with heavy exposure to volatile markets.

Approaching pre-retirement in your late 50s and 60s, the emphasis can be a little more on protecting your capital and balanced growth – remembering you could live a long time. Certainly, more of peoples' portfolios are usually allocated to defensive investments such as bonds, cash and term deposits – but many still drive for growth with their long-term capital. The goal at this stage is to shield your short- and medium-term savings from significant market downturns, ensuring you don't lose a substantial portion of the super balance you plan to spend just before you need to start drawing on it.

Once you reach retirement, your strategy shifts again, this time focusing on maintaining a steady income stream. Defensive assets often take centre stage in the short- and medium-term portions of your portfolio, as preserving capital becomes a key priority.

However, with people living longer in retirement than ever before, there's a growing recognition of the need to keep some exposure to growth assets. Many funds are adapting their strategies to reflect this reality – seeking to strike a balance between stability and growth. Maintaining exposure to growth assets helps your portfolio keep pace with, or even exceed, inflation, ensuring your money lasts and continues to grow throughout your retirement years.

One of the main benefits of lifecycle investment options is that they offer a set-and-forget approach. The super fund automatically adjusts your investments as you age, reducing the need for active management or frequent rebalancing. This makes them ideal for those who prefer a hands-off approach to their superannuation strategy.

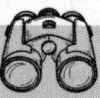

CHOOSING THE RIGHT INVESTMENT OPTION

The key to choosing the right investment option within your super fund is understanding where you are in life, your risk tolerance, investment timeframe and retirement goals. If you have many years left before retirement, you may be more comfortable with higher-risk growth assets, whereas if you're closer to retirement, defensive options that protect your capital might be more appealing. Most super funds allow you to switch between investment options as your circumstances change, so it's important to regularly review your strategy and adjust it to fit your needs.

CHOOSING THE RIGHT SUPER SOLUTION: PROFIT-FOR-MEMBER FUNDS, RETAIL FUNDS, PLATFORMS AND SMSFS

When it comes to choosing how to manage your superannuation, Australians often find themselves deciding between profit-for-member funds, retail funds, platforms and SMSFs (self-managed super funds). While all options serve the same ultimate purpose – growing your retirement savings – their structures, fee arrangements and levels of control and flexibility can differ significantly. It's essential to understand these differences so you can make a conscious choice that suits your financial goals and personal circumstances, as each solution offers distinct advantages depending on what you're aiming to achieve. Again, there's no right answer – only your answer.

Profit-for-member (industry) funds

Profit-for-member funds operate as not-for-profit organisations, meaning any profits are reinvested back into the fund to benefit members. This structure often results in lower fees and potentially higher net returns for members. Historically tied to specific industries such as construction, retail or healthcare, these funds are now open to all workers, regardless of occupation.

Industry funds typically offer balanced or diversified investment options, often managed by large and experienced in-house teams. Their management fees are known to be very competitive, although the gap between industry and retail fund fees has narrowed in recent years. For many Australians, these funds represent a straightforward and cost-effective way to invest for retirement. The largest industry funds in Australia are, in order of size, AustralianSuper, Australian Retirement Trust (ART), Aware Super, UniSuper, Hostplus, HESTA, Cbus Super and Care Super. And while some of the largest funds dominate in size, it doesn't always mean they're doing the things they should be doing to help people navigate pre- and post-retirement. We'll be highlighting how super funds are supporting members in the retirement phase with the Epic Retirement Tick (see pages 123–24).

Retail funds

Retail funds, typically operated by for-profit financial institutions, aim to deliver returns for both their members and shareholders. Following the 2018 Royal Commission into Misconduct in the Banking, Superannuation and Financial Services Industry, many banks exited the super industry, leaving retail funds predominantly managed by independent investment companies.

One of the key advantages of retail funds is the breadth of investment options they provide. These funds often cater to individuals seeking customised portfolios or specialised investment options, which may appeal to those with more complex financial needs or specific goals. However, the increased flexibility has until recently come with higher administrative and management fees compared to industry funds. But in recent times, retail funds have been innovating to make themselves more competitive, especially in response to fee scrutiny.

Interestingly, financial advisers frequently recommend retail funds, as they offer tailored investment portfolios, access to sophisticated tools and advanced adviser platforms. These platforms provide detailed reporting and tracking capabilities, making them valuable for clients with unique financial objectives. Advisers often work through dealer groups, which provide administrative and compliance support but are sometimes affiliated with retail platform providers – this can influence fund recommendations.

The largest retail funds in Australia are, in order of size, Insignia Financial (under the MLC brand), AMP Super Fund, Colonial First State and Mercer Super Trust. The Epic Retirement Tick highlights how retail and industry funds are stepping up to support members through midlife and the retirement phase (see pages 123–24).

Beyond these two categories, there are other options to consider.

Platforms

A platform is an online investment management tool that allows investors to buy, hold and manage a variety of investment products such as superannuation, managed funds, ETFs and direct shares in one centralised place. In Australia, investors can choose from a wide range of investment platforms, from traditional to emerging options. Popular platforms include Hub24, Netwealth, Macquarie Wrap, Praemium, BT Panorama and North (by AMP), among others. Each platform offers different features, investment options and fee structures, catering to various investor needs.

Investing via a platform is becoming a popular way to manage superannuation and other investments, particularly for those working with financial advisers.

Platforms are commonly used by financial advisers to oversee client portfolios, but they are also accessible to individual investors looking for greater control and consolidated reporting on their investments. Many platforms offer tax reporting, performance tracking, and administrative services to streamline investment management.

Platforms have a few advantages. They streamline the management of investments, providing comprehensive reporting on performance, fees and asset allocation – something an adviser will need to do their job. They often offer a wide range of investment choices, including ethical, diversified and sector-specific options. They also offer shared visibility – allowing both clients and advisers to track investments in real time, make portfolio adjustments, and ensure compliance with regulations. Platforms also allow clients to integrate superannuation with broader wealth strategies such as family trusts, direct property investments and estate planning.

However, the convenience of platforms often comes at a cost, with additional platform fees layered on top of fund management, accounting and personal advice fees. It's important to assess whether the benefits outweigh the costs in your particular situation.

The layering of fees on platforms can really add up, making them less cost-effective for people with average super balances. In fact, platforms often pale in comparison to simpler, low-cost options like industry and retail funds or index funds, which are perfectly fine for most Aussies.

There's also a subtle bias in the way platforms are pushed. Financial advisers and dealer groups often have commercial ties to specific platforms or fund providers, which can steer their recommendations. Platforms are packed with features such as detailed reporting and compliance tools, which advisers love – but a lot of these extras might be overkill for the average person.

The largest platform providers in Australia in order of scale are Macquarie Wrap, BT Panorama, Netwealth, Hub24 and Praemium.

Self-managed super funds

Australians who want complete control over their superannuation and the ability to invest in a broader range of assets such as property and derivatives may want to consider a self-managed super fund (SMSF). An SMSF gives you the power to manage your own super investments, but with that control comes greater responsibility and complexity – and not necessarily higher returns.

Unlike traditional super funds, where professionals handle the investments for you, an SMSF allows you to choose and manage your investments yourself. This means you can invest in a wider range of assets, including shares, property, funds, derivatives and even collectibles like artwork, depending on your strategy. Many Australians choose an SMSF to invest in direct property (such as rental properties, commercial properties or industrial buildings) or derivatives (options or futures), which are typically not available through regular super funds.

However, running an SMSF requires more time, knowledge and administration than a standard super fund. You need to comply with strict regulations set by the ATO, such as preparing annual financial statements, conducting audits and ensuring the fund complies with superannuation laws. If not managed correctly, SMSFs can face penalties, so it's often a good idea to work with a financial adviser or accountant.

The costs of an SMSF can also be higher, particularly if your fund has a smaller balance. Set-up fees, annual audit costs and the expenses involved in managing investments can add up quickly. For this reason, SMSFs are typically better suited to those with larger balances (generally $500,000 or more) who want a tailored investment approach and are prepared for the extra responsibilities. They can also be a more cost-effective option for couples combining their super funds, as they share the administrative costs.

Many people find themselves unwinding their SMSFs as they get older, when they shy away from financial complexity. So before setting one up, consider how you might manage it as you age. Have an exit strategy in mind.

PROJECTING YOUR FUTURE SUPER BALANCE

Here are some tools and calculators that might help you grasp how your super and the age pension can be projected to provide you income:

> The Moneysmart Superannuation Calculator (moneysmart.gov.au/how-super-works/superannuation-calculator) helps you to extrapolate how much super you'll have when you retire and understand how the fees you are paying might affect your final balance.
>
> The Moneysmart Retirement Planner (moneysmart.gov.au/retirement-income/retirement-planner) helps you to extrapolate how much income you can generate from your superannuation and the age pension combined over your lifetime.
>
> Alternatively, if you are with a major superannuation fund, you may find their retirement planning calculators a great help in understanding the income your super can generate over time.

INVESTMENTS COMMONLY MIXED INTO DIRECT INVESTMENT PORTFOLIOS

As you approach midlife, securing your financial future becomes more important than ever, and a key part of building that security is understanding how to structure a well-diversified investment portfolio to help you fund your pre-retirement or post-retirement years. At this stage, balancing risk and return is crucial to protecting your wealth while continuing to grow it. A diversified portfolio is designed to spread risk across different types of investments (asset classes), so that you aren't overly reliant on one source of returns. Let's break down the types of investments that are most commonly mixed into a diversified portfolio and how they can help you achieve a steady financial foundation.

INVESTING IN EQUITIES

Direct shares

Equities, or shares, are one of the most common, versatile and important investments in a diversified portfolio, particularly in Australia. When you invest in shares, you're buying a small piece of a company and becoming a part-owner. This ownership offers two main financial benefits: capital growth and dividends.

Capital growth sees the value of your shares increase over time, and over the long term, the equity market has always increased in value. For example, if you buy shares at $10 each and the share price rises to $15, you've made a capital gain of $5 per share. These gains aren't realised (or taxed) until you sell the shares, and if you've held the shares for longer than one year, you'll enjoy a 50 per cent discount on the CGT.

Dividends, on the other hand, are payments made to shareholders from a company's profits. Some companies, especially the more mature ones, regularly distribute a portion of their profits to shareholders in the form of dividends. This can be an excellent source of passive income for investors, especially for those approaching or in retirement who want a reliable income stream without drawing on their capital. Some dividends also often come with an extra tax perk known as franking credits.

I explained franking credits earlier in this chapter, but to recap, they can reduce the tax you pay on dividends. When a company pays tax on its profits before distributing dividends to shareholders, it attaches franking credits to those dividends, representing the tax the company has already paid (usually at the corporate tax rate of 30 per cent).

For investors, this means that when they receive dividends, they can use these franking credits to offset their own tax liability. If your personal tax rate is lower than the corporate rate, you may even get a tax refund on the difference. This makes fully franked dividends (which are common among Australian companies) highly attractive for investors looking to reduce their tax bill while earning income from their shares.

Another big advantage of shares is their liquidity – how easily and quickly you can sell an investment and turn it into cash. Unlike property or other more illiquid investments, shares are traded on the stock market, meaning you can typically sell them within a day or two if you need to access your money. This flexibility is one of the reasons why shares are a cornerstone of many portfolios – they give you both growth potential and the ability to cash out when needed.

Equities are highly liquid and offer the potential for both capital growth and income, but they also come with higher risk compared to bonds or cash. Share prices can fluctuate significantly in the short term, influenced by market sentiment, company performance and economic conditions. However, over the long term, shares have generally provided higher returns than many other asset classes, making them a key source of growth in investment portfolios. Some investors may choose to balance the risk of equities with safer investments, or they may focus on companies that pay dividends or have a history of stability.

Exchange-traded funds and index funds

One of the easiest ways to invest in the share market is through exchange-traded funds (ETFs) and index funds. These low-cost investment options give you exposure to a broad range of stocks without having to pick individual ones. You can invest in funds that track major indices such as the ASX 200 or S&P 500, or focus on specific sectors such as technology, healthcare or international markets. With a single purchase, ETFs and index funds allow you to own a slice of hundreds – or even thousands – of companies, making them a popular choice for long-term investors.

The key benefits of ETFs and index funds are the same:

- **They are a great way to buy a diversified asset**. By holding a basket of assets, ETFs and index funds, you spread your investment across multiple companies, industries and countries, reducing the risk of underperformance by any single stock.
- **They are extremely cost-effective**. Most index funds and many ETFs are passively managed, meaning they track an index rather than relying on a fund manager to pick stocks. This generally results in lower fees, which can significantly boost returns over time. However, some ETFs are actively managed or follow specific investment strategies, so costs and structures can vary.

- **It's an easy way to invest.** You don't have to become an investing expert. Both funds are ideal for investors who don't want to spend time managing individual stocks.
- **They tend to be less volatile than direct investments.** This is because they spread risk across multiple assets rather than relying on the performance of a single company or sector. This diversification helps smooth out market fluctuations, reducing the impact of any one stock or asset that is underperforming.

Exchange traded funds (ETFs)

Exchange-traded funds (ETFs) are a flexible and cost-effective way to invest in the market. Unlike traditional managed funds, ETFs are traded on a stock exchange, meaning you can buy or sell them throughout the day at market prices. They come with low management fees, though you'll need to pay brokerage for each trade. One of their biggest advantages is flexibility – since they trade like shares, you have more control over when you buy or sell. ETFs also offer transparency, as you directly invest in the individual components of an index. For example, buying an ASX 200 ETF means you own shares in all 200 companies in that index. ETFs are best suited for investors who want easy access through an online trading platform or stockbroker, as well as those using a 'core and satellite' strategy or looking for tactical exposure to specific sectors, geographies or asset classes.

WHAT IS A 'CORE AND SATELLITE' APPROACH TO INVESTING?

A core and satellite approach is a popular investment strategy where the 'core' of a portfolio is allocated to broad, diversified investments (eg index funds or ETFs), while the 'satellites' are targeted investments in specific sectors, geographic locations or asset classes for growth or tactical opportunities. Many financial advisers and self-directed investors use this approach to balance their risk and diversification.

Index funds

Index funds are a straightforward, low-cost way to invest in the market. Unlike ETFs, they are bought directly from the provider and only trade once a day at the end-of-day price. They come with low management fees, and transaction costs are typically embedded in the overall price – though minimum investment amounts may apply. If purchased through a brokerage, additional brokerage fees may be charged. While index funds offer less flexibility than ETFs, as you can only trade once per day, they still provide broad market exposure. They also tend to be less transparent than ETFs, though their underlying investments are similar. Index funds are best suited for long-term investors who prefer a simple, set-and-forget strategy rather than actively managing their investments.

Both ETFs and index funds are easy to start, and the rapidly rising popularity of these funds shows their appeal.

BONDS

Bonds are another fundamental part of a diversified investment portfolio, known for providing stability and a consistent income. When you invest in bonds, you're essentially lending money to a government, corporation or other entity. In return, the bond issuer promises to pay you regular interest (known as a coupon) over a set period and to return the initial amount you invested (the principal) when the bond matures.

One of the key benefits of bonds is the steady, predictable income they provide. The interest payments you receive from bonds can offer a more stable income stream compared to the fluctuations of dividend payments from shares. This makes bonds attractive for those who are looking to balance the risk in their portfolio with a reliable income source. The return you receive from bonds tends to be lower than shares, but they also generally come with less volatility.

Different types of bonds are available, each with varying levels of risk and return:

Government bonds

Government bonds are considered the safest because they are backed by the government. In Australia, Commonwealth Government bonds are often seen as a low-risk option, though their returns are typically lower than other bonds due to the reduced risk. State government bonds can provide a higher interest rate (or coupon) with some additional risk. Some bonds offer exposure to government-owned infrastructure assets as well.

Corporate bonds

Corporate bonds are issued by companies and tend to offer higher interest rates than government bonds, but they come with more risk because a company is more likely to default than a government. Investment-grade bonds rated BBB- or higher by credit agencies, such as those issued by banks and companies, provide a lower-risk investment.

Some investors prefer a mix of both bond types, as this provides a blend of stability and higher returns.

One thing to keep in mind with bonds is interest rate risk, or the inverse relationship between bond prices and interest rates. When interest rates rise, the value of existing bonds tends to fall because new bonds are issued at higher rates. Conversely, when interest rates drop, bond prices typically rise. This can impact the overall value of your bond investments, especially if you need to sell them before they mature.

Bonds are often seen as a safer, more conservative investment, particularly when compared to equities. Because they promise a return of your initial investment at maturity (assuming the issuer doesn't default), bonds are commonly used by those who are more focused on capital preservation – the idea of protecting the value of their investment. While bonds won't typically deliver the same level of growth as shares, they do offer a sense of security and help balance out the riskier parts of a portfolio.

Typically, the risks of bonds and equities are inversely correlated (or opposite). The economic forces that send share prices lower send bonds higher, and vice versa. Well-constructed portfolios will incorporate bonds into the risk management. A typical 60/40 portfolio will have an equity exposure of 60 per cent and a bond exposure of 40 per cent.

Like equities, bonds are generally considered liquid investments, though they are not quite as liquid as shares. You can sell bonds on the secondary bond market if you need access to your money before the bond matures. But the price you receive for selling a bond early depends on current market interest rates and the bond's remaining term.

MANAGED FUNDS

Managed funds pool money from multiple investors, with a professional fund manager deciding where to invest across a variety of assets like shares, bonds and property. These funds can be actively managed, meaning the manager aims to outperform the market, or passively managed, where they track a specific index. Managed funds offer diversification by spreading your investment across different assets, but they typically come with higher fees than ETFs or index funds due to the active management. They're a good option for investors who prefer a hands-off approach but want professional management of their money.

LISTED INVESTMENT COMPANIES

Listed investment companies (LICs) are publicly traded companies that invest in a portfolio of shares or other assets on behalf of their shareholders. LICs are similar to ETFs in that they offer exposure to a range of investments, but the key difference is that LICs are closed-ended, meaning they have a fixed number of shares on the market. This can lead to shares trading at a premium or a discount to the value of their underlying assets. LICs can provide dividend income and capital growth, and they are known for having a long-term investment approach.

INVESTING IN PROPERTY

Direct property ownership

One of the most common ways to invest in income-generating property is through direct ownership of real estate, whether it's residential or commercial. Residential properties, such as rental homes or apartments, offer the potential for regular rental income while gradually appreciating in value over time. On the other hand, commercial properties, like office buildings or retail spaces, often provide higher rental yields than residential properties, but they come with more risks, including longer vacancy periods and higher upfront costs.

Owning property directly gives you full control over your investment decisions, from choosing tenants to managing maintenance, but it also comes with the challenge of managing all those things – which anyone who's managed a rental property will know can be very painful. Direct ownership of property requires substantial capital and ongoing maintenance – and let's face it, property is relatively illiquid, meaning it could take time to sell and access your money when you need it. It does have one big drawcard, and that's the ease of tax deductibility. Many investors use tax-effective strategies like negative gearing to offset the costs of owning property, allowing them to claim tax deductions on the interest paid on loans and reduce their taxable income while waiting for long-term capital growth. It's a common way to get started in rental properties.

If you want to own property, but you don't want the pain of managing tenants and dealing with poor liquidity, real estate investment trusts (REITs) might be a better option.

Real estate investment trusts (REITS)

REITs are companies that own and manage the portfolios of income-generating properties, such as shopping centres, office buildings and industrial precincts. By buying shares in a REIT, you can gain exposure to a range of properties without the need to buy and manage real estate yourself. REITs provide regular income through distributions and can be easily traded on stock exchanges, offering liquidity – and in many cases in Australia, that income is franked. The composition and tax status of distributions can be quite complex at times, including capital gains and foreign income, so be sure you have the appetite for this.

Property syndicates

Property syndicates allow multiple investors to pool their money to invest in large-scale property purchases or developments. Managed by professionals, these syndicates offer investors a proportion of ownership in the property and allow them to share in rental income and potential capital gains. You must remember, however, that property syndicates can be illiquid, with investors often committing to the investment for several years. This makes them better suited for those comfortable with longer-term commitments and limited options for selling their stake early.

Property ETFs

Property ETFs offer another way to gain exposure to real estate markets. They invest in a variety of real estate assets or REITs and can be bought and sold on stock exchanges just like shares. They provide broad diversification across different property types and regions, and generally cost less than actively managed property funds. Property ETFs also offer liquidity and can be a simple, efficient way to diversify your portfolio with real estate exposure.

Mortgage funds

Mortgage funds allow investors to pool their money to lend to property buyers or developers. These funds provide regular income from the interest on loans and typically offer much higher yields than traditional savings accounts or bonds. However, mortgage funds come with the risk that borrowers may default on their loans. Although the loans are usually secured against property, there is still the potential for loss if the borrower cannot repay. So do your homework on the fund manager and understand your risks.

HOLDING CASH

Cash investments are the most secure and stable option in any portfolio, providing a dependable way to preserve capital with minimal risk. However, they offer little to no protection against inflation, which can erode purchasing power over time.

While cash won't deliver the same growth potential as shares or property, it provides liquidity and easy access to your funds when you need them.

There are two simple ways to hold cash: in term deposits, and in high interest, at-call cash management bank accounts.

Term deposits

Term deposits are fixed investments where you agree to lock away your money for a set period, usually ranging from a few months to several years, in exchange for a guaranteed interest rate. The main advantage of term deposits is their certainty – you know exactly how much interest you'll earn, and your capital is protected. Term deposits are less flexible since you generally can't access your money until the term expires without incurring a penalty. Term deposits went out of favour during the low-interest rate environment of the 2010s, but as rates have improved in recent years, they have come back into favour, particularly for money you want to hold in cash, but need reliable returns above the rate of inflation and don't want to feel tempted to spend it.

Cash management accounts

Cash-at-call bank accounts, often called cash management accounts, on the other hand, offer flexibility and instant access to your money, making them ideal for managing day-to-day expenses or as an emergency fund. These accounts typically offer lower interest rates than term deposits – although sometimes only marginally. Most importantly, they allow you to withdraw or deposit funds anytime, giving you complete liquidity. While they won't deliver significant returns, cash-at-call accounts are excellent for short-term needs and provide the peace of mind of knowing your money is readily available.

Both term deposits and cash-at-call accounts are safe, low-risk options that prioritise capital preservation over growth. They can be a useful part of your overall portfolio, offering security and liquidity, especially when balancing riskier investments like shares or property. You can hold both within your superannuation fund, or outside it too.

It's crucial to remember that inflation is a real risk when holding significant cash. While cash feels safe, inflation quietly erodes its purchasing power, meaning every dollar buys a little less over time. If you're holding too much cash without a strategy to outpace inflation, you risk seeing your savings lose value, especially in low-interest accounts. So it's a good idea to assess how much cash you need for immediate needs while directing surplus funds toward investments with better growth potential – so that inflation doesn't chip away at your long-term financial goals.

GETTING THE BEST CASH RATES

If you've got cash and are looking for the best interest rates on cash-at-call (or high-interest savings) accounts or term deposits, it's worth noting that the big four banks don't always offer the best deals – especially for midlife and older Australians who've already paid off their mortgages.

The big banks tend to reserve their most competitive rates and perks for younger, mortgage-seeking customers who might use multiple banking products. They also prioritise those who hold their main transactional account with the bank, as it helps them claim you as 'theirs' in banking sector surveys.

To get better rates, you'll probably have to take some action. Here's some you might consider:

- **Consolidate your accounts**: Keeping your transaction and savings accounts with the same institution could unlock better interest rates and perks. Banks large and small often reward loyal customers with special offers or better deals. Look for them.
- **Look beyond the big four for higher-interest accounts**: Smaller banks, credit unions and online-only banks typically offer higher interest rates on savings, especially for older Australians not focused on home loans. Organisations like

Macquarie Bank with its 'Accelerator' account, and ING with its 'Savings Maximiser', are just two leading the way. Online-only institutions often have fewer restrictions, like minimum monthly deposits or withdrawal limits, which you should keep your eye out for. Just ensure any bank you use is covered by the Australian banking guarantee, which insures funds of up to $250,000 with any authorised deposit-taking institution (check the website of the Australian Prudential Regulation Authority for details).
- **Consider keeping a $10 balance on your mortgage**: Some banks may offer better interest rates to customers with a mortgage, even if only a small balance remains.

Lastly, stay proactive. Regularly compare interest rates, and don't hesitate to switch banks or negotiate with your current provider. And if the thought of moving accounts sounds like a hassle, then using tools like Apple Pay or Samsung Pay can make the process easier. Just swap the underlying bank card in your phone's settings and keep tapping.

LIFETIME INCOME STREAMS

As you approach retirement, securing a reliable, steady income becomes a top priority. While growth investments like shares and property offer great long-term potential, the real challenge for most pre-retirees and retirees is having the confidence to spend their money and enjoy life without worrying about market downturns or how long they might live. Many find themselves stuck in 'preservation mode', holding back just in case markets take a nosedive. If this is you, a new option may help.

There's an emerging breed of guaranteed income streams called 'lifetime income streams', sometimes referred to as 'lifetime annuities' and 'lifetime pensions'. These products are leveraging the old concept of an annuity (a fixed-term income stream) and making it more suitable for the generation that is now arriving at retirement with a longer life expectancy, superannuation and age pension eligibility, but they don't necessarily feel certain about how much they can afford to spend.

Think about it: a pay cheque that arrives for the rest of your life, no matter how long you live, and that can rise with inflation, grow if you choose market-linked investment options, give you a discount on the pension assets test, access to your investment value at any time if your circumstances change, and, if you pass away earlier than expected, your loved ones can receive a death benefit. That's the promise of lifetime income streams. These relatively new financial products have been gaining traction thanks to a government push to ensure you never outlive your savings. For those worried about living longer than expected (which is a good problem to have!), lifetime income streams are becoming an increasingly attractive option.

New products in this space are much more flexible than previous generations of annuity-style products. Some options let you access part of your lump sum if life throws you a curveball, while others allow you to pass on a death benefit to your loved ones. Many even offer a mix of investment options so you can still have one foot in the market while enjoying a guaranteed income. It's all about giving retirees more choices and flexibility to suit their financial goals.

When you sign up for a lifetime income stream, you're 'purchasing' a financial product that offers a rate of return along with a selection of features you can choose from. Typically, the rate of return is higher the earlier you purchase it in life, as you're spreading the income over a longer period. On the other hand, the payment amounts tend to be higher if you purchase it later, as the timeframe over which you'll be drawing the income is shorter.

The features are extensive. One of the most useful is inflation protection, which means your payments will increase over time to keep up with rising living costs, which is particularly important as health care and other expenses tend to grow in retirement.

Another great perk is the favourable treatment under the age pension assets test. For qualifying products, only 60 per cent of the purchase price counts as an asset until you turn 84 (or for at least five years), and after that, it drops to 30 per cent. This can help you qualify for a higher age pension compared to holding fully counted assets like shares or property.

Other handy features include the option to redraw funds, invest in market-linked assets for potential growth, downside protection to ensure your money never goes down in the event of a market crash, and death benefits, so your loved ones can receive a portion of the funds if you pass away earlier than expected.

We're seeing more retirees putting part of their super into lifetime income streams to achieve a balance between income security and growth potential. It's a smart way to cover your everyday living costs – like housing, food and health care – while keeping the rest of your portfolio in higher-growth assets that give you access to capital and the chance to benefit from market returns. This mix of guaranteed income and growth options lets you have the best of both worlds: the security of knowing your basic expenses are covered for life with the potential for growth elsewhere.

You can purchase lifetime income streams through a financial adviser or, increasingly, directly from super funds. The biggest independent providers of lifetime income products in Australia are Challenger, AMP North, Generation Life and Allianz Retire+. These organisations offer income solutions designed to last for life, helping retirees manage longevity risk and maintain financial confidence well into their later years. While each product varies in its structure and flexibility, they all aim to provide a stable income floor – something increasingly important as more Australians face the reality of living well into their 80s and 90s.

In addition to this, many funds are beginning to offer these alongside account-based pensions, as part of the government's push through the Retirement Income Covenant, which requires super funds to develop tailored strategies for retirees.

This is certainly a space to watch. With super funds rolling out new, integrated solutions that include lifetime pensions, the growing focus on secure retirement income is set to drive greater interest and engagement from both consumers and financial advisers, ushering in a whole new conversation about income layering.

BUSTING THE MYTHS

There are a few myths floating around about lifetime annuities. Let's clear these up.

'The age pension is my guaranteed income, so I don't need a lifetime income stream.' Sure, the age pension is great, but most people find it's not enough to fully cover their lifestyle and living costs. Adding a lifetime income stream can provide that extra layer of security and may even help you get a higher age pension with the 40 per cent asset test discount.

'I won't get exposure to growth assets with an annuity.' Not true anymore! Many lifetime income streams now include investment options that allow you to tap into growth assets, often managed by some of Australia's top fund managers. You can still diversify while enjoying that guaranteed income.

'I can't access my money if I need it.' Modern lifetime income streams offer options that let you draw down some capital if your situation changes and you need access to cash. Flexibility is the name of the game now.

'If I die early, my loved ones will get nothing.' Not anymore! Death benefits are a key feature in many of today's lifetime income streams. You can set things up so that if you pass away earlier than expected, your family can claim part of the remaining funds.

'I don't need to think about this until later.' The sooner you explore your options, the better. Some lifetime income stream products can be purchased with a larger lifetime benefit if you buy them earlier in life. Lifetime income streams can play an important role in planning a retirement you can enjoy without worrying about running out of money.

'You need to invest a huge amount to make it worthwhile.' Not necessarily. You don't need to put your entire retirement savings into a lifetime income stream. Many people use them as just one layer of income, combining them with other investments or the age pension to create a balanced income strategy that fits their needs.

> **'They're expensive.'** Lifetime income streams mean you are putting in place an insurance policy and transferring any risk back to the provider. The cost may also depend on factors like your age, the amount you invest, whether you choose features like inflation protection or death benefits, and the interest rates at the time.
>
> So while they can feel 'expensive' compared to other traditional investments, the value lies in what you're getting in return: guaranteed income, reduced risk of outliving your savings, and, in some cases, favourable age pension treatment.

9. CONSIDER YOUR FUTURE ELIGIBILITY FOR THE AGE PENSION

If you're in your 40s or 50s, the age pension might seem like something too far off to worry about. But understanding how it works could help you make smarter decisions about your savings, planning and spending in your Prime Time. The age pension is a critical source of income for many retirees, and if you plan strategically, it can play a valuable role in your own retirement.

As of 2025, three in five Australians over 67 will access some form of age pension, and more than 44 per cent of retirees depend on it as a major source of income. While this reliance is expected to reduce as more Australians retire with superannuation savings, the age pension is here to stay.

There's no need to worry about a stigma, either. Australians with average super balances of between $250,000 and $400,000 per person will likely access a part or full age pension at some stage during their retirement. And many people who start with a million dollars in super may find that over time it whittles away, and they too become eligible. In fact, you might even plan your finances so that you qualify for it, as it can provide a powerful layer of income.

Let's break down how the age pension works, how much you can receive and how the system interacts with your other assets, including superannuation. The more you know now, the better you can plan for your future.

HOW MUCH DOES THE AGE PENSION PAY?

At the time of writing, the full age pension (including supplements) provides the following amounts.

Pension rates	Fortnightly	Annually
Single	$1149.00	$29,874.00
Couple	$1732.20	$45,037.20

Included in these pension amounts are two supplements – the pension supplement, which is designed to help with the cost of prescriptions, rates, telephone and internet connection; and the energy supplement, which is designed to assist with energy costs.

Supplements	Single	Couple
Maximum pension supplement (fortnightly)	$83.60	$126.00
Energy supplement	$14.10	$21.20
Total	$97.70	$147.20
Annual total	$2540.20	$3827.20

AGE PENSION ELIGIBILITY CRITERIA

To be eligible for the age pension, you must meet three core criteria: age, assets and income.

1. Reaching age pension age

You can only start receiving the age pension once you reach the qualifying age, which is currently 67.

2. The assets test

The assets test assesses the value of the assets you hold (excluding your principal residence). This includes your home contents, cars, boats, financial investments (inside and outside super), deprived assets and any other assets.

Your family home is exempt from the assets test, so even if you live in a mansion in Sydney's Northern Beaches, you could still qualify for the pension. This exemption is an important consideration when planning your financial strategy for retirement.

The assets test applies thresholds, and if your total asset value exceeds these thresholds, your pension may be reduced or eliminated. The tapering system works as follows: for every $1000 that your assets exceed the threshold, your age pension is reduced by $3 per fortnight. This allows for a gradual reduction in pension payments rather than an all-or-nothing cut-off.

Full pension thresholds:

Your situation	Homeowner	Non-homeowner
Single	$314,000	$566,000
A couple, combined	$470,000	$722,000

Part Pension thresholds:

Your situation	Homeowner	Non-homeowner
Single	$697,000	$949,000
A couple, combined	$1,047,500	$1,299,500

WHAT IS A DEPRIVED ASSET?

A deprived asset is an eligible asset you have given away in the last five years that still qualifies as an asset under the assets and income test. Each year, those looking to qualify for the age pension have a maximum amount they can gift without triggering the deprived assets rules:
- $10,000 annual limit
- $30,000 over five years.

The rules have a few nuances, however:
- Spouses can gift assets to each other without triggering deprived assets.

> - The limits apply to a couple as a whole, not to each individual in the relationship.
> - Deprived assets rules are also relevant for aged care means testing.

3. The income test

The income test measures the income you generate from various sources, such as work, rental properties and investments. Here's a breakdown of how the income test works.

Work income

You're allowed to earn a certain amount from employment without reducing your age pension, thanks to the pension work bonus. You can earn up to $300 per fortnight (or $7800 per year) from wages or eligible self-employment without affecting your pension. Additionally, you can accumulate extra credits through the Work Bonus Income Bank, allowing you to earn up to $11,800 per year without impacting your pension.

Furthermore, you can also earn $212 per fortnight as a single person or $372 per fortnight as a couple (this is called the pension income test free area) before any reduction in your age pension occurs (as at March 2025).

If you earn more than these thresholds, your pension is reduced at a rate of 50 cents for each dollar over the limit.

Real estate income

Income from rental properties is also assessed under the income test. The age pension income test considers your net rental income after deducting eligible expenses like interest on loans, rates and maintenance costs. If your property generates negative income, you cannot use this to offset other income; it will simply be treated as zero.

Deemed income from investments

The government uses deeming to calculate your potential income from financial assets such as superannuation, shares, managed funds and cash deposits. Deeming assumes you earn a certain return on your investments, regardless of their actual performance.

- Singles:
  - The first $62,600 of financial assets is deemed to earn 0.25 per cent.
  - Any amount above $62,600 is deemed to earn 2.25 per cent.
- Couples (combined):
  - The first $103,800 of financial assets is deemed to earn 0.25 per cent.
  - Any amount above $103,800 is deemed to earn 2.25 per cent.

These deemed amounts are added to your income from other sources to calculate your adjusted taxable income, which is then compared to the income test thresholds. *All pension limits quoted are current as at March 2025.*

APPLYING FOR THE AGE PENSION

Applying for the age pension can be a bit of a hassle, but it helps to know you can get a head start by applying up to 13 weeks before you're eligible. And here's a tip: if things are dragging on, reaching out to your federal member for assistance might help move things along!

If your initial application is unsuccessful, don't stress. You're allowed to reapply every 12 months. And if you qualify but later decide to return to work, you can still keep your pensioner concessions for up to two years, which is a nice safety net.

PLANNING YOUR PRIME TIME AND EPIC RETIREMENT WITH THE AGE PENSION IN MIND

Understanding how the age pension works, especially its interaction with the assets and income tests, allows you to plan more effectively for your future. You may choose to adjust your investment strategy or manage your superannuation withdrawals to remain within the pension thresholds, ensuring you can maximise your income from both the age pension and your own savings.

By taking these factors into account, you can structure your finances in a way that leverages the age pension as a valuable part of your overall retirement income strategy.

Rent assistance

If you qualify for the age pension, or another form of social security, you will also qualify for Commonwealth Rent Assistance, a subsidy that can be used to pay rent on a house or apartment. It can also be used to pay site fees for a land lease or relocatable home, site fees for parking your caravan at a caravan park, or fund non-government-funded residential aged care.

The government subsidises the rent over base thresholds at a rate of 75 cents in the dollar. There is a cap on the amount of rent that will be subsidised.

Rent assistance rates	Your fortnightly rent is more than ...	To get the maximum payment, your rent must be at least ...	The maximum rent assistance fortnightly payment
Single	$149.60	$432.27	$212
Couple	$242.40	$508.80	$199.80

Concession cards and benefits

Once you reach age pension age, which for many Prime Timers is a while away, there are two powerful little concession cards that help with the cost of living and health expenses. You should know these exist, and think about whether you'll be able to access cheaper government services and health care because of them later in life.

The Pensioner Concession Card

This is the most powerful concession card for older Australians, and it's only available to people who are eligible for $1 or more of the age pension. It gives you access to heavily subsidised prescriptions, and a low cap on how much you can spend on prescriptions each year before they all become free. You can also access bulk-billed visits with your doctor. And many discounts are offered by the states, such as rebates on power and water bills, car registration, rates and public transport. You'll also be able to access long-distance rail travel at significant discounts.

The Commonwealth Seniors Health Card (CSHC)

This is a nice consolation prize that most self-funded retirees can access. The CSHC is available to those who are of pension age and meet an income test amount specific to the card, which is quite high. You use your adjusted taxable income as the assessable amount.

When you qualify, you can access cheaper prescriptions, a lower cap on the Medicare safety net, and bulk-billed doctor visits – if your doctor offers them.

> You can find a lot more information on the age pension, and the clever, perfectly legal strategies you might consider to improve your eligibility for it, in my other book, *How to Have an Epic Retirement*. I don't go into as much detail about it here because there are so many other things to consider to make the most of your Prime Time.

UNDERSTANDING THE SWEET SPOT WHERE THE AGE PENSION AND SUPER COMBINE

There's this strange little anomaly in our retirement system that's truly worth understanding. It's the fact that people with less superannuation can actually end up earning more retirement income, just by knowing how to use the systems of retirement. It's the sweet spot where both singles and couples with a lower superannuation balance leverage the age pension alongside their superannuation income stream to earn more in retirement income than someone with a far larger superannuation balance can at the same drawdown rates.

I wish more people understood it, because the income generated from layering superannuation, the age pension and working can form quite a reasonable income, if you're not living the high life. This begs the question, is it worth the grind to become a self-funded retiree, when starting retirement with a more modest super balance can still secure a moderate income?

To break down how to find the sweet spot, or the amount of money to hold in superannuation when you hit pension age and meet the conditions of release, there are three things to understand.

The first thing to pay close attention to is the pension assets and income test thresholds for receiving the full age pension. This is at the heart of what we call the sweet spot – every time these thresholds change, the sweet spot shifts as well.

Right now, the limits for the full pension are $470,000 in assets for couples and $314,000 for single people. If you have more than this, your pension will be gradually reduced through the tapering system.

There's an interesting quirk in the two tests at the moment. Couples are a little better off than singles. For couples with the maximum allowable assets for the full pension – $470,000 – their deemed income is still below the income test free area, meaning they won't trigger the income test. However, single people face a slightly tougher situation. Although the asset limit for a full pension is $314,000, if you have more than $301,000 in assets, your deemed income will exceed $212, which is the income test free area for singles. As a result, your pension will be reduced by 50 cents for every dollar over the limits.

The taper rate is the second thing you need to understand. There are two different taper rates, one for the income test and one for the assets test. The taper rate on the assets test is activated when your assets exceed specified thresholds, reducing your fortnightly pension by $3 for every additional $1000 in assets above the limit. For instance, if you have $1000 over the asset threshold, your pension decreases by $78 every fortnight, which is calculated as 26 multiplied by $3. To counteract this reduction, you would need to earn a return of more than 7.8 per cent on any additional superannuation funds you possess.

The income test also has a taper rate, but it works a little differently. For every dollar of income earned over the income test threshold, your pension is reduced by 50 cents. This means that if your income exceeds the threshold, every additional dollar reduces your pension, potentially leading to significant reductions in the support you receive.

When considering both taper rates, it may be more beneficial to strategically manage your assets and income. For instance, if you're close to the asset or income test thresholds, it might make sense to spend some of your superannuation on experiences such as holidays or home renovations, or to invest in quickly depreciating assets like cars or boats. This could help you maintain a higher total income and enjoy a better quality of life.

The third thing you need to understand is the impact of earning additional income on your bigger financial picture, particularly from working. If you are looking to the pension to deliver a significant portion of your retirement income, then you'll want to understand the pension work bonus and the pension income test free area, which when combined will offer you up to $11,800 in money you can earn from working before your pension income is reduced.

Let's look at some examples.

Tom and Maria, who are both one year into retirement, have a super balance of $470,000 and they have drawn 6 per cent or $28,200 per year as an income stream. They combine this with the full age pension of $45,037.20 to achieve a comfortable income of $73,237.20. Their super fund earned 8.5 per cent in balanced and growth investments last year, so they haven't gone backward; in fact, their super balance is now a little above their starting balance, at $481,750.

Why does this work? Tom and Maria's assets sit right at the cut-off point for the full age pension, and they don't trigger the income test because the deeming rate is used to calculate income on financial assets. Their deemed income is $326.88 per fortnight on $470,000 and the income test free area for couples is $372.

They're planning a trip to see their daughter in Singapore this year and will draw the $11,750 in excess earnings they hold in super as a lump sum to pay for it. They want to try to keep their super balance at or around the assets test caps, because every $1000 they have in assets over $470,000 takes $3 off their fortnightly pension. They've both kept tinkering with work too, knowing they can earn $7800 per person without impacting their age pension.

A self-funded retired couple with $1.3 million in income-generating assets would need to draw a 5.5–6 per cent income stream from their superannuation to be able to match this level of income. It's worth noting that if they gradually spend down some of their capital, they may eventually become eligible for a part pension as their assets decline and the pension is indexed over time. Some retirees strategically aim for this 'sweet spot' – spending down their super at a controlled rate to maximise their income while later qualifying for age pension support.

Here's a similar scenario. Priya is 68 and single and draws a 6 per cent income stream from her super balance of $314,000, the cut off-point for the age pension. This gives her a superannuation income stream of $18,840. She combines this with a full age pension of $29,754 to form a layered retirement income of $48,594. And, with $7800 from working, this gets her close to the ASFA comfortable retirement benchmark of $51,814. Similarly, her superannuation fund returned her 8.5 per cent last year, and she wants to manage the tapering of her age pension, so she's decided to do a small renovation of her bathroom to make her house a more suitable place to age in, spending the $7850 in additional funds that remain in her super fund above the threshold. She could consider using it in other ways too, such as drawing it as a lump sum or an increase to her income stream.

Understanding this sweet spot can be tricky, but it's something that should give people approaching retirement with a smaller super balance much greater confidence – and that's important. Most super funds offer advice on these types of strategies at no extra cost. You're probably paying for the advice in your annual member fee, so ask! Tell them I sent you.

Lesson 6
Learn the new lessons of midlife money management: time, income and spending

You're now at the point where you understand your financial foundations:
- How to save more than you earn
- How to invest those savings and build assets through compounding
- How to pay less tax – legally – and put those savings toward investments too
- How to pay off your home, and how that home plays into your bigger financial picture over time
- How to use superannuation to make your money grow faster
- How to invest, and what your options are for creating better or more appropriate investment returns.
- How the age pension works as a layer of retirement income you can count on.

And you know that when you put this knowledge into practice, even if you get there late, you'll build wealth a lot quicker.

Now it's time to learn about the next phase.

If you've got this far into the finance section, you know the rules start to shift as you reach midlife. This phase of life isn't just about reaching immediately for retirement anymore. It's about designing the life you want to live and embracing the freedom and the flexibility of your prime time years.

The only way you can do that is by understanding how much life you've got ahead, what you'd like to be doing, what you can afford to be doing, and how to make more active choices. Life is probably going to go through several phases, each with different driving forces, and you need to be in the driver's seat as this happens, conscious of the money you have and the choices it gives you.

Here's the reality: if you want to keep working, but less than you have been, and only on things that you're passionate about, then you'll have to learn the other three lessons that become important in midlife:

1. Planning for a longer life with phases
2. Layering your income streams
3. Purposefully allocating your spending.

When you approach your finances with these new midlife lessons, you're not just managing money. You're making active choices about what's important. Let's dive in and make these lessons work for you.

1. PLAN FOR A LONGER LIFE

One of the most important things to think about when planning your finances in midlife is just how long you're likely to live – and it's probably longer than you think. Over the last 50 years, we've added an extra 15–25 years to our life expectancies, and today's 50-year-olds who make it to 65 can expect to live well into their 90s. For men, the median life expectancy is 89, for women it's 91, and for couples, there's a strong chance one of you will make it to 95 or beyond. And people with above-average health and wealth should expect to live longer than the medians.

Here's a snapshot of the adjusted life expectancies for a 50-year-old in Australia today, considering health advancements and lifestyle factors.[19] This approach gives a realistic guide to longevity, helping to plan for the right mix of finances, health care and lifestyle choices as you age.

	25th percentile	50th percentile	75th percentile	90th percentile
Male	85	89	95	98
Female	87	91	97	100
Couple	92	95	98	101

Note: These figures are for people who are aged 50 in the middle of 2025, assuming they live past 65. Based on the 2020–22 Australian Life Tables with 25-year improvement rates are rounded up.[20]

ABOUT LIFE EXPECTANCY PERCENTILES

Life expectancy percentiles show how long you or your partner are likely to live compared to others. These estimates help with planning your retirement savings and ensuring they last as long as you do. Here's what the percentiles mean:

- **25th percentile:** At this level, there's a 75 per cent chance you'll live longer than the stated age, and a 25 per cent chance you won't. This is the 'conservative estimate'.
- **50th percentile (median):** This is the midpoint of the life expectancy as it stands today, where half of people live beyond this age, and half don't.
- **75th percentile:** At this level, 25 per cent of people should expect to live longer than the stated age. This is a 'longer-than-average' estimate.
- **90th percentile:** Only 10 per cent of people are projected to live beyond this age. It's the 'super long life' estimate.

So why does this matter for your midlife planning? Because it's not just a number – it's a huge chunk of extra time that you'll need to plan for. You'll be living longer, healthier, more productive years, and that means your vision of life has to change. And your money needs to last you longer, too. Instead of winding down financially in your 70s like the generations before us, you could be planning for a Prime Time and an Epic Retirement that stretches 30–45 years or more, depending on when you kick off your Prime Time. That's a lot more time in which you'll need to cover your living expenses, lifestyle goals and eventual healthcare needs.

The great news is that you can expect to spend most of those extra years in good health. On average, Australians today spend about 88 per cent of their lives in good health, so those extra years aren't just tacked onto the end – they're why we have a Prime Time today. But as you get into the last 7–10 years of life, those health care costs will start to creep up, and it's vital to factor those in when you're working out how to manage your superannuation, investments and income streams.

Planning for a longer life is about adjusting your expectations. It's about making sure your financial resources can support you, not just for the next 10–15 years, but for 30–40 years – through all the phases of life ahead. Part of this planning involves shaping your assets, income and spending, and you should also be rethinking how long you want to work and the role work will play in your life in the decades to come.

I want you to embrace your Prime Time with confidence, knowing you won't have to fear running out of money. With a solid plan, you can gradually shift from full-time work into a lifestyle with the balance, fun and fulfilment you're looking for, maybe even keeping work in the mix if that suits you.

CONSIDER THE NEW PHASES OF LIFE

It's really important to consider all the phases of life that lie ahead. We talked about them earlier, but now you need to use them to map out your spending and your income, and prepare to put your planning into action.

Remember that you have the power to choose which of these early phases are important to you and when you want to embrace them in your life. But the later phases of passive retirement and frailty will probably not be periods you get to choose the timing of.

Set-up years

This is the phase that occurs before you make lifestyle your main focus, and it's a critical time for getting your finances in solid shape. Here, you're working to pay off your mortgage and any other outstanding debts, and hit savings targets both inside and outside superannuation. It's also the time to assess your asset allocation: if too much of your wealth is tied up in your home, you might consider reallocating some of it to assets that can later generate passive income streams.

The goal is to build both your income streams and your financial confidence, so you're ready to transition smoothly into a lifestyle that offers more balance and flexibility. In this set-up phase, you might be building a pool of assets to support part-time work leading up to retirement, while also strengthening your super for later years. It's the perfect time to think about reshaping your work, aligning it with the life you want to live in the years ahead.

Lifestyling years

This is the phase where you finally get to start choosing *you*. For many, real lifestyle flexibility begins when the mortgage is paid off and the big costs of raising a family start to wind down. With those expenses lifting, you'll likely find extra funds sliding back into your pocket – funds that can now support the lifestyle you want, whether that's travel, hobbies, new projects, or simply enjoying a bit more freedom. This phase is all about putting yourself first, using that freed-up cash flow in a sensible way to start living the life you've worked so hard to create.

You may still be working and building up your superannuation and investments, but during these years you may opt to do more 'lifestyling'. For some this is the time for a long sabbatical, while for others it's an opportunity to take time out to study something new. Or you may want to simply take some trips or short breaks that can fit in comfortably around your work, which is probably still full-time. And you'll be able to spend more time on hobbies and other things you're passionate about.

Part-timing phase

This is a growing phase before full retirement that can go on for years. It sees you enjoying some real work–life balance – working a few days per week, and spending your non-working time digging into the lifestyle and the leisure that a modern Prime Time brings. I hope by this point that you're doing work you're passionate about, and that it forms just one part of your life.

Your work income may or may not be enough to cover your chosen lifestyle during this phase, so you may have to draw an income from investments. If you're under 60, that will need to come from investments held outside superannuation. If you're over 60, you've got some choices.

If you don't want to resign or 'retire' but you want a supplementary income stream from your super, you might consider drawing a transition to retirement pension. If you meet the conditions of release (turning 60 and ceasing your employment), you can move your super into the retirement phase, making it tax-free, and start enjoying the drawdowns. And remember, you still have the freedom to take up a part-time or casual role, or even to later return to full-time work if you choose. Or you can keep on working, knowing that once you turn 65, you can put your superannuation into the retirement phase and enjoy tax-free earnings unconditionally.

The key to this phase is mixing things the right way for you – enjoying your work and enjoying your lifestyle.

Epic Retirement

Once you meet the conditions of release for superannuation and fully retire from work, you enter what I hope will be your Epic Retirement. This is an exciting time. It's a time when you don't have to work but you can still choose to do work-like activities: volunteering, various pursuits and providing care are common parts of people's days. It's my hope that you make it to this stage in good health, ready to chase your retirement dreams using the time that opens up. During this phase, most people find their income comes from a combination of superannuation, investments, annuities and the age pension, if they're eligible. Investment priorities during this phase are usually chiefly within superannuation, where you can for the first time generate income and growth tax-free, and draw down funds without restrictions.

Investments in active retirement can be done more cautiously by some, or at least put into risk buckets with a change in focus to income generation. You want your money to last and to allow you to live a comfortable, even more exciting existence.

After you leave your Prime Time, there are still two more stages of life to be accommodated financially and functionally. You need to keep that in mind as you plan for the whole second half of your life.

Passive retirement, or our ageing years

This phase typically extends across the last 7–10 years of our lives, according to actuaries. It is often marred by health issues, or dominated by a need or want to be closer to home, family and health care. Your lifestyle spending normally drops a little as you spend less time heading overseas on grand adventures, but at the same time, your need for health care, home help and other services rises, and you need to be prepared for that. Academics point out that in our 70s and 80s, our financial cognition can slip a little, so it's important to be financially prepared before you reach this phase, even if this is something many people don't like to hear. Depending on your risk profile and financial literacy, your priorities can shift to more balanced or even conservative investments in this phase. And we see many people today unwinding complex financial structures for ease of management in their later years. It really is a personal choice as to how tricky you want things to be during these years.

Frailty

This refers to the last years of your life, when care needs often spike and your ability to look after yourself gradually dissipates. It can be a frightening time, and for most people, it's when their financial literacy falters. Women, who are on average expected to live longer than men, often face these years alone, making it even harder for them. So it makes good sense to be prepared. In Australia, 2025 has brought rather significant changes to the aged care and home care systems, increasing the costs of care, but also providing more certainty to the sector for the years ahead. As a result, more of our care services have turned towards being user-pays. However, beyond these services, and the ongoing costs of housing, food and incremental and likely local leisure, there is little to spend on during our frail years. So investing in this phase is passive and usually maintained in a fund or portfolio that can be managed by your powers of attorney.

2. LAYER YOUR INCOME STREAMS

As you move through the next stages of life, it's almost certain that your sources of income will shift. In your earlier years, most of your income probably came from a regular pay cheque. Sure, you might have had a side hustle or some investments ticking along, but for most people in this stage of life, the bulk of their income is still actively earned from work.

But as you transition from your full-time career into your Prime Time's various stages, and eventually into retirement, there's a noticeable shift from active income, earned through work, to passive income, generated from investments, super, annuities or other sources.

The good news? You've got a lot of choice in how to make this transition work for you. First, you need to be clear on:
- The financial goals you want to hit
- The work–life balance you're aiming for
- Where your passive income will come from.

Then it's about sitting down and making sure you understand those income sources, and that the investments you plan to rely on are securely in place, so you can move through the next phases with confidence. This shift happens at different times for different people. For some, they might start to leverage alternative layers of income in the tail end of their set-up phase, while others won't start drawing on passive income until their lifestyling phase, or they wait until their part-time retirement. Whenever it happens, knowing how to manage this transition from active income sources (like wages) to passive income sources (from investments and super) is key to maintaining your financial stability and peace of mind in retirement.

Let's learn more about it.

BUILDING LAYERS OF INCOME

In your Prime Time, you'll need to think of your income sources as layers that together create a stable financial foundation, rather than looking at a single pay cheque. Each layer serves a unique purpose and contributes to your overall income. The idea is to gradually add and strengthen these layers over time, so that when one layer – such as your salary or wage income – begins to decrease, others are there to support you. There are a few different types of layers to learn about.

Work or active income

This is your salary or wages from employment or working. Many people transition to part-time work or freelance roles during their Prime Time, allowing for greater flexibility while still earning an active income. The layers we commonly see are:
- Full-time work
- Part-time or casual work
- Gig work
- Small business income
- Consulting, directorships and advisory income
- Side hustles
- Entrepreneurial projects and ventures.

I want you to think about doing work you enjoy as you move through your Prime Time, both for the financial benefits and for the fulfilment it brings you.

Passive income outside superannuation

Most people build up assets outside super that can provide them with a source of passive income until they can access their super. The goal is usually to maintain the capital and drive predictable income from

it. These types of investments can provide a steady stream of income with less active involvement, offering financial flexibility as you begin to shift your focus from full-time work – particularly if you plan to step your work back before you access your superannuation. The types of passive income you'll commonly hold include many of those we covered in our investment lesson:
- Financial investments: equities, ETFs, bonds, LICs and managed funds
- Cash accounts: term deposits and high-interest savings accounts
- Rental properties: houses, apartments and commercial property
- Business income: earnings from a business where you've moved into a more passive role
- Other investments.

Superannuation income

For Australians, superannuation becomes a critical income source once we meet the conditions of release for technical retirement. Understanding how to manage and draw from your super effectively can make a big difference. Most people draw their money in one of four ways:
- TTR income stream
- Account-based pension
- Lifetime income stream/lifetime annuity
- Lump sum drawdowns.

Age pension

Then there's the age pension. It can be a valuable income stream that supports you in your later life – a guaranteed layer you can rely on. So take your time to understand your eligibility for the age pension, and how much of your cost of living it is likely to provide, well ahead of time. For some, access to the government age pension clicks in as soon as they cross eligibility at 67, while others have to burn through some of their assets or wait until their income declines to qualify.

Either way, it's great to know it's there and to know at what point you might trigger your access to it.

Concessions

If you become eligible for an age pension, you might find there are other government benefits or entitlements you can tap into alongside it. Australian pensioners get access to the Pensioner Concession Card, which includes some great cost-of-living reductions and healthcare concessions, including reductions to rates, car registration costs and electricity supplements, and a cap on the cost of prescriptions and doctor visits.

In Australia, there's a second, more accessible concession card for those who don't qualify for the age pension, but who meet certain income criteria, called the Commonwealth Seniors Health Card. The CSHC chiefly offers discounts to medicines and caps on your overall healthcare costs each year.

Savings and emergency funds

It's always wise to have a safety net you can tap into in case of emergency. So I want you to think about maintaining a layer of cash savings or accessible investments that you can use for unexpected expenses or to supplement your income during market downturns. The size of your cash layer really depends on your risk profile and the amounts you already have accessible to you with any other investment strategy (like bucketing), but simply having one can really help you sleep at night and maintain your financial confidence, even when investment markets wobble.

HOW THE LAYERS SHIFT AND GROW THROUGH YOUR PRIME TIME

Now that you've got a feel for each income layer, it's time to think about how they'll work together across the stages of your own life, giving you a reliable, adaptable income – and, most importantly, inspiring you to live your best Prime Time. The aim is to let these layers evolve as you do, shifting to match your changing priorities, goals and visions.

In your set-up phase, almost all your income will be coming from working, and will be used to pay down your mortgage and build up your financial assets. And any money from investments will be compounding to make those investments grow fast.

In your lifestyling phase, you might start to tap into money that was previously flowing into paying down debt, to enhance your lifestyle.

In your part-timing phase, your work income drops, and you might need to start to draw on the income from your financial assets to sustain your lifestyle.

Then, in your true Epic Retirement, everything you earn comes from passive income sources.

The journey is different for everyone! So you need to decide how it will work for you given your unique financial situation.

Think of it as creating a rough plan for your income layers rather than locking in exact figures. Start with estimates for how you'd like your income sources to look over time. You'll adjust and refine this as life unfolds, but having a flexible outline helps guide your financial decisions now and later.

Here's a table to help you sketch your ideas.

	PHASE 1	PHASE 2	PHASE 3	PHASE 4
	SET-UP	LIFESTYLE	PART-TIME	EPIC RETIREMENT
Active earnings income layer				
Employment				
Consulting/directorships				
Side hustles				
Entrepreneurial projects				
Investment income layer				
Rental income				
Dividends from financial investments				
Cash investment income (bank accounts etc.)				
Superannuation layer				
Account-based pension				
Lifetime income stream				
Lump sum drawdowns				

	PHASE 1	PHASE 2	PHASE 3	PHASE 4
	SET-UP	LIFESTYLE	PART-TIME	EPIC RETIREMENT
Age pension layer				
Concessions layer				
Savings and emergency funds layer				
TOTAL PROJECTED INCOME BY PHASE				

3. PURPOSEFULLY ALLOCATING YOUR SPENDING

As we step into our prime time years and eventually into retirement, our spending habits naturally shift, and this becomes another 'choose-your-own-adventure' moment. It's essential to understand and adapt to these changes.

The goal isn't to lead a penny-pinching life during your Prime Time or Epic Retirement. Instead, it's about embracing a fresh perspective on spending – one that reflects the unique opportunity of being part of a generation that's had superannuation for most of their working lives, and doesn't want to copy the generation before them. It's time to build an understanding of your spending choices and give you the confidence to spend wisely and make your money work for every stage of the life you want to live.

To do that we need to look back before we look forward and plan. Traditional retirement theories, like those rooted in Franco Modigliani's Life-Cycle Hypothesis from the 1950s, suggested that spending naturally declines as we age.[21] This made sense for older generations who, without the benefit of superannuation, often had to rely heavily on the age pension, leading to more and more frugal spending habits in later life. Modigliani's theory suggested that people would save during their working years and then gradually spend those savings in early retirement, with spending tapering off as their needs shifted primarily to basic necessities.

But today's gen X and baby boomers, who've now had superannuation for more than three decades, have been rewriting the rules. With more robust superannuation balances than ever, and longer life expectancies, people have developed a greater focus on maintaining a fulfilling lifestyle throughout their retirement.

Instead of their spending tapering off early in retirement, many are choosing to front-load their spending during the early years of retirement – taking big trips, pursuing hobbies, and enjoying the fruits of their labour. And then, the good news is that so far, many are maintaining that lifestyle-driven spending well into their 70s – they might even hold it into their early 80s – we'll have to watch and see. The focus has shifted from mere subsistence in later life to enjoying our Prime Time and our Epic Retirement to its fullest, and that's reshaping the traditional lifecycle of saving and spending. And each generation is likely to spend more than the one that came before it, as quality of life and expectations of the good things improves further over time.

We don't know exactly how it's going to play out yet, but what we do know is that people with more financial security (the superannuation generation) are shifting the narrative on retirement spending. Modern retirees who are financially secure are saying they aren't keen to downshift their spending drastically as they get older. They're interested in maintaining a consistent, enjoyable lifestyle well into their later years. And then, once their health declines, they expect their in-home services and home care expenses to be more heavily user-pays than previous generations, and we're seeing newly implemented aged care legislation support that, so the spending probably won't fall.

If you agree with this, then we need to talk about how we budget for the phases of life ahead of us, and challenge the old theories of retirement spending declines for today's Prime Timer. Then, just like we did with our income streams, we need to work through how our own budget might change and adapt through the various stages of our Prime Time and Epic Retirement. Most importantly, I want you to understand more clearly than ever how you can enjoy the money you've saved over all the good years ahead.

Whether your Prime Time starts when you're 48, 50 or 55 (depending on when your kids start to take on more financial independence), you will find there's a period of cash-flow relief in your life that you may not have enjoyed for decades. And when you feel that, I want you to get serious about reconsidering how your money will work – for the rest of your life.

I think this is the window for significant change to your budget, allowing you to capture the extra dollars that start to appear and pour them into your phased approach to your Prime Time and, later, to your Epic Retirement.

RESETTING YOUR BUDGET AS YOU ENTER YOUR PRIME TIME

The best time to revisit your budget is when your cash flow starts freeing up, such as when your kids become more independent. If you've been covering school fees or activities, take note of that money flowing back into your pocket. Finished paying off the mortgage? Capture those freed-up funds. Downsized your home? Enjoy the savings on power, utilities and rates. Rather than letting this extra cash slip into impulse spending, put it to work shaping the life you truly want.

Now's the time to think through your spending, savings and goals. Set up a framework that aligns with the lifestyle you envision for your prime time years, aiming for financial flexibility that lets you start designing that lifestyle sooner. With a solid budget in place, you'll be in a stronger position to gradually reduce the work you don't enjoy, take on meaningful projects, or enjoy more lifestyle options without financial strain.

This approach also makes your transition through the next phases – whether it's lifestyling, moving to part-time work, or easing into an Epic Retirement – far smoother. The goal? To let your mix of fulfilling work, compounding investments and passive income support a lifestyle that's sustainable, and to let it adapt.

When your finances are set to work in the background, you can focus on the experiences, interests and connections that matter most, knowing you're well prepared for whatever's next.

BUDGETING FOR YOUR PRIME TIME CHALLENGES

Right-sizing your cost-of-living budget in your 50s as your set-up phase begins, and harnessing the savings/surplus in your budget throughout your Prime Time and retirement, does challenge the old, conventional retirement budgeting theories often espoused by the industry. These theories have traditionally suggested that you should rewrite your cost-of-living budget as you retire and expect to cut your costs to 80 per cent of your pre-retirement cost of living.

I think we should want to make these smart 20 per cent cost-of-living changes earlier, knowing that these savings are better deployed toward paying off the mortgage sooner, building up our superannuation earlier, saving for some lifestyle and pre-retirement years, and really enjoying the best years of our lives. Your capacity to save early will be key to the quality of the Prime Time you get to enjoy – really.

When you recalibrate your budget for Prime Time, it's my view that you should trim your spending, build your savings up in the set-up phase, and then redeploy some of these funds toward your lifestyle as you hit your goals. And you don't then expect to cut your budget again when you retire. Instead, you budget to a level that will allow you to live a lifestyle you can accommodate, and you plan to carry that average cost of living right through the active and possibly even the passive phases of life ahead, knowing the line items might change on your budget but the topline amounts spent probably won't. And there will be a line of savings that you create when you budget, which initially is used to pay down debt and save for the future, that can later become discretionary spending if you can afford it, so you enjoy your life every step of the way.

BUDGETING FOR THE PHASES OF PRIME TIME

We've talked ad nauseam about how the phases of our Prime Time can come together. But now we need to explore how our cost-of-living and lifestyle budget shifts during each phase, to put things into perspective.

1. Set-up phase (could be anywhere from late 40s to early 60s)

In the set-up phase, you're likely at the peak of your earning power. This is your moment to double down on saving and investing, capturing every bit of surplus income into debt repayments and investing. For many, paying off the mortgage is within reach. After that's done, any funds freed up should be channelled into building a strong income-producing asset base, within superannuation and outside it, to support both your Prime Time and Epic Retirement.

Aim to capture any boost in cash flow, whether it's through lower household costs as the kids become more independent, or paying down the mortgage – and allocate it with purpose.

If your kids have left home, downsizing may be another opportunity to reduce costs and free up capital for lifestyle investments outside super, but not before you're 55 if you want to access the downsizer concession.

2. Lifestyling (mid 50s to mid–late 60s)

As you enter the lifestyling phase, you're likely free of major expenses like mortgage payments and education costs. With those hefty financial goals achieved, take a bigger look at the line item in your budget that was dedicated to savings in your set-up years, and the other line item dedicated to paying your mortgage, and consider spending more on what truly brings you happiness. These are your lifestyle years after all.

For many gen Xers and late boomers, this phase is all about balance. You might have a healthy-ish super balance but aren't ready to retire or even step back just yet. You're in this unique sweet spot – still working, but with more flexibility and hunger to shape your life outside of work.

This is what makes lifestyling so special: it's your chance to blend your career with more of what you love, whether that's reshaping your work to better fit your values, travelling more, engaging in other pursuits, or simply having more time for yourself.

3. Part-timing (mid–late 50s to mid 70s)

Stepping into the part-time phase can be an exciting shift. For those who enjoy their work, easing off can make it sustainable for years. For others, part-timing is a way to gradually reshape their view of work and transition smoothly into retirement without the shock of suddenly stopping.

As you step back, the focus naturally shifts to lifestyle choices. Many people take on part-time roles, consulting, or a side hustle that aligns more with their passions. But you'll also notice the cost of enjoying life tends to rise in this phase – travel, hobbies and family time can all add up. Balancing this with your income is key.

The approach depends on your age, financial set-up and goals. For some, work might cover essential costs; for others, it funds extras like travel and leisure, or just provides added meaning. However you shape it, part-timing offers the flexibility to enjoy life on your terms while keeping finances in check.

Under 60: planning for the transition years

If you're under 60 and thinking about cutting back on work, it's important to plan ahead and be realistic about what you can afford. Since you won't be able to access your super just yet, you'll need to rely on savings, investments or other income sources to fund this period if your part-time wage doesn't cover your expenses. So careful budgeting is key here. You want to make sure you've got enough to cover your everyday living costs, lifestyle goals and any one-off expenses, like that long-awaited holiday. With a solid plan, you can enter this phase feeling confident and excited, knowing your finances are set up to support the life you want to lead – without the stress. And let's face it, you can always do more work if things don't go to plan.

Over 60: leveraging superannuation

Once you hit 60, more doors open to your long-saved income streams. And that might give you more confidence to spend.

You can take advantage of a TTR strategy, allowing you to draw from your super while still working part-time, without fully retiring. Or, if you're ready, you can move into the retirement phase of superannuation and access your super tax-free, turning it into an account-based pension and drawing on lump sums, which could give you more flexibility and a larger income line in your budget. If you're between 60 and 65, you'll have to meet the conditions of release by ceasing work; or you can wait until you're 65 and access your super unconditionally. Either way, this is your chance to really shape your part-timing budget by understanding your ideal cost-of-living and lifestyle choices.

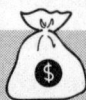

GETTING COMFORTABLE WITH SPENDING IN RETIREMENT

As we get older, our emotional relationship with money tends to evolve. Studies in behavioural economics show that many retirees hold onto their savings tightly, driven by a fear of outliving their money – despite often having more than enough. This fear, along with the uncertainty around how long retirement will last, can lead to overly cautious spending. But research also suggests that clearly understanding your financial situation and setting a plan aligned with your changing needs can help ease those worries.[22] Good financial literacy, regular financial check-ins with your super fund, and getting financial advice that's suitable for your situation can boost your confidence, allowing you to enjoy the money you've worked so hard for without the constant fear of running out.

4. Entering Epic Retirement

As you enter full and active retirement – what I like to call Epic Retirement – the focus shifts to fully enjoying life without work, ideally without scaling back your lifestyle. This phase is all about maintaining a comfortable level of spending, thanks to a healthier and more financially secure outlook than previous generations.

Today's retirees aren't typically slowing down as quickly. Instead, many are healthier and more active, wanting to keep their spending and lifestyle up well into their 70s and beyond. Their budget has also shifted: no more saving for retirement or paying down debt; now, those funds go straight into experiences.

Your Epic Retirement is about embracing this stage with energy, enjoying every aspect of the life you've built and sustaining it for as long as possible.

5. Passive retirement/ageing (late 70s or early 80s and beyond)

In the later stages of retirement, lifestyle spending tends to naturally decline. By this point, you may feel less inclined to travel or take part in high-cost activities, and your focus might shift more toward things closer to home, such as maintaining your comforts and staying on top of health care. It's a gradual change, one that's expected as you slow down a bit, but it doesn't mean your lifestyle has to take a hit. You'll still be able to enjoy comfort, just with a few tweaks to where your money is going.

It's important to anticipate rising costs in health care and home maintenance. In fact, many people find that even though their discretionary spending decreases, the amount they spend on health and maintaining their home tends to grow. That's why it's important to keep an eye on your budget and make sure it adapts to these shifting priorities, helping you stay secure and comfortable, even as things change.

6. Frailty

As passive retirement progresses, most people experience a phase known as 'frailty', where health and physical abilities begin to decline more significantly. This stage typically occurs in the later years of retirement and sees a sharper change in the things you spend money on. You still have to keep a roof over your head, and the electricity on, but there's little to no travel to speak of in this phase.

Frailty often comes with increased health challenges, such as chronic illness or reduced mobility, which can lead to higher medical and care-related costs. You'll likely face more frequent medical treatments, medication expenses, and possibly the need for home modifications to accommodate changing needs. Home-help services or in-home care may also become necessary, and while the government has pledged to make these services more user-pays, particularly for those who aren't financially disadvantaged, they should remain affordable as your other living expenses decline. Importantly, the government has also committed to covering care costs, ensuring access to the necessary support regardless of wealth.

> **CHOOSING YOUR OWN ADVENTURE IN YOUR PRIME TIME**
>
> Not everyone will be able to – or want to – experience every stage of their Prime Time. For some, the financial reality may mean they can't afford to stop working until they're eligible for the age pension. For others, it's a choice – they simply don't want to give up work. The great thing about your Prime Time is that your need to meet social expectations fades. You're past all that. Now it's about choosing your own adventure, picking the phases you want to enjoy, and planning for them. Just make sure to always live within your means, and focus on making the most of what you have.

HOW DO YOU ENJOY YOUR PRIME TIME IF YOU DON'T HAVE A LOT OF MONEY?

Enjoying your Prime Time doesn't have to be all about having a lot of money. It's about planning for the future, making the most of what you have today and finding fulfilment in the things that truly matter to you. It's also about not waiting for retirement to have that plan, instead putting the actions in place and starting to build up your lifestyle elements alongside your financial confidence, earlier in life.

Think about it. Even if money's tight, you can still try to capture the savings as your kids become more independent and eventually leave home. You can still try to pay down a mortgage before you plan to step back from your full-time work to part-time. And you can still try to contribute more to superannuation, allowing it to compound for your future. Some people, those in more challenging financial situations, might not be able to go part-time until an income layer from the age pension becomes available – that's actually part of the lessons on layering that I want you to learn. But at least you know *when* you can, and you *can make choices* about how to live your life to its fullest.

Here are a few ways to embrace your Prime Time even if your financial resources are limited:

1. Prioritise the set-up phase

Even if it feels scary, I want you to embrace your set-up phase and learn about your money. Put in place the financial foundations: your budget, your super contributions and investment settings, and your best tax-minimising strategies. Understand how your spending and income can afford to shift over the years ahead and build a view of what your prime time years could look like. Even if they are more frugal years than others, having confidence in what you *can* do and where you're headed is key. Every situation can be improved with smart strategic effort.

2. Learn about the pension early on

The age pension might not be available until you're 67, but it is available. In fact, it's an amazing layer of income for those who need it, and learning about it can bring you a sense of calm as you plan for your Prime Time and Epic Retirement. Dig in and understand it, even if it feels complex.

3. Embrace experiences, not things

The best memories aren't tied to price tags. They come from moments shared with the people you love and the experiences you have. Instead of focusing on buying things, focus on experiences. Whether it's having a BBQ with friends, enjoying a scenic walk, or visiting a free event in your local area, these experiences will bring you more joy than material possessions ever could.

4. Find joy in the little things
Sometimes the greatest happiness comes from the simplest pleasures. A cup of coffee on your porch, a good book, or a morning walk in nature can give you a sense of meaning. Slow down and truly appreciate these experiences. Live in the moment a little more and allow yourself more joy in your life.

5. Get involved in your community
Communities are full of opportunities to connect, share and grow – all without spending much. Whether it's joining a local club, taking part in free or low-cost community events, or volunteering for a cause that matters to you, being part of a community can bring a deep sense of fulfilment and purpose. And many communities have options that can be pursued while you keep working. Truly!

6. Travel doesn't have to be expensive
If you love the idea of travel, remember that you don't need a big budget to explore. You can plan local trips, discover hidden gems close to home, or even consider house-swapping or budget-friendly options like camping. It's about the adventure, not the price tag.

7. Rediscover old hobbies or pick up new pursuits
Now's the time to dive into hobbies and pursuits that you love or explore new interests you've always wanted to try. Whether it's gardening, painting, learning to cook new recipes, or even getting crafty, these activities don't have to cost much, but they can bring you immense joy and satisfaction.

8. Prioritise your health and wellbeing
Good health is priceless, and staying active doesn't require an expensive gym membership. Take walks in the park, do yoga at home,

or find a fitness buddy to keep you motivated. Prioritising your mental and physical health will help you enjoy this phase to the fullest.

9. Make the most of what you have

Even if money is tight, there are often ways to maximise your resources. Look into any government support or discounts you might be eligible for, like the age pension or concessions. And consider simplifying your expenses, such as downsizing or cutting back on non-essentials, to free up more for the things that truly bring you joy.

10. Get creative and think outside the box

Living on a budget can spark creativity. Whether it's cooking up affordable, delicious meals, taking picnics, swapping skills with friends, or finding creative ways to repurpose things around the house, you'll find that being resourceful can be surprisingly fun and rewarding.

Ultimately, your Prime Time isn't about how much money you have but about how rich your life feels.

Lesson 7
Review your big financial picture and your budget

NOW THAT YOU UNDERSTAND ALL THE FINANCIAL FOUNDATIONS, AND YOU'VE learned the main lessons of your Prime Time too, it's time to make an action plan. There will be debts you need to demolish, decisions you need to make about your assets, and actions you need to take to get you in the best situation possible.

I want you to get out the big financial picture you created at the beginning of the book and ask yourself these six questions.

1. WHAT ARE THE DEBTS I NEED TO DEMOLISH?
It's important to look at any debts you're carrying and assess their impact on your long-term goals. Prioritise non-deductible debt like credit cards, personal loans and your home mortgage first, as these don't offer tax benefits and can weigh down your financial freedom. Clearing these debts helps free up cash flow, letting you use those funds for lifestyle or investment goals as you move into your Prime Time.

2. WILL I EVER BE ELIGIBLE FOR THE AGE PENSION?
This is an essential question. Remember, your primary home is exempt from the age pension assets test. Any choices you make around reallocating equity from your home to income-generating assets could affect your future eligibility.

3. ARE MY INCOME-GENERATING ASSETS OPTIMISED?

Take a close look at how your assets perform. Are they diversified, providing steady income, and well positioned for long-term growth? Small adjustments now could yield better security and returns down the road.

4. IS MY HOME THE RIGHT SIZE FOR THE YEARS AHEAD?

Think about whether your home matches the lifestyle you envision. Consider the portion of your total wealth tied up in your home compared to what's actively generating income. It's about finding the right balance and fit.

5. DO I HAVE ENOUGH ACCESSIBLE FUNDS OUTSIDE OF SUPER?

Given that access to super is restricted until retirement age, ensure you have sufficient liquid assets outside of super. This supports lifestyle choices, unexpected expenses, or a gradual transition into part-time work if that's in your plan.

6. IS MY SUPER INVESTED APPROPRIATELY?

Look at the structure and performance of your super investments. Are they aligned with your risk tolerance and timeline? Adjusting your investment approach within super could drive your compounding harder, sooner.

Activity: BUILD YOUR FUTURE BUDGET

Next, I want you to build a future-focused budget. This is the tool that brings together your income and your expenses, so you can see them in one place.

You'll use the analysis of your budget you did when you created your current big financial picture, though this time I want you to get forward-looking. But before diving into the numbers, it's important to think about some of the ultimate goals of budgeting. Budgeting is about giving you confidence in your income and your expenses. It should give you power, because you know exactly where your money is coming from and going each month, and it allows you to be more purposeful about how that money is deployed. And it should allow you to set goals for your money, because you know what's going on.

Budgeting for the future, then managing your budget, can sound painful, but it's about becoming more aware of your money and how it really works in this next phase, which you can now see is different to the last phase.

There are three key parts to shaping your prime time budget. Each needs to be thought through and understood:

1. **Build your cost-of-living and lifestyle budget:** This is the baseline – the amount of money you want to cover your essential expenses and your discretionary lifestyle, travel and leisure activities through the different phases of your life.
2. **Set out your one-off expenditure budget:** You'll need to account for larger, irregular expenses like home maintenance, buying a new car, or accessing care as you age. These are the big-ticket items that pop up occasionally but need to be planned for.
3. **Plan for lifestyle lump sums and epic experiences:** Finally, this is where you map out the larger lifestyle goals, things like taking a sabbatical, buying a caravan, or celebrating big life events. These are the significant one-off sums you'll want to have available at different phases of your Prime Time.

With these three components in place, you'll have a well-rounded budget that not only covers your everyday needs but also allows room for the experiences and milestones that make life rewarding.

STEP 1: BUILD YOUR FUTURE COST-OF-LIVING AND LIFESTYLE BUDGET

Your goal here is to map out how your *current* spending differs from *what you plan to spend in the future* – category by category. Some expenses might increase, while others may decrease. For example, will you spend less on work-related expenses like commuting, or adjust your food and entertainment budgets when you're not eating lunch at work? Will you increase the amount you budget for travel every year? Your future budget should give you a clear picture of how much money you'll need each year to meet your cost-of-living and chosen lifestyle needs.

As you review it, remember that in the next stages of life, it's not just about getting by but enjoying the things that matter to you. Identify your non-negotiables (like housing, utilities or health care) and priorities (like fitness, travel or family time). This budget should reflect both what you need to live and what you want to spend on to enjoy your life. For example, if staying fit is essential, budget for gym memberships, nutrition and training. If visiting your children or grandkids is a priority, factor in the cost of those trips. Make sure your future budget aligns with these lifestyle goals.

Once you've adjusted each spending category, you'll arrive at an annual amount – the amount you'll want access to each year to meet both your needs and your core lifestyle goals. This number will act as a cornerstone for all your financial planning moving forward.

As you move through the rest of your life, your cost-of-living and lifestyle budget shouldn't change much. The only time it might change is if you significantly downscale your home or expenses somehow (or for some reason upscale them). So we'll use the same cost-of-living budget through every phase in your budget.

FUTURE BUDGET TEMPLATE

The prime time future budgeting template is on your big financial picture spreadsheet. Download it from becwilson.net/primetime_resources

	Current spending	Future budgeted amount (in today's dollars)	Difference (make some notes to remind you)
Housing expenses (household utilities)			
Fresh food			
Household goods and services (utilities, cleaning, gardening, internet, phones)			
Clothing and footwear			

	Current spending	Future budgeted amount (in today's dollars)	Difference (make some notes to remind you)
Car, public transport and other transport costs			
Personal health			
Entertainment and leisure			
Insurances			
Work-related expenses			
Family and friends			
Travel and experiences			
Credit card payments			
Long-term savings			
Total			

YOUR ANNUAL BUDGET SHOULD INCORPORATE DISCRETIONARY SPENDING

Build into your budget the joys and pleasures that go beyond your basic living expenses. It's the money set aside for lifestyle choices, leisure activities and experiences that make life fulfilling, whether that's dining out, pursuing hobbies, enjoying entertainment, or indulging in annual travel adventures.

Building your discretionary budget

Think about your annual travel costs: Whether it's a yearly trip to visit family or an overseas adventure, travel is often a major part of living well. Plan for regular getaways and travel goals, factoring in flights, accommodation and spending money. If travel is a priority, make sure it's a core part of your discretionary budget.

Map out your pleasures: Think about the experiences that bring you joy – dining out with friends, catching a show, or indulging in a spa day. Decide how often you want to enjoy these and allocate your budget accordingly.

Factor in hobbies: Hobbies often provide a sense of purpose and joy. Whether it's a golf membership, art supplies or weekend hiking and camping trips, make sure your budget supports these passions.

Plan for spontaneity: It's essential to leave some flexibility for the unexpected, such as a last-minute holiday or spontaneous outing. Building a buffer for these moments allows you to say yes to exciting opportunities without financial stress.

Balance enjoyment with sustainability: The key is to balance today's pleasures with tomorrow's needs. Ensure your discretionary spending aligns with your long-term goals, so you can continue enjoying life without worrying about overspending or running out of funds.

Category	Notes or details
Annual travel	Flights, accommodation, spending money for trips (domestic/international)
Dining out and entertainment	Restaurants, movies, concerts, theatre
Hobbies and leisure activities	Golf membership, art supplies, gardening, sporting equipment
Health and wellness	Gym membership, personal training, wellness retreats, spa treatments
Weekend getaways/short breaks	Occasional trips within driving distance
Spontaneous spending	Buffer for last-minute plans, extra treats or surprises
Gifts and celebrations	Birthdays, holidays, family celebrations, special occasions
Miscellaneous fun	Any other unplanned discretionary spending

STEP 2: SET OUT YOUR ONE-OFF EXPENDITURE BUDGET

Throughout life, there are bigger, irregular expenses that come up when you least expect them. These aren't the everyday costs – they're the big-ticket items like home maintenance, replacing your car, a scheduled surgery with costs not covered by private health insurance, or accessing care as you age. They don't happen every year, but when they do, they can take a big bite out of your finances if you're not ready for them.

That's where your one-off expenditure budget comes in. It's about being smart and planning ahead so you're not caught off guard when these expenses arise.

Here's what you need to plan for:

Home maintenance and upgrades
Your home is going to need some work over the years, whether it's a roof repair, updating the heating system or general maintenance. While these jobs might not come up every year, they're still significant when they do. Plan for both the routine fixes and those unexpected repairs so you've got a safety net in place.

Car replacement
Your car won't last forever, and whether it's time for a new one or an upgrade, you'll need to have the funds ready. Think about how long your current car will last and when you'll need to make that switch. You might have a couple of upgrade cycles in your life ahead to factor for.

Health, home care and aged care services
As you grow older, one-off, unforeseen health expenses can add up, whether it's getting a cochlear implant, dental implants, or a knee replacement and modifying your home to suit how you want to age or paying for care in the home. Planning ahead for these expenses is pretty important. It's not fun to think about, but having a buffer for unexpected health and care needs will give you peace of mind down the road.

Here's how to plan for one-off expenses:

Anticipate when they'll hit
Take a good look at your situation. How old is your car? When was your home last renovated? Do you think your home will one day need a lift or a ramp? How much do you want to have in a buffer account for your health and ageing needs? These questions will help you figure out when these bigger expenses are likely to pop up.

Save a little each year
Instead of waiting for these expenses to catch you by surprise, set aside a bit each year for the bigger stuff or allocate it in your capital. That way, when the bill comes in, you've already got it covered.

Keep things flexible

Not all one-off expenses can be perfectly predicted, so it's smart to keep some flexibility in your budget. Having a bit of breathing room means you won't be stressed out when something drops.

Planning for one-off expenses means you're setting yourself up to manage life's bigger, less predictable costs with ease. It's not just about covering the everyday stuff.

Category	Estimated cost	When will this happen?
Home upgrades or maintenance	$45,000	Roof in 2026
Car replacement	$50,000	In 2030 and 2035
Health and home care	$30,000	Amount set aside for an emergency surgery and/or X months of home care and support services
Total	$125,000	

STEP 3: PLAN FOR LIFESTYLE LUMP SUMS AND EPIC EXPERIENCES

Finally, this is the fun part, where you map out the big lifestyle goals you want to tick off during your Prime Time and in your Epic Retirement too. These are the one-off lump sums you'll want available to enjoy some of life's bigger moments, like taking a sabbatical, buying a caravan, or celebrating those major life events with family and friends. They're the significant experiences you've been dreaming of for years, and it's important to plan for them. They deserve a place in your financial plan.

Here's how to think about it:

Map out your goals

Think about the big experiences you want to prioritise over the coming years of your Prime Time and Epic Retirement. Is it travelling abroad for a six-month sabbatical? Taking a few months off to explore Australia in a caravan? Going to live in the UK for the birth of a grandchild? Whatever it is, write it down.

Set a timeline
When do you want to make these dreams happen? Are they part of your pre-retirement lifestyling, or are you saving them for your epic retirement years? Getting a clear idea of the timing will help you budget accordingly.

Allocate lump sums
Estimate the one-off amounts you'll need for these goals. This might be $50,000 for a sabbatical or $40,000 for a new caravan. Whatever the case, build those numbers into your future planning.

Enjoy the journey
These lump sums are about creating memories, ticking off bucket-list items, and enjoying the freedom that Prime Time gives you. Don't hesitate to plan for them and make sure they're achievable within your bigger financial picture. You probably also want to map your epic retirement expenses out, because you'll be envisioning these at the same time.

By planning for these lifestyle lump sums, you're ensuring that the best moments of life don't happen by accident. Instead, they're part of a deliberate plan to live your Prime Time, and one day your Epic Retirement, to the fullest.

Category	Estimated cost	When will this happen?
Sabbatical	$50,000	Targeting 57–58
Caravan purchase	$40,000	Targeting 62
Anniversary celebration	$30,000	50th wedding anniversary: 75
Extended overseas trip to celebrate retirement	$60,000	Targeting 65
Total	$180,000	

You can bring all these together in the prime time budgeting spreadsheet, reflecting how they might work in each phase. My template helps you simplify the process.

Lesson 8
Work out how much is 'enough'

It's time to stop and think about the biggest question of all: 'How much is enough?' Before we dive into the details of working this out, it's important to first explore the five key principles that shape how we approach this question.

1. PLAN IN THE RIGHT ORDER

The first and most important step in understanding how much is enough is knowing the right order to plan in.

The idea of shifting to a more flexible lifestyle or even retiring early can be thrilling, but it requires careful planning to make it work. Now that you understand the phases of your Prime Time and your Epic Retirement and the financial considerations for each, it's time to think about the right order of priorities when building your plan.

This approach is particularly useful for those who want to enjoy their prime time years, transitioning into part-time work or semi-retirement before fully retiring. It might feel counterintuitive, but here's the key: you plan and save for retirement first. Why? Because setting up a strong foundation for your later years allows you to take full advantage of compounding inside the low-tax environment of super. Once that's secured, you can layer on the earlier years and make space for flexibility, freedom, and part-time living.

2. THINK ABOUT YOUR RETIREMENT FIRST

Setting your goals around a Prime Time or early retirement doesn't mean you can skip the basics of long-term retirement planning. If anything, you need to think even more carefully about ensuring your money lasts – especially when you have decades ahead for which you'll need to fund your living and lifestyle ambitions.

Many people who want to retire early get excessively focused on building savings outside of super, but stop and think about it – that would have them neglecting the enormous tax advantages that super offers (and boy oh boy they're good!). Here's why that's a mistake in my opinion.

We pay less tax when we contribute to super and we also pay less tax when our super generates income and returns. That means the earlier you get money into super and compounding for you, leveraging those lower tax rates, the bigger it will grow.

And, once we've retired officially, by reaching 60 and giving up work; or by accessing our super unconditionally at 65, we can withdraw our super tax-free. This makes it one of the most efficient vehicles for funding retirement.

Your goal should be to build your super early and let time and compounding do their thing. Maximise concessional contributions (such as salary sacrifice and voluntary contributions) and non-concessional contributions while you're earning. Once you know your long-term retirement is covered, you can shift focus to what you'll need to fill the gap in your prime time years – the years before you can access super and want flexibility.

3. FILL THE GAP BEFORE SUPER

Here's the tricky part about early retirement: unless you're past preservation age and meet the conditions of release, your super is off-limits. That means you need a plan to fund your prime time flexibility until you can access it.

You can fill the gap in two sensible ways – you can build a pot of money you can spend down; or you can build a sustainable investment portfolio that can provide you with a steady income.

Let's consider both.

Build a pot of funds

If your plan is to head into the lifestyling or even part-time phase of your Prime Time at 55 you might want to focus on saving the amount you want to have in income, for the years you want to have it. So, if you need $70,000 per year, and you want to go five years early, then you'll need five times $70,000. And it makes good sense to invest this conservatively, unless you're okay with having to change your plans if the markets fall apart.

Build an investment portfolio

The other option is to build up an investment portfolio that's designed to deliver a steady income through dividends and other distributions that won't run dry before you hit the preservation age of 60. This is a strategy that will need some careful planning – and maybe benefit from some good-quality financial advice to ensure you've chosen the right kinds of investments for your goals. Then, if you choose to build an investment portfolio outside super, you'll no doubt want to work out how to shift these funds or assets into your superannuation once the window where you can access them is in sight. That might be through contributions, transfers, or tax-effective strategies that set you up for the retirement phase.

In either case, tax planning is crucial. Any income you earn outside super is taxable, so it's important to minimise capital gains and manage your effective tax rate.

4. DEMOLISH YOUR DEBTS

If you're serious about an early retirement, one of the most powerful things you can do is eliminate recurring expenses – starting with your mortgage.

Housing is typically the single biggest cost for Australians. Paying off your home before retirement doesn't just give you peace of mind; it slashes the amount you need to fund your lifestyle. Without a mortgage, you need far less income, and every dollar you save on repayments is effectively tax-free and can be deployed toward savings or lifestyle.

For example, the average Australian mortgage costs around $3900 a month. To cover this in early retirement, you'd need nearly $1.2 million in investments at a 4 per cent withdrawal rate. Compare that to a mortgage-free lifestyle, and your income needs drop significantly.

It's not just about the mortgage, either. Beyond your mortgage consider:

- Can you downsize your home to free up equity?
- Are there other big-ticket costs you can clear before you retire?

Reducing your expenses doesn't mean giving up the good stuff; it's about clearing the big hurdles so you can spend more on what you truly value.

5. MAKE FLEXIBILITY YOUR FOCUS

Chasing a period of life with greater choice and flexibility isn't just about quitting your full-time job, it's about creating options. Whether it's stepping back to part-time work, changing careers, or focusing on hobbies and passions, financial independence is all about choice.

The key to flexibility is building a solid foundation:

- A well-funded super for long-term security
- A pot of funds that lets you live well before you reach preservation age
- Minimal debt and streamlined expenses for peace of mind.

When you focus on all of these considerations, you're not just planning for your Prime Time – you're setting yourself up for a life that's rich in freedom, purpose and opportunity. You're setting yourself up to have choices.

Now it's time to put rubber on the road – and show you how to work out how much is enough.

SO – HOW MUCH IS ENOUGH FOR YOU?

It's a big question, and it's not as simple as just putting a number on it. When you're asking yourself this question, you're really asking three different questions, based on the three big lessons we've just learned about midlife.

1. **Time**: How long am I likely to live, and how will my life take shape?
2. **Spending**: What will I want to spend each year – and how will that change over time?
3. **Income**: What will my income sources be, and how will they shift over time?

And if you have a partner, you're asking for both of you – it's about your whole household. As couples step into their Prime Time, they pool their resources and actively shape the life they want together. They also come to recognise when more money won't add more fulfilment, just excess, and that's when they unlock the power of *choice*. I've said it before and I'll say it again: the power of choice in the second half of life is the greatest superpower you can have, *and I want you to have it*. So let's look at those three questions in detail, using a workbook format, so you can decide for yourself if you have 'enough'.

THE DEFINITION OF 'ENOUGH'

The *Cambridge English Dictionary* defines 'enough' as: 'As much as we need or want.' But in reality, 'enough' is a personal concept that varies from one person to the next. For you, it might mean:

- **Covering basic living expenses.** Ensuring your everyday costs (housing, food, utilities, health care) are comfortably met
- **Achieving your lifestyle goals.** Making affordable the activities and experiences that bring you joy, whether that's travel, hobbies or spending time with loved ones
- **Maintaining financial security.** Having a safety net for unexpected costs, so you don't run out of money
- **Planning for the long term.** Making sure your finances can support your quality of life, even if your needs change down the line.

Ultimately, 'enough' is about feeling secure and confident that you can live the life you want, without the constant worry of running out of money.

TIME: HOW LONG AM I LIKELY TO LIVE, AND HOW WILL MY LIFE TAKE SHAPE?

Think about your best-case scenario for life expectancy and how you want to live through the various phases of your life, starting with the set-up phase and going through pre-retirement lifestyling, part-time retirement, full retirement and into the ageing years. As part of this, consider key financial goals, like paying off any outstanding debts, to give yourself more freedom and choice in the later stages of life. And think about the timing of when you might want to reduce work or switch to more fulfilling roles, even if it means taking a pay cut before fully retiring.

Let's work through it as an exercise. First, think about how long you might live and then consider how long you'll spend in each phase. Remember, you may choose to jump one or more of these stages.

Here's the latest life expectancy data again to remind you. Simply circle which one you're aiming for.

	25th percentile	50th percentile	75th percentile	90th percentile
Male	85	89	95	98
Female	87	91	97	100
Couple	92	95	98	101

Note: These figures are based on the 2020–22 Australian Life Tables with 25-year improvement rates. Figures were rounded up.[23]

HOW MANY YEARS WILL YOU SPEND IN EACH PHASE?

Contemplate the shape of your life in the table below.

Lifestyle phases I have ahead of me	Number of years I plan on being in each phase
Set-up years	
Pre-retirement lifestyling years	
Part-time retirement years	
Epic retirement years	
Passive retirement years/ageing	

WHAT DEBTS DO YOU NEED TO HAVE PAID OFF BEFORE YOU GET TO HAVE MORE CHOICE IN YOUR LIFE?

It's time to tally up the debts that need to be paid down in your life before you can reach new levels of financial freedom. List them out so they're top of mind and set yourself a feasible goal for demolishing the debt, either by paying it off or pragmatically downsizing to a mortgage you can afford to get rid of.

Debt to be dealt with	Amount	Goal
Home mortgage (example)	$175,000	Pay off $35,000 per year for next five years to accelerate paydown of the mortgage by December 2030.

WHAT WILL YOUR SPENDING GOALS BE AND HOW WILL THEY EVOLVE?

Get really clear on your annual spending targets, both for everyday living expenses and larger bucket-list or one-off items. Will your spending stay consistent or change as you move through each phase of life? Do you have specific dreams, like a sabbatical, a big trip or a home renovation, that need special planning? And don't forget to budget for the longer term, including how your spending might shift in the later stages of life when health and other care-related costs may increase as lifestyle expenses, like travel, taper off.

To get a clearer picture of your future, it's crucial to break down your budget for each phase of your life. Think about:

- **Cost of living**: How much you'll need annually to cover everyday living expenses (food, utilities, health care) for each phase of your life
- **Lifestyle spending**: Your annual budget for things like travel, hobbies, and dining out
- **One-off expenses**: Major expenses like home repairs, a new car, children's weddings, contributions to the bank of mum and dad, or health care

- **Bucket-list items**: The big, one-off lifestyle splurges like a sabbatical, caravan or overseas trips.

By the end of this, you should have two key numbers for each phase:
1. **Annual budget**: The total amount you'll need each year, by phase
2. **Lump sum needs**: Larger, one-off amounts you'll want to tap into for big life events and experiences.

Lifestyle phases I have ahead of me	Annual cost of living and lifestyle budget	Lump sum needs during that phase
Set-up years		
Pre-retirement lifestyling years		
Part-time retirement years		
Epic retirement years		
Passive retirement years/ageing		

INCOME: WHAT WILL MY INCOME SOURCES BE, AND HOW WILL THEY SHIFT OVER TIME?

Identify the layers of income you'll have at each phase, whether it's from work, superannuation account-based pension, lifetime annuity, investments or the age pension, and how they will change over time.

Think about whether you can afford to go part-time before full retirement and supplement that income with other sources like a TTR income stream, savings, or even a part pension. Finally, consider how you'll ensure you have enough income to meet your long-term goals, including funding your Epic Retirement and maintaining financial security for as long as you live.

Each of these considerations needs some solid thought, and it's important to think about when you'd like these things to happen in your life so you can put a plan in place. You want to feel confident that you're set for your Prime Time, that your Epic Retirement is within reach, and that you've thought ahead to your later years as well.

The best way to visualise it is to map out your income layers in each phase.

Income sources by phase	Phase 1: Set-up	Phase 2: Lifestyle	Phase 3: Part-time	Phase 4: Epic Retirement	Phase 5: Ageing
Active earnings income					
Investments income					
Superannuation account-based pension					
Lifetime annuity/income stream					
Age pension					
Savings and emergency funds					

With this plan in hand, you'll know when it's time to step into your next phase of life, fully prepared and excited for what's ahead.

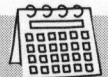

KNOWING WHEN YOU CAN ACCESS DIFFERENT LAYERS OF INCOME

If you're planning for your Prime Time and retirement, you need to be cognisant of some of the pivotal 'ages' or milestones in Australia's retirement system that are essential for unlocking access to your super, qualifying for age pension payments, and optimising your financial strategy. The government says you can't access your superannuation until 60, but there's no rule that says you can't retire before 60, if you can afford it.

Age 60: preservation age. The first critical milestone is reaching 60 years of age, the preservation age for Australians born after 1964, and when you can access your superannuation under certain conditions. At 60, you have the option to cease work and transition your super into the retirement phase. As we've discussed, you can either draw it down as a lump sum or start an account-based pension for a regular income stream.

Once your super is in the retirement phase, income drawn from it is tax-free, as long as the total is under the $2 million transfer balance cap. Any funds exceeding this cap remain in the accumulation phase, where earnings are taxed at 15 per cent, unless you're over the $3 million limit for the proposed Division 296 tax.

You can re-enter the workforce after shifting your super into the retirement phase. If you do, any new contributions will go into a separate accumulation account while you continue receiving a tax-free income stream from your retirement account.

Remember, at 60, you also have the option to keep working and access up to 10 per cent of your super each year using a TTR income stream. This option allows for an income stream but not lump sum withdrawals.

And don't forget: depending on your state, at 60 you may qualify for a Seniors Card, which offers discounts on public transport, goods and services – though few 60-year-olds feel like 'senior citizens' until they enjoy those savings!

Age 65: full access to super. The next big turning point is 65 years of age. At this stage, you can access your superannuation without any work-related conditions. You're free to withdraw your super as a lump sum or start an account-based pension income stream, regardless of whether you're working or retired.

Many people at 65 seek advice on whether to withdraw a lump sum to pay off any remaining debts or adjust their investments to match their risk appetite. At this age, you can also continue contributing to super – even if you're still working – through concessional and non-concessional contributions, up to the age of 75.

Age 67: age pension eligibility. Age 67 is the official age pension age for Australians born after 1957. Once you reach this age, you may be eligible to receive age pension payments, subject to income and assets tests. The pension provides a valuable financial safety net and can work alongside your superannuation and other investments to support your retirement lifestyle.

Age 73: last chance to use the bring-forward rule. If you're thinking ahead to tax efficiency or estate planning, age 73 is your final opportunity to trigger the full three-year bring-forward rule for non-concessional (after-tax) contributions. This rule lets you contribute up to $360,000 in one year by bringing forward two future years of caps. Once you turn 74, you're still allowed to make contributions, but you won't be eligible to bring forward future years. So, 73 is the last realistic age to move larger sums into super to reduce the tax impact on your estate or simply get more into the tax-free retirement phase.

Age 75: last chance for personal super contributions. Age 75 is an important milestone in the super system because it marks the cut-off age for most types of personal contributions, like concessional and non-concessional contributions. After 75, you generally can't make these personal contributions, except for special cases like downsizer contributions. You can, however, still receive employer contributions beyond the age of 75 if you're working.

SEE THE PRIME TIME STRATEGIES PLAY OUT

We've created a free booklet of mock case studies to show how the planning and budgeting strategies from Prime Time can work in the real world.

Developed with financial adviser David Lane, the Queensland State Manager and Senior Financial Adviser at Ord Minnett, these realistic examples walk through key money moves in your 50s and 60s – from part-time transitions to super drawdowns and retirement income planning.

They're not real-life examples, but they're realistic and relatable – and designed to help you explore what's possible in your own Prime Time.

Download your copy now at becwilson.net/primetime-resources

Lesson 9
Get appropriate financial advice for your situation

FINANCIAL ADVICE IN AUSTRALIA CAN FEEL LIKE A MAZE RIGHT NOW. THE INDUSTRY has been undergoing a huge shake-up for over seven years, and there's more change on the way. The most progressive companies are evolving the way they offer advice, trying to make it easier for people to access the services they need and make pricing easier for both the consumer and their teams. Over time, new legislation will hopefully bring in more accessible, affordable advice that average Aussies can use. But let's take a look at the advice landscape as it stands and what choices you have.

GENERAL ADVICE

Think of general advice as helpful guidance. It's the type of advice provided by superannuation call centres and workplace super advisers that gives you factual info about things like contributions, investment options, the age pension and income strategies for retirement.

The people giving this advice have to have formal training, an RG146 qualification at a minimum, but keep in mind – it's factual information as well as 'what people in similar situations might consider', and it's not tailored to your personal situation, objectives or needs. This type of advice is great if you've got a simple situation and you're just starting to explore your options and want to understand how things work, but if your situation has any complexity, you'll need more than this. Many funds let you ring their general advice hotline as many times as you like to have questions answered – it's worth knowing if you're trying to get your head around how superannuation works.

INTRAFUND OR SUPER FUND ADVICE

This is where things get more personalised but remain focused on super. Intrafund advice, or super fund advice, is provided by appropriately qualified advisers from your super fund, but their advice usually sticks to topics within the fund itself, like your investment options, contributions, insurance inside super and potentially any Centrelink entitlements. Some funds allow their advisers to give a broader scope of advice, but others are stricter. Most super funds offer this service at no extra cost, but in reality you're paying for this through your annual fees. Some charge a fee for helping set up your retirement accounts or giving specific and detailed retirement advice. Any additional intrafund advice fees can usually be deducted from your super balance.

Just remember that intrafund advisers can't provide advice for a couple unless you're both with the same fund. And if you need advice on things outside super, like other investments or joint financial strategies, you'll need to seek out an independent financial adviser.

A NEW CATEGORY OF ADVICE

One of the big shifts coming to the financial advice landscape is the introduction of a new class of adviser (who will probably get a fancy name). This type of adviser is intended to offer a more accessible, personalised form of advice that sits between general advice and independent financial planning. The goal is to offer affordable, targeted advice to people who don't necessarily need the full works of a personal financial adviser but want simple retirement advice – and more guidance than general advice or intrafund advice can offer.

Super funds are expected to play a key role in this space, with many already working on plans to offer this new type of extended advice directly to their members in addition to or in combination with their existing intrafund offering. This new layer of advice will focus on helping you make specific decisions about your super with the benefit of the adviser being able to understand your wider household financial picture – helping you choose the right investment options, adjusting your contributions, or planning your transition into retirement. The government is currently working through the details of what types of advice they will allow funds to provide, and whether they will allow the costs of providing this advice to be 'collectively charged' to members. There is no formal timeline for it to be rolled out at this stage, so watch this space.

FINANCIAL PLANNING AND ADVICE

Financial planning and advice is where things get specific and tailored to you, taking into account your partner, your assets inside and outside super, and your big picture. Advisers do one of two things: they either help you address a single issue, limiting their scope to the information they need to advise on it; or they take a holistic look at your financial life – your goals, cash flow, assets, and risk profile – and build a comprehensive strategy. The latter might cover everything from super and investments to insurance and retirement income streams. The strategy is usually provided as a standalone service.

Many advisers will also offer a service, either through their own company or through a sister company, to help you implement their strategic recommendations – guiding your investment options into either model portfolios or custom-built portfolios, setting up tax structures, and regularly rebalancing your activity. They'll check in with you yearly (or as needed), adjusting the strategy to keep you on track. As you approach retirement, their focus shifts to transitioning your super, managing your pension and layering your income streams.

It's important to understand how advisers structure their services so you can decide exactly what you want to sign on for and pay for, and can go looking for the right types of advisers to provide that type of service.

SINGLE ISSUE FINANCIAL ADVICE

This is when you go to an adviser for help with one specific problem, like how to invest an inheritance, or reassess your risk profile for investing. Advisers can only legally provide you with single-issue advice if you request it as a customer, limiting their scope. Otherwise, legally they have to take in your whole financial picture under legislation that obliges them to act in your 'best financial interests'.

Increasingly, savvy financial advice firms are building their offerings into a menu of services that allow people to get single-issue advice for a predictable price – as long as your situation is not complex. So if you think your need is 'one off' and you don't want to build and pay for an ongoing relationship with an adviser, ask about single-issue advice.

I should point out that some smaller or more premium advice firms avoid single-issue advice, as the process of engaging a new client for advice is complex and time-consuming, yet clients expect to pay less and don't want an ongoing relationship with the firm. That said, new legislation is on the way to make single-issue advice easier for advisers to deliver and therefore it will hopefully become more accessible as time goes by.

COMPREHENSIVE FINANCIAL ADVICE

This is the full-service option everyday people seek out. A financial adviser takes a deep dive into your finances, looking at your current position, goals and risk tolerance, to develop a personalised strategy. Many people struggle to define their goals upfront, and that's okay – part of the adviser's job is to help you figure that out.

While it sounds like a straightforward and repetitive process, advisers still have to do a lot of groundwork to provide comprehensive and appropriate advice. Legally, they need to gather detailed information about your finances, do a 'know your client' assessment, and document the entire advice process.

Some of the more common reasons people seek comprehensive advice include:
- Planning for retirement (anytime from about midlife) by working out how to save, invest and project future income

- Dealing with major life changes like a death, inheritance, divorce or buying a new home, where everything needs a financial rethink
- Getting 'on track' financially by focusing on saving, tax strategies, and making sure debt and investments are working long-term
- Hands-off investment management, where the adviser builds a strategy, makes investment recommendations, and manages those investments on your behalf
- Managing life risks through insurance, like life or trauma cover, especially as life circumstances change, such as paying off a mortgage or becoming an empty-nester.

The adviser's role isn't just about the numbers. It's about helping you see the big picture and guiding you toward your goals with confidence. And when you get this type of advice, you might still decide to implement it yourself – managing your own investments, maintaining your relationship with your existing or a new super fund yourself, and reshuffling your own mortgage through a mortgage broker or bank of your choice. If you prefer to stay with a high-performing fund, let your adviser know as early as possible. Many advisers tend to recommend investments they can actively manage for an ongoing annual fee, so being clear about your preference upfront can help ensure your strategy aligns with your goals.

FINANCIAL ADVICE FOR HIGHER NET WORTH CLIENTS

This type of advice is usually a blended combination of strategy and implementation. Customers seek out an adviser, usually one that has an appropriate research and implementation capability within their operations, and they work with them on an ongoing basis, getting regular strategic advice on their contributions, cash flow and structuring; ongoing management of their investments; and rebalancing of their portfolios. Some high net worth advisers specialise in certain areas, like stockbroking, funds management and/or wholesale investing. While these specialists still follow the same rules as personal financial advisers, they focus on specific needs or client types. If you are managing an above-average-sized portfolio, usually more than $1.5 or $2 million, it's good to know these services exist.

TOOLS AND CALCULATORS

Many super funds now offer calculators and planning tools that let you play around with your numbers and see how things might pan out. These tools can be a great way to get hands-on with your finances before speaking to an adviser. Plus, some funds encourage you to use these tools as a first step before calling their advice lines.

DIGITAL ADVICE AND ROBO-ADVICE

The rise of digital advice platforms and robo-advice means you can get detailed financial advice online. These tools collect your information and give personalised recommendations based on your goals. It's a DIY approach that's becoming more popular, and it's worth exploring if you want a more hands-on way to manage your financial planning.

HOW DO YOU FIND A FINANCIAL ADVISER THAT'S RIGHT FOR YOU?

The first thing you need to work out is whether you really need independent advice, or whether you're happy taking advice from your superannuation fund's advice team or an advice firm they recommend to you. This will all depend on how well your super fund is performing and what your goals are. As you've just read, superannuation funds increasingly offer multiple levels of advice, including offering comprehensive advice that can rival the services of independent financial advisers. In fact, you'll probably find that many funds have put in place trusted partnerships with national advice firms to provide their members with the comprehensive advice they need at affordable prices.

If you're considering independent advice – whether it's to switch super funds, move toward a platform, or even set up a self-managed super fund – start by looking within your local community for a reputable adviser who specialises in the types of investments you're interested in. A great way to begin is by identifying the most successful people in your circle who share your values and investing ethos. Reach out to them and ask them who they trust for financial advice. Aim to gather recommendations from two or three people you respect and know personally.

This is the best way to find someone who is skilled but also aligned with your goals. And if they've been serving your community for a long time, chances are they've built their independent advice business on a foundation of providing reliable, long-term financial guidance with a strong reputation to match. Resist the temptation to seek advisers in Facebook groups or to take advice from people who haven't invested time and effort in establishing their credibility in their community. (You'll note that everyone on the internet has 'a mate' that does this and they'd love to introduce you to them, but be very wary! Plenty of people pay 'mates' online for leads and not all of them are reputable.)

You should meet with at least two or three advisers in person when weighing up your options, then choose one who feels like the right fit. Assess them in terms of their technical expertise, communication style and cost. Most, if not all, will offer a free initial appointment. Keep in mind that they won't be able to provide you with proper advice on your situation until after you've completed a fact-find and they've prepared a statement of advice. This is usually when you'll receive a quote for their services, outlining both the upfront and ongoing costs. If you're worried about ongoing costs, make sure you ask for detailed information. Nothing will be done after this point until you pay them for their advice services, which is when they start properly working on your strategy. All the good learnings and advice come after that. But you have to make a choice about which adviser to go with before you pay. They can't give you any personalised financial advice for free – it's against the law for advisers to provide advice without compensation.

One interesting thing to point out is that most, if not all, advisers are tied to a dealer group – the company that defines their preferred product list, and sets the standards and procedures they follow. This affiliation can heavily influence the products and services the adviser recommends to you and the way they do business. Many of these organisations have also built up companies that 'manage investments' and provide research and build model portfolios for them. Be aware of who the dealer group is, how that relationship works, and what the limitations of their preferred supplier or product list are, and contrast that with your investment and advice objectives. Ask your adviser how they are paid and whether their firm offers any incentives or bonuses that could influence their recommendations.

HOW MUCH DO FINANCIAL ADVISERS CHARGE, AND WHAT DO YOU GET FOR YOUR MONEY?

How long is a piece of string? Well, you need to work out how you want it cut. Here's a snapshot of how advice fees work.

INTRAFUND OR SUPERANNUATION ADVICE

First up, let's talk about superannuation advice. Your fund provides this as part of your ongoing fees, so while it might feel like it's free, you're actually paying for it through those 0.2–1.5 per cent management fees. If you're not using it, you're missing out on something you're already paying for. Some funds let you access this advice as often as you like, while others limit you to one meeting per year. And many will charge for more specific retirement services like setting up your account-based pension. Don't be afraid to ask – they'll tell you. And certainly don't be afraid to use the services on offer.

SINGLE-ISSUE ADVICE

Next, let's look at single-issue advice. This is where financial advisers focus on helping you with just one specific area of your finances, rather than providing a full financial plan. It's a changing space at the moment. Advisers offering this type of service have recently started using a pricing menu to calculate fees, working out the cost by adding up the different services you want to access. While you might not always see the full breakdown, advisers use these menus internally to ensure they can price their services fairly and consistently.

Their menu of services might include specific tasks like:
- Risk profile assessment: $400–$600
- Superannuation investment strategy: $1000–$2000
- Drawdown strategy: $1200–$2000
- Estate planning advice: $1500–$3000 (depending on complexity)
- Cash flow management: $500–$1500
- Insurance review: $800–$1500.

These prices vary by adviser and region, but this kind of modular approach allows you to get tailored advice in the areas where you need the most help, without committing to a full financial plan, which can sometimes be more than what you need. It's a flexible and cost-effective option, especially for people who already have a good handle on their finances but need expert guidance on a specific topic.

COMPREHENSIVE ADVICE

Now, onto comprehensive advice. This is a bit trickier to explain.

Most financial advisers offer the first meeting for free, no matter what your situation. It's a chance for them to get to know you and for you to figure out if their services are a good fit. After this, they'll present you with a proposal, outlining their fees and what they'll deliver. They can't give you any actual advice until you sign off on this. When reviewing the proposal, look for two key things:

1. The advice fee

This is the upfront cost for the deep dive into your finances and the preparation of a detailed statement of advice (SOA). The fee is usually based on how complex your situation is. Expect something like this:
- Simple advice (single issue or straightforward situation): $1500–$3000
- Complex advice (more detailed but without complex structures): $3000–$5000
- Comprehensive advice (deep dive into everything if you have complex investment structuring): $5000–$10,000.

Some advisers (particularly high net worth advisers) will waive this fee if you sign up for ongoing advice and implementation services.

2. Ongoing or future costs

If you seek independent advice, that often leads you to set up and maintain a long-term investment strategy, as well as a platform or SMSF, which comes with ongoing fees. These break down into three main areas:

1. **Strategy/ongoing advice fees**: Payment for monitoring and adjusting your strategy over time, these are often charged as a percentage of the funds under management, usually around 1–1.2 per cent.
2. **Platform fees**: The cost of using an investment platform (like HUB24, AMP North, BT Panorama or Macquarie Wrap), typically around 0.2–0.5 per cent of your funds under management; premium advice groups usually integrate this service as core and so don't charge for it.
3. **Fund management fees**: These cover the cost of managing the actual investments and can range from 1–1.5 per cent, depending on how your adviser structures things. Some funds charge this through a sister company or a partnering firm, or you might fund them purchasing managed investments with separate management fees. These fees will be in your SOA, but they're often not in bold, so make sure you ask what they mean.

You can minimise some of these costs by choosing advisers who use lower-cost investment options like ETFs, but make sure you're aware of the different layers you're paying for, and ensure you have an appetite for it. Ask the right questions upfront.

Some advisers serving high net worth individuals will choose to offer a blended fee for their comprehensive service offering, often quoted at up to 1 per cent of the portfolio, rather than charging individually for each service. Others charge a fixed fee per account, and when you add them up across multiple accounts (SMSF, family trust etc.), they often come to close to 1 per cent of the portfolio value.

PAYING FOR FINANCIAL ADVICE OUT OF YOUR SUPER

Did you know you can use your superannuation to pay for financial advice? This is possible under Australian superannuation laws, and it can be a useful way to cover advice fees without affecting your cash flow. Paying for advice from your super is often more tax-effective, as it uses pre-tax dollars, which are generally taxed at a lower rate than personal income.

There are a few things to keep in mind if you're considering this:

- The advice must relate directly to your superannuation or retirement planning, such as investment strategies, contributions or pension options. Broader financial advice unrelated to super generally cannot be paid from your super balance.
- You can pay for independent financial planning advice. This means you can seek advice from an external, independent adviser, as long as the advice relates to your super.
- Your super fund's trustee needs to approve the deduction, and each super fund has different policies. Always check with your fund to confirm if they allow payment for external, independent advice.

GETTING THE MOST OUT OF YOUR ADVICE APPOINTMENT

A good adviser should help you understand your whole financial picture before making any recommendations. If they don't, you need to ask more questions or rethink whether their approach is right for you.

Here are some smart questions to bring to your first appointment, whether you're meeting with a comprehensive financial adviser or a retirement specialist from your super fund. They're designed to help you feel more confident, more informed, and more in control.

Meeting with a comprehensive financial adviser? Here's what to ask:

These are the kinds of questions that help you get the full picture, not just about products or investments, but about their approach, values and what kind of support they actually offer.

1. **Do you offer full retirement planning and projections, or just investment management?** There's no wrong answer here, just the right fit for your needs. Make sure their focus matches your goals.
2. **Does your firm have a preferred product list or a specific investment philosophy?** Ask them to explain how it works – you're allowed to understand how your money is being managed.
3. **If I move to a wrap account, will I have to leave my current super fund?** Make sure you know how this might affect fees, performance, tax, and your insurance arrangements.
4. **Can you model different retirement scenarios for me?** For example: keeping vs selling an investment property, switching super funds or not, and different drawdown or tax strategies. A good adviser should be able to map out what's possible.
5. **Do I need ongoing advice, or is this a one-time plan?** Ask about the costs and whether ongoing fees are genuinely necessary for your situation.
6. **If I want to keep my super where it is, can you still help with retirement planning?** Some advisers only work with clients who move their investments. Ask this early to avoid wasting time.
7. **What are all the fees involved?** Request a direct comparison to your current set-up, so you can see whether their advice and product recommendations truly add value.

Tell 'em I sent you! Good advisers love working with clients who are informed, curious, and ready to plan wisely for their future.

Talking to a super fund adviser? Here's what to ask:

Super fund advice is often included at no extra cost, but it can be limited to your current fund. These questions will help you figure out how much help they can give, and whether it's enough for what you need.

1. **Can you help me build a full retirement plan, or just provide advice about my super with your fund?** This tells you whether they offer holistic guidance or are limited to your current account.
2. **Can you help me understand how long my super might last based on different retirement ages or income goals?** Scenario modelling is gold – you want to see if they can walk you through what's realistic for you.
3. **Can you explain how my investments are set up right now and whether they suit my stage of life?** Good advisers should be able to explain this clearly, in plain English, and talk through options if they're not quite right.
4. **Can you show me how much I'm paying in fees, and whether there are better-value options within the fund?** A quality fund adviser should be open about fees and keen to help you find the right fit.
5. **What happens to my insurance if I change investment options or move to retirement phase?** Insurance can change when you move accounts or switch strategies – it's important to understand the impact.
6. **Can you help me plan how to draw down my super in retirement, including when and how to start an income stream?** This is where fund advisers often shine – make sure they offer help with setting this up clearly.
7. **Can you explain the tax side of things, such as how my super income is taxed in retirement?** A good adviser will talk about the transition to retirement phase and what it means for your tax position.
8. **Will I be able to come back for more advice later if my situation changes?** Super fund advice is often free or included, but it's good to know what ongoing support is available.

Good luck! And remember, advice should leave you feeling more confident, not more confused. So use it for that. And if it doesn't it's simply not good advice.

Lesson 10
Take a modern, proactive approach to your legacy

WHEN YOU THINK ABOUT YOUR LEGACY, YOU PROBABLY THINK ABOUT YOUR WILL, your financial assets, your binding nomination (the legal document directing your super fund trustee on how to distribute your superannuation and any life insurance benefits) and the things you'll leave to your loved ones. But it's so much more. Your legacy really is the passing on of everything you've worked for, the values you've lived by and the impact you've had on the people you care about most. I want to challenge you to think about legacy not as something you deal with at the end of life but as something you can shape and define right now, both financially and emotionally.

You may also be able to use this knowledge to help your parents better navigate their own legacy and end-of-life planning, given you're probably going to have to help them do that sometime in the future, if you haven't already.

THE AVERAGE AGE OF INHERITANCE IS OLDER THAN YOU THINK

Did you know that the average age at which Australians inherit from their parents is now 58–59? The median estate size across the country is close to $500,000, with about 20 per cent of estates

> exceeding $1 million and 7 per cent more than $2 million. As life expectancy continues to increase, more people are receiving their inheritance while they're preparing for retirement rather than in their younger or middle-aged years, when it could have provided a financial leg up.
>
> This shift has led many to rethink legacy planning. If you have more than enough to last your lifetime, you might consider helping your children and grandchildren financially while you're still alive. Whether it's contributing to a first home, paying off a chunk of their mortgage, funding a big family holiday or supporting your grandchildren's education, these life-changing investments can ease financial stress when it matters most.
>
> Take some time to think about it. Explore your own thoughts on what a modern legacy might look like.

WHAT DOES LEGACY MEAN TO YOU?

Before we dive into the nuts and bolts of this topic, let's take a moment to reflect: what does legacy actually mean to you? For some, it's about passing on financial security to the next generation. For others, it's leaving a lasting impact on their community, supporting causes they're passionate about, or making sure their family is taken care of emotionally and financially. Legacy can mean creating a sense of continuity, as in helping your children and grandchildren live better lives because of the financial and community foundations you've built.

But legacy is deeply personal too. It's about the stories you share, the values you instil, and the memories you create with those you love. And here's the thing: you don't have to wait until later in life to start building your legacy. You can shape it now. One thing you definitely want to ensure is that your end-of-life choices and paperwork don't damage your legacy or leave behind broken relationships, fights over money, or feelings of greed, sadness or jealousy.

For many people, legacy feels like a mechanical process. You sort out your will, power of attorney and advance care plan so that your family knows your wishes. But it's more than just this. The decisions you make when drafting these documents can have a big impact on those left behind, especially if those choices are made without considering how they might affect family dynamics. Even if your intentions are good, handling things poorly, unfairly or without respect for the values you've tried to instil in your family over your lifetime, can undo the legacy you've worked so hard to build.

Let's look at Tom's story. He was a successful small business owner with two sons, Michael and David. Michael had worked in the family business his whole life, while David had chosen a different career path. Tom always intended to leave the business to Michael, and assumed that David, being financially independent, would be fine with receiving a smaller share of the estate.

Tom didn't discuss his plans with his sons in detail, thinking everything would be clear in his will. But when Tom passed away, David was shocked to learn he was receiving less than his brother. He had always assumed that, despite their differences, his father would treat him and Michael equally. The sense of being valued less strained the brothers' relationship, leading to resentment and arguments over what was 'fair'. They fell out, stopped talking, grew apart. Their families never fully connected after that, and their children never really bonded.

This conflict could have been avoided if Tom had approached his legacy differently. By having an open conversation with both of his sons while he was still alive, he could have explained his intentions, addressed their feelings and taken time to understand what his family legacy could be – beyond the money. Tom's legacy was not just financial. It damaged the bond between his children and later between their families. In the end, the lack of communication created division, which wasn't what Tom had wanted.

But that's legacy too, and it's a reminder that how you handle your end-of-life decisions is just as important as the values you hope to pass on.

By contrast, there's Nancy and her husband Sean, who spent their late 50s and 60s spending every spare minute with their grandchildren. Nancy was the big driver of what I think is their real legacy. When she wasn't working, she spent her time encouraging the grandkids to read stories and imagine the characters, showing them how silkworms turned into butterflies, and what happened when grasshoppers landed in big spider webs. She played cricket in the garden with them and they baked scones together on Sundays. She taught her grandkids to live in the moment, exploring the world rather than being on their iPads alone. And as those kids have grown up, they look forward to her company and the fun things they do together: hiking trips, picnics, country visits and exploring the great outdoors. Her adult children have watched on in amazement, grateful for the help in raising curious kids. At the same time, she's been even-handed, making sure she spreads her efforts among the families of her three children, interested in all of them. And she has looked for ways to help them all financially too.

Nancy's father died when she was 59, and there was a healthy inheritance that she and her husband didn't really need, so she helped each of her adult children with a living legacy – a gift of $60,000 offered on the condition it be used to relieve their mortgages a little. If Nancy and Sean are financially secure in 10 years' time, they want to do that again – to help. She knows that when she goes they'll probably inherit more, and she's trying to be fair about the way that's handled. But she doesn't want the money to be what she's loved for, or even part of the story of her relationship with her children and grandchildren when she's done – she wants the love to be.

These stories are a reminder that a legacy isn't just about dividing assets. It's about what we choose to prioritise and how those decisions affect the people we love. Love, fair treatment, communication, empathy and thoughtful planning can help prevent misunderstandings and ensure your legacy is more than just the money, that it brings your family closer together rather than driving them apart.

LEGACY VERSUS LIFESTYLE: IT'S GOT TO BE YOUR CHOICE

It's important to consider the balance between enjoying your life now, leaving a legacy for others when you die, or sharing your assets with loved ones along the way. Often, people feel pressured to save for the future, ensuring they leave something behind for their family. But there's a conversation worth having about spending the money you've saved during your lifetime on yourself while you're fit and healthy, whether it's for travel, hobbies, or experiences that truly enrich your life.

There's also a time to talk about what you want to spend on your ageing, allowing yourself funds for later-life community living and care that will make your older years more pleasant, rather than only focusing on building a financial legacy for your loved ones. A lot of people's children deny the value of this if they have to trade off an inheritance, something which angers me. After all, you've worked hard for your money, and there's real value in using it to live your later years in high spirits, good company and relative comfort as opposed to being alone and lonely.

Spending on yourself doesn't mean being irresponsible or selfish; it's about finding a balance. Living your best life now can still be done while planning for your family's future. In fact, choosing to spend money in ways that create lasting memories with your family, or investing in your wellbeing and happiness and maintaining your independence and community later in life, are also part of the legacy you leave. At the end of the day, your family should want to see you happy and fulfilled as much as they want financial security in the future. And if they don't, they might need some healthy reframing.

So think about the joy you can get out of life in the present, while also considering what will be left behind. Your legacy isn't just the money. It's also the time you've spent with loved ones, the values you've shared, and the experiences that will stay with them long after you're gone – really!

YOUR APPROACH TO YOUR LEGACY

Take a minute to consider these questions:
- What brings you joy right now, and how can you spend in a way that really does enrich your life?

- How will you balance enjoying your savings today while still securing your family's future?
- What kind of legacy do you want to leave beyond money? What values and memories will matter most to you and your family in your lifetime?
- When do you want to share your financial legacy – with your loved ones while you're alive, or after you're gone? Or perhaps a little of both?

WHAT DO YOU NEED TO THINK ABOUT AND WORK THROUGH?

When you start planning your legacy, there are a few key areas to focus on. These range from legal and financial decisions to emotional considerations, all of which need careful thought to ensure your wishes are carried out the way you envision. Here are the main components of legacy planning.

THE BINDING DEATH NOMINATION FOR YOUR SUPERANNUATION

One of the most important aspects of legacy planning is ensuring your superannuation is distributed according to your wishes after you pass. Unlike your other assets, which are covered by your will, your super isn't automatically included in your estate. This is where a binding death benefit nomination comes into play.

As mentioned, a binding nomination is a legal document that directs your super fund trustee on how to distribute your superannuation and any associated life insurance benefits when you die. If you don't have a valid binding nomination in place, the trustee of your super fund has the discretion to decide how your benefits are distributed, and this may not align with your wishes. A valid binding nomination gives you control over who receives your super, whether it's family members, a spouse or another beneficiary.

Australian law only allows certain people to be nominated for your superannuation. You can nominate:

- Your spouse or de facto partner
- Your children (including stepchildren)
- Financial dependents
- Your estate (via your legal personal representative).

When planning your nomination, it's important to consider the superannuation death tax (covered in more detail later in this section), which can affect the amount your beneficiaries receive. If your super is left to a spouse, a dependent child (under 18) or a person with whom you have an interdependency relationship, it will generally be tax-free. If your super is left to an adult child or non-dependent beneficiary, part of the payout may be subject to tax. This is because the taxable portion of your super (which includes your concessional contributions and their investment earnings) may be taxed at up to 15 per cent plus the Medicare levy when paid to non-dependents.

To minimise the impact of this tax, some people choose to make withdrawals from their super once they've retired, then use their non-concessional contributions to 'recontribute it' in a way that will make it tax-free for their beneficiaries. It's worth discussing tax strategies with your financial adviser to help your beneficiaries maximise their inheritance.

There are two types of death nominations. The first is a binding nomination, which, if it's valid, must be followed by the trustee of your fund. Usually such nominations need to be renewed every three years, otherwise they become invalid. Some funds have perpetual nominations now – ask about it. The second is a non-binding nomination, which gives the trustee an idea of your preferences but they aren't required to follow them.

'How do you make one?' I hear you asking. You simply contact your super fund to request a binding nomination form and nominate your beneficiaries, ensuring they fall into one of the eligible categories. Then you sign and date the form in the presence of two witnesses who are over 18 and not nominated as beneficiaries, and submit the form to your super fund, keeping a copy for your records.

Just like your will, it's important to keep your binding nomination up to date. You should review it regularly, especially after major life changes such as marriage, divorce or the birth of a child. If your nomination lapses (typically after three years), the trustee may have discretion over your super, so make sure to renew it on time.

WILLS AND ESTATE PLANNING

A will is the cornerstone of any legacy plan. It's the document that specifies who gets what when you're gone. But it's more than just a list of assets. It also ensures that your estate is distributed in line with your wishes, and with the least amount of fuss. You need to decide how your assets will be divided among your loved ones, and who you want as the executor to make sure those wishes are honoured. It's essential to review your will regularly, especially after significant life changes.

How to make a will

You don't need an overly complex or expensive will, but it's essential to have one that's up to date, valid and enforceable. Here's how to go about it.

Choose an executor

The executor is responsible for carrying out your wishes as outlined in your will. They'll manage your estate, pay off any debts, and distribute your assets according to your instructions. Choose someone reliable and trustworthy, as they'll need to handle legal and financial responsibilities after your passing. It's not an easy job, so it is best to choose someone who is good at detail, and has the time and capacity to work through things.

Consider sensible tax planning

Speak to a solicitor or financial adviser about structuring your estate in a tax-efficient manner. Planning for tax efficiency in your will can ensure that your beneficiaries maximise their inheritance, especially if you are passing on investment properties, shares or other income-generating assets.

List your assets and beneficiaries

Make a clear list of your assets, including property, bank accounts, investments and personal belongings. Decide how you want to distribute these assets, whether to specific individuals or to be divided among beneficiaries. Consider any special bequests for sentimental items. If you have complex assets, tax considerations may impact how you allocate them, so think about whether certain assets should be distributed through a trust to minimise tax for your heirs.

Appoint guardians for minor children

If you have young children, your will is the place to name a guardian to care for them in case something happens to you and the other parent. This decision is critical and requires discussing your intentions with the person you want to appoint as a guardian to ensure they are prepared for this responsibility.

Sign and witness your will

For your will to be legally binding in Australia, you must sign it in the presence of two adult witnesses who aren't beneficiaries. These witnesses must also sign the will, confirming they've seen you sign it.

Keep your will safe and updated

Store the original will in a safe place, such as with your solicitor or in a safety deposit box. Make sure your executor knows where to find it.

Review your will

You should review your will periodically and update it when significant life changes occur, like a marriage, divorce, the birth of a child, grandchild, or a major financial change or shift in the family structure such as divorce of your children.

ENDURING POWER OF ATTORNEY (EPA)

Your enduring power of attorney (EPA) ensures that someone you trust can make decisions on your behalf if you're unable to. This person will manage your financial and legal affairs (you can also appoint an EPA to manage health-related decisions), so it's critical that you choose someone who is responsible and who understands your values and financial intentions. This is especially important as you age, as there could be periods when you are physically or mentally unable to make decisions for yourself.

How to set up an EPA

Choose your attorney(s)
The person or people you appoint as your enduring power of attorney will make financial and/or legal decisions on your behalf if you're unable to. Choose someone you trust, such as a family member or close friend, who understands your values and can act in your best interests. You can appoint more than one attorney and set out how they should act together, either jointly or severally (independently).

Decide the scope of the EPA
You can choose what powers to grant your attorney. This can be broad (for example, managing all your financial affairs) or specific (dealing only with your property). You can also decide when the power comes into effect – either immediately or only if you lose the capacity to make decisions.

Complete the relevant forms
Each state and territory in Australia has its own forms for setting up an EPA. You'll need to complete the correct form for your location, outlining the powers you are giving and to whom. You can usually find these forms online through your state or territory government website. In some cases, a solicitor can help draft the document.

Sign and have the EPA witnessed
You'll need to sign the EPA document in front of an eligible witness (such as a solicitor or justice of the peace). The witness must not be the attorney themselves, their spouse or someone who benefits from your estate. Some states have additional witnessing requirements, so check the specific rules in your area.

Register the EPA if needed. In some states, like Queensland, if the attorney will be managing real estate or property, the EPA must be registered with the Land Titles Office. Check your local requirements.

Provide copies to key people
Give copies of the signed EPA to your attorney, family members and your solicitor, if you have one. Make sure everyone involved knows the scope of the powers and when they take effect.

ADVANCE CARE DIRECTIVE
This document (your living will) lays out the plan for your worst-case scenario, where your health takes a serious turn or you have a debilitating accident, but you keep living and need care. It goes well beyond financial and legal details, ensuring that your medical and healthcare preferences are honoured if you can't express them yourself. Whether it's about the kind of treatment you want, your thoughts on life support, or how you'd like your final care to be managed, an advance care directive is essential. It takes the emotional burden off your loved ones, sparing them from having to make difficult decisions during a challenging time, and it gives them peace of mind knowing they're following your wishes.

How to create an advance care directive
Think about your wishes for medical care
Start by considering what types of medical treatment you would or wouldn't want if you become seriously ill and can't communicate your wishes. This can include decisions around life support, palliative care, and specific treatments like resuscitation or feeding tubes.

Discuss your wishes with loved ones and doctors
It's important to communicate your decisions to your family, loved ones and doctors so they understand your values and preferences. This can prevent confusion and stress later on. If possible, include your future EPA (medical) in these conversations to ensure they know how to act on your behalf.

Complete the advance care directive documents
Each state and territory has its own forms and requirements for creating an advance care directive (or equivalent). Some are simple statements of your preferences, while others are legally binding documents that require witnesses or even doctors' signatures. You can usually access these forms through your state or territory health department.

Sign and witness the document
For the directive to be legally binding, you'll need to sign it and have it witnessed according to your state/territory's rules. It may require a doctor's signature as well.

Store the document securely and share it
Once the document is signed and witnessed, store it in a safe place, such as with your solicitor or alongside your will. You should also provide copies to your doctor, attorney (if appointed) and close family members. It's essential they know where it is and how to access it if the need arises.

Review your advance care directive regularly
Just like a will, your advance care directive should be reviewed and updated as your medical conditions or preferences change. Make sure to inform your family and doctors if any changes are made to your plan.

FAMILY DYNAMICS AND COMMUNICATION
This is the tricky bit. No matter how well you've planned, things can still go sideways if family dynamics aren't taken into account. It's not always about dividing everything equally; sometimes it's about being fair and having things align with your values – and those aren't always the same thing. It really is important to remember that the way in which you communicate your plans with your loved ones, both before and after your death, can make or break the harmony within your family. That's why having open, honest conversations about your intentions, and explaining your reasoning behind certain decisions, is so important. It might feel uncomfortable at first, but it

can save your family from misunderstandings or even disputes later down the track.

Once you've considered your end-of-life wishes, it's worthwhile, having 'the tough talk'. Here's a facilitation checklist with questions and talking points. You might also use the checklist to help your parents navigate their own journey.

The 'tough talk' checklist: the end-of-life talk no one likes to have

1. **Wills and assets**
   - Do you have a will, and if so, is it up to date?
   - Have you appointed an executor? Does that person know where your will is stored?
   - Have you listed all your major assets? How do you want them distributed?
   - Are there any specific sentimental items (like heirlooms or jewellery) you want to leave to particular people?

2. **Funeral preferences**
   - Do you have specific wishes for your funeral or memorial service?
   - Would you prefer burial or cremation?
   - Have you prepaid a funeral or set aside money for this?
   - Are there any special readings, songs or traditions you'd like to include?

3. **End-of-life care**
   - Have you drafted an advance care directive (living will)?
   - What are your preferences if you are unable to communicate? For example, would you want life-prolonging treatments like resuscitation or ventilators?
   - Do you have a 'do not resuscitate' (DNR) order in place, if that's your preference?
   - Who have you appointed as your enduring power of attorney (for health and finances)? Have you discussed your wishes with them?

4. **Financial and legal planning**
   - Who will manage your finances if you become incapacitated?

- Are there specific accounts or assets your family needs to know about (bank accounts, investments, properties, insurance policies)?
- Have you considered how you want your debts or mortgage to be handled?

5. **Medical and care planning**
   - What kind of medical care would you want if your health declined significantly or you were in a terrible accident?
   - As you age, do you prefer to stay at home or would you consider retirement/assisted living or aged care?
   - Do you have savings set aside for aged care or do you intend for your house to be sold or reverse-mortgaged to fund care?

6. **Family communication and legacy**
   - Have you communicated your wishes to all your family members to avoid misunderstandings later?
   - Are there values or lessons you want to pass on to your children or grandchildren?
   - How do you want to be remembered? Is there a message or legacy you'd like to leave behind?

7. **Digital assets and accounts**
   - Have you made a list of your online accounts (email, social media, banking and so on) and shared it with someone you trust?
   - What should happen to your digital presence after your death? Should accounts be deleted, memorialised or passed on?

8. **Financial support for dependents**
   - If you have dependents, how will they be supported financially if something happens to you?
   - Do you have life insurance, and have you communicated the details to your beneficiaries?

9. **Charitable giving and contributions**
   - Are there any causes or charities you want to support through your estate?
   - Have you included this in your will or estate planning?

10. Family relationships
- Are there specific family dynamics you want to address to prevent future disagreements?
- How can you make sure that your end-of-life decisions don't lead to conflict or confusion among your loved ones?

CONSIDER GIVING DURING YOUR LIFETIME

Our lives are longer than they ever have been before. That means inheritances are being received later and later, when they can have less impact on the lives of your loved ones. It is for this reason that many people are choosing to give gifts or financial assistance while they're still alive. This allows you to see the impact of your generosity and to give guidance or support while you're here. Whether it's helping a child or grandchild with a house deposit, funding the grandchildren's education, or donating to causes you care about, lifetime giving can be a meaningful part of your legacy. But you also need to weigh it up against your own financial security – don't compromise your comfort for the sake of generosity.

PLAN FOR THE BIG DEATH TAX

Australia does not have an inheritance or death tax, but it does have a Superannuation Death Benefits Tax to be aware of that can take a bite out of your estate. You really should understand it and know how to navigate it if you have to.

HOW DOES IT WORK?

When super is left to a non-tax dependent – usually adult kids – part of it may be taxed. Super is split into two main components, the tax-free component, which includes your after-tax (non-concessional) contributions. This part is not taxed when passed on to beneficiaries.

Then there's the taxable component, which includes employer contributions, salary sacrifice and investment earnings. This part is taxed when passed on to a non-dependent. But the taxable component can be made up of two different elements:

- The taxed element – usually taxed at 15 per cent
- The untaxed element – taxed at 30 per cent.

That 30 per cent rate often applies when there's a life insurance payout inside the super fund, or if you're in an older government or defined benefit scheme where contributions weren't taxed going in. So while many people expect their kids to pay 15 per cent tax on the taxable part of their super, it could actually be up to 30 per cent on part of it, and that can make a huge difference on large balances.

It's worth understanding how your super is structured, and considering strategies such as withdrawal and recontribution in retirement to reduce the taxable portion before you pass it on.

Withdraw your superannuation before death

If you're retired and have full access to your super tax-free, you can consider withdrawing some or all of your super while you're alive. Once it's out of the super system, you can gift it to your loved ones or invest it in assets that won't attract the same level of tax. This can help you avoid the super death benefits tax altogether. But keep in mind that you'll lose the tax benefits of keeping your money in super, so it's something to weigh up carefully with a financial adviser.

Recontribute to reduce the taxable components

If you're over 60 and meet a retirement condition of release, you can use a withdraw and recontribution strategy to reduce the taxable component of your superannuation. When you withdraw from your super, the withdrawal is tax-free. You can then recontribute that money back into your super as a non-concessional contribution (which is from after-tax income). This recontribution converts the taxable portion of your super into a tax-free portion, reducing the potential death benefits tax your beneficiaries would otherwise face.

However, be mindful of the non-concessional contribution caps, which limit how much you can contribute without incurring extra taxes. Currently, the cap is $120,000 per financial year or up to $360,000 over three years if you're eligible for the bring-forward rule. Also remember that after age 73 you can no longer bring forward up to three years of non-concessional contributions. And after age 75, you can't make non-concessional contributions at all, so the timing is crucial.

Nominate your dependents

Superannuation benefits paid to dependents, like a spouse or minors, are entirely tax-free. So another option is to ensure your super is directed to dependents by using binding nominations or reversionary pension options. This way, the tax won't apply and your beneficiaries will receive the full benefit.

This and the other aforementioned strategies are where a financial adviser can be a great help, allowing you to structure your super in a way that protects your legacy, minimises tax, and ensures your beneficiaries get the most from what you leave behind.

MANAGE YOUR SENTIMENTAL ITEMS

Not all legacies are financial. In fact, it's often the other items, such as family heirlooms, sentimental possessions, memorable pieces of art or furniture, or special mementos, that can carry as much, if not more, emotional weight than a lump sum of money. So it's important to consider how you want these to be passed down, who you want to pass each item to, and whether there are stories or family traditions you want to preserve with your gift.

It could be important to take the time to give these gifts more personally and thoughtfully, with explanations to the loved ones receiving them. It certainly can strengthen family bonds and leave a more personal legacy than if jewellery or treasured items are just handed on after death with no storytelling or emotion.

VALUE FINANCIAL EDUCATION, AND INSTIL IT IN FUTURE GENERATIONS

I often say to my dad, 'I'd much rather have you around forever than inherit your money. With you here, I can learn how to invest from a legend.'

This is one of the most meaningful legacies you can leave: the knowledge and skills your loved ones need to make their own money grow and later to manage any inheritance you pass on to them. More than money, it's about instilling the values and practical know-how they need to make wise financial decisions.

One way to begin this process is by making money a positive conversation topic throughout your life, normalising discussions about saving, investing and managing wealth. This doesn't mean overwhelming young people with technical jargon, but rather integrating financial principles into everyday conversations. Whether it's teaching your kids the basics of saving pocket money or explaining how you budget for family expenses, these small lessons add up over time.

Leading by example is another powerful way to pass on financial wisdom. Show your children or other loved ones how you manage your finances, whether it's investing in shares, paying off debt or saving for a major purchase. Let them see your decision-making process, and don't be afraid to share mistakes you've made along the way. This transparency builds a real-world understanding of money management that can't be learned from textbooks alone.

As they grow older, encourage them to take ownership of their finances. This could start with them managing their own savings or investments, making decisions, and learning from their experiences. You can support them along the way by offering guidance, but letting them figure things out will help build their confidence. Additionally, gifting books, recommending podcasts, or even introducing them to a trusted financial adviser when the time is right – all these things can help them deepen their knowledge independently.

The key is to make financial education an ongoing part of life, rather than something saved for later. And when major life events occur – buying a house, starting a family or planning for retirement – these are perfect opportunities to guide loved ones through more complex financial lessons and considerations – ones they might not learn from anyone else in their lives.

Bonus lesson
Reconsidering your insurances

As you head into a new phase of life, you've got a lot to manage, but I'm going to add one more thing to the list: your personal insurances. Many of us set these up earlier in life, at a time when we first took big risks, like buying a home and taking on a mortgage. Those policies were often in place to protect our loved ones and ourselves in case of sudden death, serious illness or permanent disability, ensuring debts would be covered and our partners wouldn't need to work until the kids were grown.

But as you get older, your kids become independent, you pay off more of your debts and your risks shift, so your insurances should shift too. In fact, for the first time in your Prime Time, you might find that you can downscale some of those policies. To do that, you need to reconsider what risks you still face and what you want to insure yourself against now.

Let's go through each type of personal insurance, revisit why you took it out in the first place, and help you figure out what your current and future needs might be.

LIFE INSURANCE

Most of us took out our first life insurance policy when we got our first mortgage. They tend to go hand-in-hand. This policy is designed to pay off your house and provide enough capital for your family to maintain their standard of living if you are to die suddenly. As I mentioned earlier, people often set the policy for an amount that covers their debts and provides an annual income for the family to live on.

For most Australians, life insurance premiums are charged to their super balance, so you might not notice it being deducted each year. However, it does reduce your superannuation's growth over time, so it's worth reviewing your policy every few years to ensure it's still right-sized for your current risk needs.

As you reach your Prime Time, two key factors may change your need for life insurance:

1. **The size of your mortgage**: If you now have a much smaller mortgage or have paid it off entirely, you might want to reconsider whether you still need this coverage.
2. **The age and independence of your kids**: If your kids are now independent and making their own way in the world, you likely no longer need to insure for years of income to support your partner in raising the family.

It's also worth reconsidering why you might want to keep this insurance, and how much you'd want to leave for your partner or family if you were to pass away. As you get older, life insurance premiums typically increase, so it's important to assess whether the cost is still worth it, considering your current financial situation and whether your loved ones will need that lump sum.

As you accumulate more assets, you may find that you no longer need as much life insurance coverage. If your partner or family would be well supported by your other financial resources, this could be the right time to think about reducing or even cancelling the policy altogether.

INCOME PROTECTION INSURANCE

Income protection insurance covers you if you can't work due to illness or injury. It's tax-deductible and usually held outside of your super. It can be pricey, so it's often taken out by people in higher-income roles, or those in jobs with a higher risk of losing their income due to injury or similar reasons.

That said, there's a point where this type of insurance might not make as much sense. As you get further into midlife, you might find you're in a position to cover yourself with passive income from investments or dip into savings if you need to take extended time off work. At that stage, you'll need to weigh up whether it's worth paying for an expensive policy to protect your income, or if you're comfortable relying on your savings if something happens.

Also, don't forget to check the waiting periods and benefits of your policy. Most income protection plans have a waiting period (like 30 or 90 days) before payments kick in, and they usually only cover part of your income. Make sure these terms still line up with what you actually need.

TRAUMA INSURANCE

Trauma insurance gives you a lump sum payment if you experience a major health event like cancer, a heart attack, stroke or other sudden illnesses, things that tend to become more common in the second half of life. It's not the cheapest policy, but if you've had it from early on, it's worth considering keeping.

Take the case of a woman who went into hospital with pneumonia and a collapsed lung. While there, she asked about an issue with her arm that had been bothering her for years. The doctors checked it out and it turned out to be a melanoma. Thankfully, it was caught early and treated successfully. Her trauma insurance paid her a tax-free lump sum of $110,000, giving her financial peace of mind while she recovered. She also had income protection insurance, which kicked in after her sick and annual leave ran out, covering 70 per cent of her wages during her time off work.

Trauma insurance is typically taken out alongside life insurance. If you make a trauma claim, the payout usually reduces the benefit from your life insurance if something were to happen later. For example, if you claim on your trauma insurance and then pass away within a year, the life insurance payout will be lower by the amount you received from the trauma policy.

Here's the thing: trauma insurance is one of those policies where the chances of claiming increase as you get older. The likelihood of facing a significant health issue rises with age, so the value of this cover becomes more apparent. Insurers know this too. They'd love for you to cancel it as you get into your 50s because your risk (and their potential payout risk) goes up. So if you've paid premiums for years, cancelling now could mean losing out on something you're more likely to need sooner or later.

TOTAL AND PERMANENT DISABLEMENT (TPD) INSURANCE

TPD insurance is designed to protect you financially in the event of your worst nightmare: becoming totally and permanently disabled. This kind of situation goes beyond just worrying about paying off the house or providing for your family. It's about ensuring there's money available to cover your own care – possibly for the rest of your life. That's the real fear: not being able to take care of yourself and needing to pay for someone else to do it.

TPD insurance can be expensive, but it's one of those policies where you're weighing up the cost of future care. You're asking yourself, 'If I couldn't work or live independently, how would I pay for the care I need?' It's not a pleasant thought, but it's a real one, worth considering.

It's rare for someone to hold all four types of insurance – life, trauma, income protection and TPD – throughout their life. At some point, you might start thinking about pivoting from one policy to another to better manage the risks you face today, depending on your situation. For instance, as you reduce your need for income protection or life insurance (maybe the mortgage is paid off and the kids are independent), you might decide to keep or increase TPD cover instead, to ensure that long-term care is accounted for.

Ultimately, it's another choice you have to make in midlife.

Part 3
WORK, PURPOSE AND HAPPINESS

Do you enjoy your work? Do you feel like you have a strong sense of purpose that guides your decisions on what to do with your time, money and energy? Do you know what feels meaningful and important to you? Do you know what really brings you joy? And has it changed in midlife?

'Pfffft!' I hear some of you saying! 'I have a career and a family and it gives me a perfectly fine sense of purpose, thank you!' Others, however, just leaned in a little bit, feeling curious.

Scientists have been digging into the ideas of happiness, fulfilment and meaning in midlife for over a hundred years, trying to figure out how it all works. While there's still plenty of debate, there are a few things most gerontologists and psychologists in this field agree on:

- Happiness dips in midlife in almost all Western countries
- Our priorities shift as we start to realise that time isn't limitless
- The templates we used to rely on for the second half of life just don't hold up anymore
- Work in its many forms can be good for you.

I want to look at these in more detail, before we dive into six big lessons around work, purpose and happiness that I think everyone should understand.

THE DIP IN HAPPINESS IS REAL

As I mentioned earlier, researchers looked at over 500,000 people over a long period of time, asking them each year, 'Are you happy?' What they found is pretty interesting: happiness is usually at its peak in our 20s and early 30s. Then it drops to its lowest point in midlife before climbing back up as we get older. This is called the U-shaped curve of happiness.[24]

This U-shape makes a lot of sense. In our 20s, life often feels like it's on track, with goals and milestones that match what we and society expect. But as we hit midlife, things get more complicated. You're dealing with more responsibilities. You've often got a big mortgage, you're raising kids, and you have higher expectations of yourself, some of which might not actually turn out the way you'd hoped. And that can all pile up and lead to a dip in happiness, usually between the ages of 48 and 55 according to the researchers.

But here's the good news: this low point often sparks change. As people go through this tough time, they start rethinking their lives and making adjustments that bring them more happiness in the here and now.

TIME AND PURPOSE MEET IN MIDLIFE

The second big finding worth discussing is the idea of meaning in life, and more significantly, how meaning in life becomes more important in midlife because that's often when we start to perceive that time might one day run out, and that drives us to reflect on what really matters to us. As we move through the middle years, the focus tends to shift from chasing external achievements – those things that we have 'societal rules for' in the first half of life, like career success, financial security and social status – to seeking deeper, more personal fulfilment.

And, according to scientists, there's more urgency once we reach midlife and start to see our time on this earth as limited.[25] In fact, they've created what they call 'socioemotional selectivity theory', which says that as we perceive our time to be limited, our motivations change, activating the goals related to emotional meaning. The science says that once these emotions click in, they have the power to change our entire goal hierarchy to make us more focused on the people who matter to us, seeking emotion and meaning rather than being future-oriented, and craving new knowledge and expanding our networks.

In midlife, many people begin to ask themselves bigger questions, such as 'What's my purpose?' and 'Am I living the life I truly want?' This search for meaning becomes more important as we realise that time isn't endless and that the choices we make now will shape the quality of our second half of life. It's not just about what we achieve but what we enjoy, what we spend our time doing, and how those things align with our core values and bring us a sense of purpose.

Finding meaning in midlife can be a powerful motivator for change, pushing us to re-evaluate our priorities and focus on what truly brings us joy and satisfaction. Whether it's through relationships, work or personal passions, the pursuit of meaning helps guide us toward a more fulfilling and contented life as we get older.

LIFE TEMPLATES REALLY ARE BROKEN

The reality of midlife in today's world is that we could live a long time. A 50-year-old today, with a life expectancy adjusted to modern longevity expectations, has a one in four chance of reaching the age of 95–97 in Australia.

And the changes to life expectancy have happened pretty quickly – for most of us, in our lifetime – meaning that all the templates for how to live our midlife and strive for retirement are out of date and rapidly becoming irrelevant to all of us. The world has changed.

We used to expect life to move through three phases: childhood, adulthood and retirement. Then we split off adolescence from childhood, and ageing from retirement. Now, social scientists are calling for all of us to split a new phase out of adulthood, before retirement, which some are calling our 'encore adulthood'.[26] 'Prime Time' sounds much sexier to me, so I'm going with that.

All the norms are broken in this phase of life and it feels like one big experiment for those in it. There are no longer clean lines between work and retirement; in fact, we're all learning that there doesn't have to be if we look after our bodies and minds and find work we really enjoy. We can, if we can afford to, choose the pace at which we want to downshift – if we want to downshift at all, that is. And, we can, if we can afford to, enjoy a better lifestyle before we formally retire, working more flexibly alongside it.

We have to get ourselves in a position where we understand what we want to do, and where we can afford flexibility so we can live the life we want to.

WORK IS NO LONGER 'BAD'

The role of work throughout our lives has shifted. When we were young, work was often seen as a 'necessary evil', something you did to earn a wage until you could retire, and then the usual pathway was to grow old, wind down and finally check out. Choosing a job was more about salary and status than following any real passion, and it was common to stick with the same role in the same company, climbing the ladder year after year.

Then along came the push for work–life balance, as if work and life were polar opposites that needed to be kept separate. Work again was seen as the bad side of the balance. But here's the truth: when you love your work, balance isn't always the point. Sometimes, imbalance is exactly what fuels us.

Today, I think we're finally moving to a different way of thinking about work – thinking about it across our whole life.

New generations are choosing careers earlier that they actually enjoy, and they're shaping their lives around purpose, fulfilment and relationships that matter. Happiness is a priority for them. Today's Prime Timers might just be the last generation to join this party. Many started their careers chasing status and salary, sticking with what they were good at or what provided stability. Others have been in industries that have changed so much they barely recognise them anymore. But now, they're reaching a stage where they can actually afford to (or are being forced to) reconsider their path, and my hope is that they can find meaning in whatever comes next.

And there's a whole new phase of our lives where we can choose to work, which some call the 'third act' of our career. The first act might have been all about building skills, gaining experience, and maybe chasing some status and stability. The second act was about using those skills and building a life, often focusing on family, responsibility and career progression. Now, in this third act, we have the chance to work on our own terms, to find fulfilment, to focus on what genuinely interests us, and even to pursue those passion projects we may have put aside before. It's a time to bring purpose and joy into our work, without the same pressures that drove us in earlier stages.

True, if you didn't start out in a field you loved but became successful, it's tough to make a change, especially during those peak responsibility years when everyone's depending on your income. But midlife brings turning points, those windows that open as you start reaching a level of financial freedom. When that happens, the reason for working can finally shift. At this stage, work can take on a whole new significance. It becomes less about the pay cheque and more about fulfilment, purpose and, yes, a bit of fun too.

As the vibe around work shifts, science is also revealing the benefits of staying engaged in work we find interesting. In 2013, a large French study of 429,000 people found that each additional year of work was linked to a reduced risk of dementia.[27] Researchers suggested that the cognitive demands of work help keep the brain active and sharp. Around the same time, the long-term Terman study, an eight-decade review of over 1500 lives, showed that people who remained engaged in meaningful work or activities lived longer than those who fully retired.[28]

And in 2017, research on purposeful ageing by the Stanford Center on Longevity found that nearly 80 per cent of older adults who pursued work in new fields or launched their own ventures reported higher levels of physical and mental health, along with a more enriched sense of life.[29]

Ultimately, there are six big lessons about work, purpose and happiness I think everyone should understand in their Prime Time. We're going to work through them:

1. Recognise the outdated models of work and retirement – understand your true options
2. Choose your path out of the workforce
3. Rediscover what brings you joy and fulfilment
4. Seek fulfilment outside of work
5. Recognise transitions and embrace the journey they offer
6. Remind yourself that curiosity, learning and flexibility are crucial.

Lesson 11
Recognise the outdated models of work and retirement: understand your true options

IF WE ACCEPT THAT THE OLD TEMPLATE FOR THE SECOND HALF OF LIFE IS BUSTED, that work is no longer 'bad' and that many of us want more meaning in midlife, then it's time to embrace a completely new set of expectations for our midlife. But it's not a one-size-fits-all deal. This new phase of life is, again, a bit like a choose-your-own-adventure story, where you get to decide what your journey looks like. And there are three parts to it.

1. **Understanding your triggers**: What triggers us to move into our Prime Time, a time when we make changes in our life more consciously, prioritising our own needs and wants? It might be a significant event in life such as being retrenched, losing a loved one, suffering a critical health incident, or your kids leaving home. It could simply be a slow, burning frustration or a hunger to adapt. Or it could be a simple decision to make a shift while being consciously aware of what you want to do next.
2. **Contemplating the shape of the Prime Time you want to live**: Once you've decided you need or want some change in the way you live your life, it's then up to you to shape it, looking hard at your skills, passions and values to guide how you

might get the most out of life, and considering how you'll mix-and-match the phases of life and types of fulfilment you want in the years to come.
3. **Recognising your power to get off the ladder**: In the first half of life, many of us are taught to see work, career and purpose as a ladder that we're constantly climbing, and that not moving up is a failure. The wisest executive coach I know helps leaders in the second half of life to see things differently. He encourages us to view life as a lattice rather than a ladder, where we have the power to choose our direction based on our values, interests, and what truly brings us joy. Remember that and explore whether you're ready to change, use your skills differently, and be happier.

REFRAME MIDLIFE AS A TRANSFORMATION, NOT A CRISIS

Don't see any part of your life journey as a 'midlife crisis'. That old-fashioned concept belonged to a world where life and careers were seen as ladders to climb, and stepping off (or being pushed off) felt like failure. Instead, reframe this stage in your own mind as a life lattice, with every direction being a possibility, and embrace your power to choose what brings you joy, meaning and, of course, the income you need from working.

Many who've been triggered to re-prioritise in midlife – whatever the reason – look back and say, 'That time was transformational,' or, 'I'm so glad I went through that'. Those who use this opportunity to carve out their own path emerge happier, more fulfilled and more in tune with what matters.

I want you to remember that Prime Time is not retirement. This phase of your life can contain all the elements of work, saving, leisure, lifestyle and fulfilment that make us tick. It helps to step back, look at life through the next stage and remix things to fit your priorities, without the pressure to 'give up' anything – unless you choose to.

1. UNDERSTANDING YOUR TRIGGERS

For many, Prime Time seems to arrive out of nowhere. It can be sparked by feelings of burnout, inner death or other life events that push us toward change – events that often are not positive, giving us things we have to work through. In a long life, there will always be disruption, transitions, times when our sense of meaning and purpose changes. I wish we all talked about them more to make them easier to traverse. With that in mind, here are some of the common triggers that kick off Prime Time.

FEELING DEAD INSIDE

Maybe you've felt it, a sense that you're just going through the motions every day, doing what needs to be done but without any real motivation. Life might seem like it's lost its spark, or like your routine has become a never-ending rut. I call this trigger 'inner death' because that's exactly what it feels like. The excitement is gone, nothing ignites your curiosity, nothing gives you a sense of achievement, and your passions feel neglected. You might even feel like your life is focused on things that just don't seem to matter anymore. This can show up as tiredness, boredom, frustration, a lack of curiosity or just plain emptiness.

Many people recognise these feelings but assume the only way out is to retire, simply because that's the only life template they know – work until you're worn out, then retire. But that template is outdated. We've got more options now, and retirement doesn't have to be the default answer. Simply noticing your inner death can be a powerful trigger, allowing you to move into a phase where you start to design a life that excites you, that you gradually lean into and let unfold.

BURNING OUT

Burnout is a reality for many in midlife. Plenty of career-driven people burn out at a hundred miles an hour, after relentlessly pursuing success, status and financial security for decades. The result is often a period of complete and utter exhaustion, and it leaves people questioning whether it's all worth it. But burnout can be a powerful driver of change, pushing you to reassess everything: your career, work–life balance, and what you want from your life in the future. It often sees proactive people make changes that prioritise their wellbeing and happiness, leaving behind some of those obsessions with status and success.

GETTING RETRENCHED OR MADE REDUNDANT

It's not uncommon to get retrenched or made redundant in midlife. Often, you're one of the more expensive employees, thanks to all those years of experience, so when a business needs to cut costs, letting go of senior staff can seem like the easiest option. And let's face it, companies are under pressure to adapt more quickly and operate more efficiently than ever before.

But it *can* be about more than just the money. By midlife, you might have suffered a bit of that inner death, where the spark that once drove you has faded. This can leave you feeling less curious, maybe even increasingly inflexible and less willing to learn new things, something that others may not want to accommodate in their teams. This combination of being seen as costly and perhaps less adaptable can make you a target during restructuring, even in an age-friendly workplace. It's something to be cognisant of if you want to keep working.

But being retrenched doesn't have to be the end of the story. In fact, it can be a turning point. You can let it eat you up, or you can let it fire your energy for the next steps. Sure, the initial shock can be soul-crushing, especially as it chips away at your confidence and leaves you wondering who you are and what got you into this position. But once you get past that, it can open doors to new opportunities you might never have considered otherwise. It's a chance to reassess your priorities, rediscover things that truly excite you, and design a new chapter in your life that really does align more closely with your passions and values today, and less with the path you chose much earlier in life.

FACING A MAJOR HEALTH INCIDENT

By midlife, most of us have had a run-in with a chronic disease or critical health condition at least once. Depending on the issue and how you cope with it, it can be completely derailing – or it can trigger you to reassess and rebuild your life around what you can do, enjoy and achieve in the next phase. The period when you're suffering can be horrible to live through, but many say afterward that it offered them a valuable time of reflection, as you have no choice but to live through it and wonder if you'll get to shape your life afterward.

I don't want to trivialise your health – it's the most important thing you have. But if you get another shot at life after a significant health incident, it can be inspiring, empowering you to make all kinds of changes and live your life for the people, passions and values that matter most to you.

STARING INTO YOUR EMPTY NEST

Your children leaving home is one of the more obvious triggers for Prime Time. It can come suddenly if they up and leave for university or head overseas. Or it can come slowly, with your kids inching their way out of the nest, allowing you to become more independent as they do too.

It can be a really significant time in life. You are no longer a primary caregiver, and for some this comes as a shock even if it has happened over a long period of time. You can wallow in the loss, feeling lonely, sad and wondering at your purpose, or you can embrace the extra time and space to focus on yourself, recognising the opportunity this brings to think about the next phases of your life.

I personally think that for parents, our Prime Time can't really start until the kids start to find their independence, both financially and functionally. This usually sees your spending on the kids drop as they start to pay for their own clothing, food and, eventually, housing expenses. And their education expenses, if that's been a priority for you, disappear eventually too. That freer cash flow allows people to prioritise their own savings goals, as they head into the set-up phase of their Prime Time, and perhaps start to explore a bit more lifestyling too.

DIVORCING

The ending of your most significant relationship in life can rip you to pieces and completely up-end your priorities. I've watched friends lose years of their midlife to the trauma of going through divorce, which can be an awful time, and one of deep reflection. For some, divorce forces them to confront and then reconstruct their life all over again in a very short space of time. For others, it's like a weight has been lifted. Once you accept the ending of the relationship and the loss of a partner, divorce can be an awesome catalyst for midlife change and growth, pushing you to reimagine your life and seek out new opportunities for happiness and fulfilment.

LOSING SOMEONE IMPORTANT

Whether you've lost a parent, a child, a sibling or a friend, the death of a loved one can be a terrible trigger for midlife change. This is one life event that really leans into 'socioemotional selectivity theory' because when you lose a loved one, you often become more aware that your time on earth is limited, and you want to grasp and enjoy every single minute you have left. The science says this changing perception of life can drive a shift in what motivates us.

BECOMING A CARER

About 4 per cent of women and 3 per cent of men in Australia who retire early and unexpectedly do so to become carers for a partner or parent. Becoming a carer for a loved one in midlife can be physically exhausting and emotionally overwhelming. It often forces you to reassess your priorities, time and energy, shifting your focus from your own needs to someone else's. While this responsibility can feel like a heavy load, it also brings a sense of purpose and meaning that can be deeply fulfilling, even with the challenges.

People in this position often reach out to me to ask how they can have an Epic Retirement or Prime Time when they can't even find themselves amidst their caregiving duties. It's a tough gig, but every carer has both the need and the opportunity to push for balance. This means maintaining their physical health, mental wellbeing and social connections, so they don't lose themselves while caring for a loved one.

REACHING A MILESTONE AGE

That big milestone birthday can be an important turning point for some. Turning 50 or 60 can be a line in the sand that people draw, prompting themselves to take stock of their life: what they've accomplished, what they still want to achieve, how they want to spend their next years. For some, it's a wake-up call to start living more authentically, make major lifestyle changes, or chase some of those goals that got lost along the way.

GETTING A FINANCIAL WAKE-UP CALL

A major financial event, like a sudden loss of income or even reaching a financial goal (like finally paying off the mortgage), can trigger a midlife shift of gears. It might see you reconsidering how you spend your time and your money, knowing you've hit the goal that allows you to move into a lifestyling, part-time or portfolio life that prioritises experiences, relationships or personal fulfilment rather than accumulating more wealth.

YEARNING FOR GREATER MEANING OR PURPOSE

As you move through midlife, it really is far more common to start questioning the deeper meaning and purpose of your life and begin to feel a yearning for change. This existential trigger can lead you to look around for more fulfilling work, volunteer opportunities, or activities that align with your core values. It might also inspire you to explore spirituality, mindfulness or other practices that help you connect with a greater sense of purpose.

RELOCATING OR MAKING ANOTHER MAJOR LIFESTYLE CHANGE

Many people find that a big move in midlife allows them the space and time to trigger change. It might be moving to a new city, a shift to live by the beach or in the country in midlife, downsizing to a different place, even retiring to another country. The disruption of your usual routine and environment can open up different perspectives and opportunities and encourage you to embrace an alternative way of living.

ENTERING A NEW RELATIONSHIP OR ENDING AN OLD ONE

Starting a new romantic relationship or ending a long-term one can be a huge trigger for change. A healthy new relationship often brings with it fresh energy, new experiences, and a renewed sense of finding oneself. On the other hand, the end of a relationship can be a time of deep reflection, healing and personal growth as you navigate life on your own and rediscover your individual identity. Either one can be the trigger for Prime Time.

So, if you're feeling triggered, like life has lost its spark, or things have to change, this might be a wake-up call. It might in fact be the beginning of the journey into your Prime Time of life. Recognising this can be the first step toward making changes, whether that's exploring new hobbies, reconnecting with passions, learning something new or even considering a major work–life overhaul. The key is to embrace it. This phase of life can be your best yet.

DO YOU REALLY WANT TO RETIRE EARLY, OR ARE YOU JUST TIRED?

A lady named Lisa wrote to me prepared for a big debate: 'I think you're wrong about early retirement. I heard you say that retirement is not a 50-year-old's project. I myself am planning to retire before 50 (along with my husband). I can't think of a better lifestyle where I'll be in charge of my own time to spend with family, learning new things, exercising, travelling, volunteering and possibly working if I feel like it. I truly believe there is much more to life than the corporate 9 to 5 grind. I just don't understand why anyone would say it's a bad idea.'

I couldn't resist probing. Lisa is 46 and hates her busy, professional job. She told me that every Friday she feels excitement as the week comes to a close, and then, on Sunday afternoon, dread creeps in for the week ahead. Her three kids are in their mid to late teens. And she's starting to reconsider her own sense of life.

Lisa's situation is really, really common. She could change jobs, but she fears her industry would only give her more of the same. So, at 46, the only light at the end of the tunnel she and her husband can see is aiming hard for an early, Epic Retirement and putting their foot to the floor trying to get there. They've been saving one of their executive salaries almost fully for two years to reach it.

But I challenged her. Maybe she wanted to embrace her Prime Time instead and use that money as a buffer to reinvent herself.

Most people like Lisa who aim for retirement in their 40s or even early 50s find when they get to early retirement that it isn't what they are looking for at all. They enjoy the first big holiday and maybe the first year or even two, when everything feels fresh and new, but then they look around and all the other 50-year-olds are busy – there's no-one to play with. And while they've spent those years relaxing and overcoming burnout, they haven't grown their knowledge, purpose and passions. They fill their time with travel to keep up the excitement, and realise travel is expensive if you do it all the time. Then they get bored, lonely, even a bit stale, and go looking for work – and then they find that hard too.

Their alternative is to recognise that they are in a classic midlife transition, at the bottom of that U-shaped curve of happiness. And they *could* embrace it, recognising where they are at, and working through the process of releasing their feelings of burnout and re-seeking their sense of purpose. It might mean using some of their savings to take a midlife sabbatical or even a gap year, investing in developing their skills and knowledge, spending time looking for things they are (or can get) passionate about, and getting ready for this exciting next stage of their life – packed with work they enjoy doing and people they like spending time with. Not all of us need to have a midlife identity crisis to kick it off, but many of us do without realising it.

> P.S. Lisa agreed. She was burnt out and had not given herself permission to explore her skills, passions and values. And that's what she's going to do next, using the money she'd saved for that early retirement.

3. CONTEMPLATING THE SHAPE OF THE PRIME TIME YOU WANT TO LIVE

Here's where the choose-your-own-adventure bit kicks in. If you're feeling triggered – positively or negatively – it's now time to redesign your life around you, and how you want to find purpose, fulfilment and passion in the next phase: your third act. It's time to make your own template for the second half of life, knowing that the existing templates are outdated and you don't want to play by those rules.

So how do we create this new template? First off, we need to acknowledge that the choices are deeply personal: what works for one person might not suit another. The best way to approach this new Prime Time is for me to lay out all the options, explain them, and then let you pick the path that feels right for you, while recognising that you'll adapt your path along the way.

Think of each of these work–life options as food for thought as you design the life ahead of you. They're like ingredients: you'll choose the ones that work best for your recipe for life. While you might want to consider what other people are doing in this phase of life, for inspiration, you might also want to block it out and run your own race.

WORKING AND SAVING

For many, one of the big early focuses of their Prime Time is building financial security. This might mean sticking with your current job to pay your super, pay off the mortgage, or save for a big-ticket item like a dream holiday or early retirement. Or maybe all three. The goal here is to balance the work grind with the rewards, ensuring that your effort today creates the freedom you want tomorrow.

TAKING A SABBATICAL OR GAP YEAR

Sometimes, you just need to hit pause. Taking a sabbatical or gap year gives you the space to recharge, travel, or simply figure out what you want next in life. Or it can be a gift to yourself, to celebrate a change of gear, to expand your curiosity and explore. This time away from the daily grind can offer fresh perspectives and a whole new sense of purpose.

It astounds me that we don't talk about doing this more. It appeals to me to do one or possibly two big sabbaticals – or sexy gap years – if I can afford it. One in my 50s, as a bit of a midlife reawakening, maybe when all my kids have left home and I've been able to save, downsize and ready myself for a half-year without income, just travelling. And another in my 60s, when I'm on the journey toward more part-time work and part-time retirement. I associate sabbaticals and gap years with travel, but there are lots of other ways to use them.

Shelley, 55, is taking a year off from her role in PR for Queensland Tourism to do her MBA, and while she's doing it she's working for a start-up in the tourism space that is developing outdoor walking treks in Tasmania. She's a passionate hiker, and she's well connected in tourism, so this move gives her a way to take a break from her everyday life and try something she's passionate about. She calls it her gap year – the reason for a 'gap' is up to you.

We can't talk about sabbaticals and gap years in midlife frivolously, though. A gap year that takes you away from your work and income can take some careful planning, because to have a sabbatical or gap year (I prefer the term 'sabbatical' because it's more realistic) you not only have to save up enough to afford your costs of living and travel, you may also need to save enough to maintain your home, care for your pets and generally put your life on pause. We have to remember that the goal of a sabbatical typically isn't to cancel everything, but to 'take time out and refresh' or to put ourselves among different stimuli.

RESKILLING AND REPOSITIONING

All too often I've heard people in their 40s or 50s, usually those suffering from inner death, say, 'Yeah, I want to learn something new and change careers. But nah! I'm too old to retrain into a new industry. I'll never get time to use it.' I despair about their view of the time they have left and the value they think they will get from learning new things and finding things they are passionate about in the second half of life.

At 48, 55 or even 60, most people have a long time left to live. So frankly, midlife can be the perfect time to reinvent yourself, whether it's picking up new skills, going back to study, or shifting your career in a new direction that's more suited to the life you want to live. Think of it as investing in your future. It's a chance to set yourself up for a fresh start, doing something that excites you and aligns with your evolving interests.

Therese, a hairdresser for her whole working life with a solidly performing home-hairdressing business, has recently at 50 made the bold step of retraining as a customs officer, knowing she doesn't want to have to stand on her feet all day doing hair to make a living through her 50s and beyond. She also admits it's hard to keep up with the hairdressing trends these days, and that's what you've got to do to be 'in demand'. So she looked for a career path that had longevity, one where she could pick up shifts and be relied upon, but that would also be flexible as her kids fly the nest and she moves into the next phase of her life. For now, she wants to maintain some hairdressing and pick up part-time customs officer shiftwork and have the choice, over time, to live a more flexible life.

CASE STUDY: NAVIGATING A DYING OR AGEIST INDUSTRY

In the advertising industry, particularly in Australia, the landscape for professionals over 50 has become increasingly challenging. Tim Burrowes, a prominent figure in the media and advertising world, highlights how the number of people over 50 in the industry is now at an all-time low. 'We're seeing people being made redundant because their salary expectations don't fit the current business model of agencies,' he says. 'Even if they're enormously experienced, they find themselves too expensive. And the reality is, they struggle to reset to what the market now says they're worth.'

For many, this transition is difficult. 'We see people waiting sometimes a year with a number in their mind before they decide to change paths,' Burrowes explains. 'But it's a number they'll never get again because that's simply not what the market pays anymore.' This gap between expectation and reality leaves some professionals in a state of limbo. Deciding to let go of either their hierarchical upward trajectory or the industry they've known all their lives feels like failing.

For those who choose to remain in the industry, meanwhile, it's often not at the same level they once held. Burrowes notes: 'The jobs they used to have just don't exist anymore. One of the knock-on effects of AI and the digitisation of business processes is that there are fewer of those really well-paid jobs.' For many industries, but particularly advertising and media, this shift is creating a massive hole.

However, Burrowes believes there's still hope for those willing to adapt. 'Where there will always be a place for us as humans is in applying critical thought based on our experience,' he says. 'This is more than just processing what already exists. It's about using wisdom to gain an edge.'

For those who refuse to innovate or adapt, however, the future is more bleak. 'Some people just want to do what they did before,' Burrowes says, 'but without innovation, they don't make much progress.

'Some professionals move into consulting, often hoping it's just a holding pattern for them until another big opportunity comes along. Sometimes, though, that big job never arrives,' Burrowes observes. 'Others start their own agencies or pivot to adjacent industries, where their domain expertise can still give them an edge.'

As Burrowes points out, industries like automotive, retail and media are in the midst of significant disruption, particularly with the rise of online vehicle ordering in automotive, automated ordering in retail and AI in media and marketing: 'It feels to me like we're in the middle of a generational shift with AI, where the true value will come from applying critical thinking and experience, not just from processing data.'

Burrowes sees opportunities for people looking to adapt and use their skills in other industries: 'For those looking for a leap out of the media or automotive sales industries, they need to recognise that sales is a transferable skill. If you can sell, you can pivot into booming industries like cybersecurity and software. There's enormous demand for technology sales.'

For those facing the harsh reality of a dying or ageist industry, Burrowes offers this advice: 'The best time to recalibrate your core skills was 20 years ago. But the second-best time is right now.' He urges midlifers to adapt.

WORKING AND LIFESTYLING

Why not find a balance where work supports your lifestyle rather than taking it over. This option is all about blending work with the things you love. It's about creating a rhythm where work is part of life, but it's not the whole story.

This is where I hope many people can get to in their Prime Time. It's not a financial reality for everyone, but it can be 'the goal'.

Fiona, 60, is a former CEO and managing director of some of Australia's largest travel companies. She recently took off on a six-month sabbatical, spending six weeks in London and three months in Lucca, Italy, in the European summer, learning the language and living like a local. She then toured Croatia and Scotland for a month on her way home, before picking up a 25-hour-per-week contract for five months. She's adamant that she is going to find balance in her next phase and work only on things she's passionate about and can make a real difference doing, alongside enjoying her life more.

DOWNSHIFTING TO PART-TIME OR CASUAL WORK

One of the best ways to get more balance in your life, and make the transition into retirement easier, is to downshift the amount of work you do each week over time. You might find you start by dropping back to a four-day work week, picking up a long weekend every week, or simply working less hours, and this allows you to do things that are becoming more important, like travelling, prioritising your health or spending time with your grandchildren. Then you might drop back to three days, or even less.

It can also be a valuable step in building your financial confidence. As you wind back the amount of work you do, you need to work through your cost-of-living and lifestyle budget and your income sources. Many people enjoy part-timing for years, seeing it as a way to 'practise for retirement' without losing all their income and reducing their super too quickly.

After 60, people who want to go part-time or casual can consider using a TTR income stream from their superannuation fund. Or, if they're over 65, they can simply put their super into the retirement phase and start drawing on it while they continue to work – without conditions.

SHIFTING TO A PORTFOLIO LIFE

The concept of a portfolio life is relatively new, and one of my favourites. It's likely sprouting from the more flexible workforce that has emerged over the last 10–15 years, with many people looking to juggle a selection of different projects they are passionate about in their 40s, 50s, 60s and even 70s in an attempt to build a more fulfilling life. This can mean mixing part-time work, consulting, volunteering and even starting a small business. The way people build out their portfolio can vary widely.

At the professional end, people from corporate backgrounds often create a portfolio of activities that reflect their skills, networks and ambitions. This might include serving on boards, taking up consulting roles, or pursuing projects that align with their expertise and passions.

At a grassroots level, the concept is much the same, although it looks a little different. People might blend a part-time job with a passion project or side hustle, while also dedicating time to volunteering or a cause they care about. It's about designing variety into their work–life mix and finding a balance that suits them.

For non-professionals, a portfolio life is just as attainable. Many people in hands-on roles such as nursing, trades, or other practical careers don't necessarily leave their industries behind. Instead, they add to their portfolio by branching into areas such as teaching, mentoring or community leadership. By sharing their real-world expertise, they inspire and shape the next generation while building new layers to their working life. For many, teaching or mentoring is just one component of their broader portfolio, sitting alongside hobbies, volunteering or part-time work.

A portfolio life can be a terrific way to transition toward retirement because it offers exposure to different social networks, perhaps seeing you take on unpaid as well as paid activities that lean into your passions. It usually allows you time to start seeking out your interests more actively than you have in your working years.

People who don't like uncertainty can find the first phases of shifting into a portfolio life quite gut-wrenching. This discomfort is not uncommon, and it's something you need to work through. Remember that if you're proactive, then over time you'll find things you love doing and new ways of making money. But to get going, you have to trust yourself to make it work and put the effort in. You also need a financial buffer.

Finally, I want to point out that saying no is just as important in a portfolio life as saying yes – as is being aware of why you're doing what you do. Is it for the money, the learnings, the people you get to work with or the passion of it all? Remember, this is a choose-your-own-adventure style of life, so you want the ability to choose.

CONSULTING OR STARTING A SMALL BUSINESS

Your Prime Time doesn't have to be a period where you pull back. In fact, it can be a wonderful time to embrace your independence, your skills and your ability to do more.

Many people start businesses in their late 40s, 50s and 60s, looking to use and share what they know on their terms. Consulting or starting your own business can give you the independence you've been craving and the flexibility you've been looking for. It's a way to stay active in your field, explore a passion project, or even turn a hobby into a new career. It can be part of setting yourself up for a portfolio life, or it can be a full-blown focus for years to come.

RETIRING, THEN RETURNING TO THE WORKFORCE

The wonderful thing about modern retirement is that it doesn't have to be permanent. Many of the people I speak to have made two, three or four attempts at retiring. They stop work with the best of intentions, take a break, then realise they are not done yet and they go back for more. Returning to the workforce can bring a new sense of purpose and keep you engaged, whether it's in a familiar role or something completely different.

And the Australian superannuation system doesn't limit you. You can shift your superannuation into the retirement phase once you meet the conditions of release, and you can go back to work later, opening a new accumulation account to put your employer contributions into (you have to keep drawing on your retirement income stream). And there's no age-limit for making employer superannuation contributions.

RETIRING AND PICKING UP A PART-TIME JOB

More people are working part-time during retirement than ever before. Employers are embracing it and retirees are enjoying it. In fact, in a recent survey of The Epic Retirement Club, more than 38 per cent of people said they intended to retire, then take up part-time work and another 37 per cent said they thought they'd like to work after retirement – but weren't sure yet.

The fact is that being retired doesn't mean you want to be idle. A part-time job can offer just enough structure and social interaction to keep you engaged, without the demands of full-time work. Plus, it can help supplement your retirement income, allowing for some extra discretionary spending money in those early years.

YOU CAN TECHNICALLY RETIRE – OR YOU CAN 'RETIRE' – UNDERSTAND BOTH OPTIONS

Retirement has two meanings. According to one definition, it is a technical term that means accessing your 'retirement phase of superannuation', where you can draw out funds tax-free and, frankly, if you meet the conditions of release, you can technically retire and pick up work afterward anyway. True retirement can also mean giving up work and shifting gears from a lifestyle perspective. Make sure you understand both concepts and know what you want.

As mentioned earlier, technical retirement is something you do to access your super, tax-free. And you don't have to give up work forever. You can technically retire your super once you reach the 'preservation age' of 60 in Australia. Between the ages of 60 and 65, you have to give up work and have no intent to return to that company – then you complete a form to transfer your superannuation into the retirement phase. It's important to point out that you can take another job after you are technically retired, or you can pick up some full-time, part-time or casual work from your old employer. It just can't be something that's pre-agreed.

Or, you can access your super unconditionally from the age of 65 and keep working.

If you don't want to retire, but you want to access an income stream from your super, allowing you to subsidise going part-time, you might want to explore a TTR account.

> The system is actually really well designed to give you choice and flexibility. You just have to decide how you want to use it.
>
> To 'retire' also has the more traditional definition of 'the action or fact of leaving one's job and ceasing to work'. In this case, you'll likely be looking at your superannuation more closely as a way of fully replacing your income sources. The same conditions apply. Once you reach 60 you can retire and access your super, tax-free. Many people in Australia, particularly those with smaller super balances, have to wait until they are closer to 67, looking to draw an age pension to supplement their superannuation income stream.

RETIRING AND BUILDING A PORTFOLIO OF PURPOSEFUL ACTIVITIES

This is similar to the concept of a portfolio life, but rather than building a portfolio chiefly rotating around more flexible work options, in retirement you're building a portfolio of passions.

Your time is yours, so why not fill it with activities that bring you meaning and joy? Whether it's volunteering, hobbies or spending time with family, this simply becomes the task of curating a life that feels rich and rewarding in ways that go beyond work.

RETIRING AND NEVER WORKING AGAIN

And then there's just retiring – nothing more, nothing less. Maybe you're ready to hang up your hat for good and you don't want any structure, any activities or any level of organisation for a while. Take some time to focus entirely on whatever makes you happiest, including simply enjoying the slower pace of life.

Hopefully by now you can start to see the possibilities for your Prime Time. It's about choosing what suits you best and creating a life that truly feels your own. There are lots of different ways of combining work and lifestyle.

FINDING MORE PURPOSE

Here are some stories of people finding purpose.

Su-en, 50, has recently finished a yoga-teaching course, doing the training over 12 weeks, and completing the lessons each weekend while working in her own dermal fillers and anti-wrinkle business on weekdays. She took the course because she wanted to be more in control of her body, strength and mindfulness, *and* she wanted to build up a sense of purpose outside her day-to-day work that she could use as she gets older. It's now a few months after the course and Su-en is teaching 1–2 classes a week at a local studio, enjoying those new skills. And she's getting paid for her passion too.

Rowena has taken several weeks out of her life in her early 50s, with one week devoted to an intensive meditation retreat as she looks to bring greater mindfulness into her everyday life. Rowena has had a long career in corporate marketing roles, but in her midlife she decided she wanted to change gears and help others in the thick of their lives better navigate their 'why'. After writing two self-help books, she now runs a 'finding your purpose' program, which she says is constantly improving as she learns more about her own mindfulness and meaning in life.

Mike, who had an enormous career in banking and was able to retire from paid work in his mid 50s, found himself taking up a volunteering role in a charity that builds and provides bikes to disabled children. Mike has a huge passion for cycling and a great love of bikes, and finds enormous meaning in his work building and delivering bikes to families that make a real difference to their children's mobility and independence. And the charity is putting his extensive business skills to good use too, asking him to help with their strategic thinking from time to time.

Bradley, a long-time executive at an ASX 20 company, was catapulted into his Prime Time in his late 40s by a family trauma. For years, he had been part of leading 45,000 staff across 42 countries, spending more than half the year on planes. But the trauma shifted his priorities. He wanted more from life than the all-consuming cycle of work, constant global travel and high-stakes management. Determined to build a life aligned with his values, Bradley and his family moved cities and re-established their roots with new schools and communities, and he began exploring roles and projects to create a portfolio life. Before long, he landed a leadership role better suited to his priorities, allowing him to spend more time at home. Alongside this, he started advising impact-driven entrepreneurs and later took on roles as a chairperson supporting the growth of multiple charities related to social development and health care both in Australia and internationally.

This was just the start of a journey into meaningful projects that ultimately led Bradley to become a coach and adviser to both listed and 'for purpose' executives and boards, helping them learn and grow on their own leadership journeys.

3. RECOGNISING YOUR POWER TO GET OFF THE LADDER

In the first half of life, many of us are taught to see work, career and purpose as a ladder that we're constantly climbing, and that not moving up is a failure. As I mentioned earlier, the very wise executive coach I know helps people in the second half of life to look at things with a different perspective, encouraging us to view life as a lattice rather than a ladder.

For much of our lives, work is seen as a ladder we must climb – promotions, pay rises, and titles are all measures of success and we can get hooked on the constant 'approval seeking' and reassurance it provides. But as we approach midlife, the ladder can start to lose its lustre as we recognise we don't need to chase approval anymore if we're somewhat financially secure and can afford to make choices. Instead of striving for the next rung, many of us begin asking, 'Is this even where I want to be?'

Enter the concept of the lattice. Instead of focusing on upward movement, the lattice allows you to explore things that interest you – taking sideways steps, pauses and shifts based on your values, interests and the life you want to create in the next phase.

The lattice mindset gives you permission to redefine success – not as climbing higher but as living authentically and meaningfully and doing things that matter to you.

If it feels right for you, ask yourself:
- What skills could I use differently?
- What roles would feel more aligned with my values?
- Would I be happier working part-time, consulting, teaching or mentoring?

For some, this might mean stepping into a more flexible or less intensive role. For others, it's about downshifting entirely to focus on hobbies, family, or travel – if you can afford to.

ADDRESSING FINANCIAL FEARS

The biggest hesitation for most to getting off the ladder is financial – after all, your 50s and 60s can be your peak earning and saving years. But they can also be the years of greatest choice and adaptation if you have the confidence to lead yourself through the change (rather than being pushed by a late redundancy). A lattice approach encourages creative thinking:
- Could part-time work or consulting bridge the gap to retirement?
- Can a transition to retirement (TTR) income stream supplement your earnings allowing you greater flexibility of work choices – maybe allowing you to take a lower paying role you're more passionate about?
- Are your superannuation and investments ready to support a gradual shift instead of a sudden stop?

FINDING HAPPINESS OFF THE LADDER

Stepping off the ladder opens the door to reconnect with what makes you truly happy. It's not about ticking boxes or meeting others' expectations anymore, it's about showing up for yourself. That can feel foreign for those who are used to striving for achievements and approval. So it helps to be conscious about it, and take time to reflect on:

- What direction feels right for you now?
- How can you use your experience to create something meaningful?
- What would a fulfilling life look like if success was measured by happiness, not status?

When you think of your next stage as a lattice rather than a ladder it can give you freedom to chart your own course – one that aligns with your values, passions and priorities. Maybe it's time to stop climbing and start exploring what you really want. And don't expect the answer to be right in front of you or easy to find – you may have to go looking.

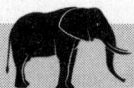

THE ELEPHANTS IN THE ROOM

I have to speak about the elephants in the room. There are three of them, and they all get in the way of living our Prime Time well, limiting or forcing choices. I can't change these for you; I can only help you understand your options. You will always have to navigate the waters you are in.

'I don't have the money to make choices': When I go on radio, people often ring up and say, 'But Bec, what about me! I don't have the money to be able to make epic retirement or prime time lifestyle choices, to take sabbaticals and stop running on the wheel of life. I didn't earn a lot in my career, I don't have a big super fund, and I can't afford to get off the work, get paid, pay bills merry-go-round, not until I get the age pension, and even then, I'll barely have enough to make ends meet. How do I seriously contemplate designing the life I want to live?'

And it's true. We all have to live within our means, building goals and making lifestyle choices we can afford. It's one of the foundations of midlife money management. If you haven't been able to save during your lifetime, then your choices in life are going to be a lot more limited. But please, resist comparing yourself with others, and instead look for things you *can* do.

If you love caravanning, maybe you can save up in midlife and go caravanning around the country, exchanging your rental property for a second-hand van and caravan park fees, and working while you travel to afford the cost of living. Or if you love animals and wish you could have worked with them, maybe you can find an animal charity you can volunteer in on weekends, or do a course to become a wildlife rescuer and contemplate helping injured wildlife, around your work obligations.

The key in midlife is to find little ways to inject purpose, meaning and happiness into your life, even if it's just a light sprinkling, around your tough financial obligations.

'Ageism is going to destroy my options': We all get it – our generation is keen to work longer than those before us. But what about ageism? It's the one social barrier that could stop us from thriving in this prime stage of life. We face the risk of being pushed out of workplaces that undervalue older workers and the experience we bring – long before we're ready.

And let's not forget, we're also at risk of telling ourselves that we're too old to keep learning, too old to keep up, and too old to keep trying. Honestly, that might be the bigger issue. Self-directed ageism is the worst type.

We've got to tackle ageism head-on, just like we're doing with sexism, racism and homophobia, by checking our own behaviours, reactions and words first. Here's how we can start:
- **Check your stereotypes**: When you catch yourself assuming what someone 'can do' or 'wants to do' based on their age, stop and ask them directly instead. You might be surprised. They might be hungry to learn and keen to step up.
- **Challenge that inner voice**: When you hear that little voice telling you you're too old to try something new, recognise it

as self-directed ageism. Remember, that old-world thinking is often based on outdated templates that just don't apply anymore.
- **Call out ageist attitudes**: When your peers, mates or even your kids say someone can't do something because of their age, challenge them. Point out that life expectancy and the opportunities that come with it have changed dramatically since the days when retirement was a brief 6–11 years. Remind them that our templates of the second half of life are broken and shouldn't be used to judge others.

'My workplace won't flex to fit me'

There's a little-known stipulation in Australian workplace laws that requires your employer to offer you flexibility from the age of 55 if they can. There's also a whole lot of other obligations you should be able to rely on from your employer, supported by legislation.

This handy list of the legislation that your employer is required to abide by might help you navigate flexibility more effectively:

- **Age discrimination protection**: Under the *Age Discrimination Act 2004*, employers *must not* discriminate against workers based on age. This includes recruitment, training, promotions and termination of employment.
- ***Fair Work Act* obligations**: The *Fair Work Act 2009* ensures that all employees, regardless of age, are *treated fairly*, with access to the same rights and protections, including leave entitlements, flexible work arrangements and protection from unfair dismissal.
- **Flexible working arrangements**: Workers over 55, or those caring for a family member, *have the right to request flexible working arrangements*, such as reduced hours, job sharing or work-from-home options. Employers must consider these requests and can only refuse them on reasonable business grounds.
- **Workplace health and safety (WHS)**: Employers are required to provide a safe working environment for all employees,

including older workers. This may involve adapting the workplace to accommodate physical needs, such as ergonomic adjustments or providing assistance with physically demanding tasks.
- **Superannuation contributions**: Employers are obligated to continue paying superannuation contributions for older workers. Since 2013, there has been no upper age limit on compulsory super payments.
- **Training and development**: Employers should offer equal opportunities for training and career development for older workers, to ensure they can continue to perform their roles effectively.

Lesson 12
Choose your path out of the workforce

It's worth pointing out that there's no magic warning light that flashes when it's time to start thinking about stepping back from full-time work. That decision is entirely in your hands – or, if you don't make it, your employer might eventually make it for you.

We know that the traditional life template – working full-time until a set 'retirement age' – has been shattered by increased longevity. Now, the real limits come down to a few key factors: how well your body, mind and spirit hold together as you age, how you balance your need for income with the fulfilment you get from your work and how your industry and employer embrace older workers.

But what's often missed in the conversation about retirement is the fact that some of us *still love working*. You might remain curious, driven and deeply interested in what you do, and that's something worth celebrating! Work doesn't have to be a chore as you age; it can continue to challenge you, keep you sharp and bring immense satisfaction.

In fact, staying engaged in work as you age can keep you healthier, mentally and physically. Studies show that people who stay active, curious and continue to learn new things tend to age more gracefully. So if work still excites you, if you're the person who's always up for the next challenge or looking to innovate, there's no reason to walk away unless you're ready.

But I do want you to be in control, understanding your journey through the next phase of working and how you want it to end. It might mean you really stick the landing well when you do retire, one day.

THE DATA TELLS US MOST PEOPLE AREN'T BEING PROACTIVE ENOUGH

The numbers make it clear: most people don't take control of their retirement journey. In Australia, only 31 per cent of people retire by choice. The rest? They're either retrenched or forced into retirement for two major reasons: declining health or needing to care for a loved one. When retirement isn't a conscious decision, it usually comes with fewer options and less control, and it can be much harder to adapt to, both mentally and financially. In fact, many report their ego and their confidence taking a huge hit, damaging the joy of retirement in its early years.

Employers I've spoken with often wish their ageing workforce would be more proactive. Many say they'd prefer employees start seriously considering financial security in midlife, so they have the freedom to explore different options as they approach financial stability. This can mean cutting down hours, changing roles, or even finding new challenges that reignite passion for the work they love. Employers would rather see people making choices based on their interests and goals, not out of necessity or because health issues have forced them to.

It's also worth noting that employers don't want to be in the position of having to push people out due to declining health or an unwillingness to keep up with new skills and technologies. Ideally, they want employees who stay curious, continue learning, and bring that valuable energy and experience to the workplace. In this scenario, you can remain engaged and relevant for as long as it excites you – if you don't become too expensive, which we all know is the other trigger for redundancy.

THINK ABOUT YOUR PRIME TIME AS A WORK–LIFESTYLE CONTINUUM

I like to think of your Prime Time as a continuum, a transition to a new stage of life where you maintain financial independence, gradually moving from active income sources to passive income sources, and getting to choose how to spend your time. For some, this might mean moving away from traditional work altogether fairly quickly, replacing it with other purposeful activities. For others, it could mean staying in the workforce but with the freedom to shift focus or reduce hours to balance other interests.

If work still excites you, it can continue to be a key part of your life. You might take on new projects, mentor younger colleagues, or innovate in areas that keep you engaged. Being passionate about your work doesn't have to end at a certain age, and it's not about fitting into a standard retirement mould. Finding the right balance between work, pursuits, community and family is what allows you to thrive.

As you move along the continuum, you can work less and enjoy more leisure time, but stopping completely doesn't have to be the end goal – unless you want it to be. The modern approach to retirement is far from traditional, and the only 'rules' you have to follow are the ones around accessing your superannuation.

The continuum gives you the flexibility to shape your own path. At one end is the traditional model of full-time work, and at the other is full retirement. But as you move along the spectrum, a range of flexible options open up: part-time work, reduced hours, or arrangements that allow you to focus more on what excites you outside of work. This could mean more time with family, pursuing hobbies, or staying in the workplace with a new role or lighter responsibilities. The choice is yours.

Eventually, you may transition into full retirement, but even then you don't have to disengage from what you love. If you step away and find you miss the structure or stimulation, nothing prevents you from returning in some form. And if you're enjoying your new-found freedom, you can continue scaling back work at your own pace. The continuum is all about finding the right balance – staying curious and active while enjoying the fruits of your hard work.

HOW DO YOU KNOW YOU'RE READY FOR YOUR PRIME TIME?

So how do you know when it's time to start shifting toward your Prime Time and, eventually, your Epic Retirement? It's about being intentional and honest with yourself. Start by assessing where you are physically, mentally and financially. Can you afford to reduce your work income? Are you still enjoying the work you do? Does your role align with your evolving interests and energy levels? Do you feel ready to focus more on personal fulfilment, or are you still excited by the challenge of work?

The key, really, is to have a plan, well before any decision is forced on you. This means setting clear goals for both your financial future and the lifestyle you want to lead in retirement.

It's really important to be proactive when thinking about retirement or transitioning to part-time work, and that starts with assessing your financial readiness, emotional wellbeing and future plans. Here's how to know if you're ready to start shifting gears.

1. YOU'VE WORKED OUT WHEN YOU'LL HAVE 'ENOUGH'

Knowing how much money is enough for you to retire or begin stepping back from full-time work is key. Everyone approaching retirement should know their 'enough number', the amount you need to have invested both inside super and outside super to retire at a lifestyle standard you're comfortable with for the rest of your life – at your target age. As you learned in Lesson 8, this includes understanding your assets, liabilities, cost-of-living budget, and how much you'll need to pursue your prime time goals and, later, your epic retirement dreams.

First, estimate how much income your superannuation can provide once you're relying on it post-retirement. Then, look at the income and capital you can draw from investments outside of super to cover any earlier years. Work out how much you can draw annually and compare it to your lifestyle and living costs.

Next, consider the age pension – will it play a role in your later years? If you're open to working during the early stages of retirement, think about how much income you might earn from flexible or part-time roles.

While many aim to replace 80 per cent of their pre-retirement salary, your personalised budget will give you a clearer figure. This number becomes your guide, helping you plan for those exciting prime time years.

Knowing your options – whether to work, retire, or mix both will give you confidence. It's about creating a flexible plan that supports your lifestyle now and into the future.

2. YOU'VE THOUGHT THROUGH HOW YOUR MONEY WILL WORK IN LATER LIFE

As you transition to part-time work or full retirement, understanding how your income streams work is crucial. You'll need to layer different income sources to create a reliable flow, especially if you're not receiving a regular pay cheque anymore.

For instance, you might decide to access a TTR income stream, drawing up to 10 per cent of your super from the age of 60 while working part-time. Or, if you meet the conditions of release, you can move your super into the retirement phase. The age pension can also supplement your income starting at 67, providing further financial support. And there's still the work that most people can do later in life too.

3. YOU RECOGNISE WHEN YOU'RE FEELING 'DEAD INSIDE' AND ARE READY TO ACT

Some people feel a strong pull toward retirement when they notice they're just going through the motions, doing the job but with no real passion or drive. This is that feeling I discussed earlier, the 'inner death', where the excitement of work fades, nothing ignites your curiosity, and your sense of purpose feels diminished. If work has lost its spark and your routine feels stagnant, this could be a signal that it's time to act on reshaping what you do with your days.

4. YOU'VE BUILT UP OTHER PRIORITIES TO FOCUS ON

It's important to nurture passions outside of work. You've probably met other people in their Prime Times who are living interesting lives, and plenty on the brink of retirement who are buzzing with excitement about upcoming trips, new hobbies and more time with family. They've cultivated interests beyond their careers, making their Prime Time and future retirement something to look forward to rather than a daunting unknown.

Become one of those people by investing in your personal passions early. It's healthy to keep learning and growing. And not all your pursuits should be career-related, because one day, your career won't be the most important part of your life.

5. YOU'RE OPEN TO SLOWING DOWN BUT NOT STOPPING

Retirement today doesn't have to mean stopping work entirely. More people are embracing flexible work arrangements, allowing them to stay engaged without the pressure of full-time work. Government legislation encourages employers to support staff over 55 with flexible options. This gradual transition – working part-time or shifting to more flexible hours – can help you ease into retirement while still maintaining a sense of purpose.

Remember, most employers should benefit from a slow, well-managed transition if they have the right attitude to supporting and engaging their team. It allows them to manage the transfer of knowledge from experienced staff to younger colleagues over time, rather than losing it all in one go.

HOW READY ARE YOU?

Think about whether you're ready to start the shift into a more flexible continuum of work and life by asking yourself these questions:
- Have I calculated my 'enough number'? Do I know when I'll have enough to retire on, and enough to fund the years before I can access my super – if any?

- How will my money work when I'm no longer receiving a full-time pay cheque? Do I understand my investment income, superannuation income and pension options?
- Am I still passionate about my work, or am I simply going through the motions? Has work lost its spark for me?
- What passions and interests outside of work excite me? Am I investing time in those now so that I can lean into them more in retirement?
- Would I prefer to slow down gradually by moving to part-time work or a flexible arrangement rather than retiring outright?

Lesson 13
Rediscover what brings you joy and fulfilment

THE SCIENCE OF HAPPINESS IS FAIRLY NEW. MOST OF THE DISCOVERIES THAT ALLOW us to understand what makes us happy and be more conscious about seeking it have been discovered in the 21st century.

While younger generations have enthusiastically embraced this knowledge, for many older generations, it can seem a bit abstract or even 'woo-woo'. But when you break down the science of happiness, it tells us a lot about how to seek joy in life and it shows us where to start looking if we've lost sight of what makes us happy, which so many people have in their midlife.

HEDONIC HAPPINESS – SAVOURING LIFE'S LITTLE JOYS

Research on happiness, which is scientifically referred to as 'positive psychology', has been spearheaded by pioneers like Martin Seligman and Mihaly Csikszentmihalyi.[30] They have identified a series of core components of wellbeing that we can use as a framework for our own lives, and they say that the pursuit of joy, meaning and purpose has a few layers. One is hedonic happiness, the fleeting and momentary types of happiness that come from chasing immediate moments of joy. If you're out of practice at enjoying life, these can be a good place to start, although remember that hedonism is a temporary feeling that is often costly and doesn't have ongoing benefits.

Here are some things to try:

Indulging in a delicious meal: Eating your favourite comfort food, like a rich dessert or a perfectly cooked steak, can bring immediate satisfaction and pleasure.

Buying a new gadget or piece of clothing: Shopping for something new can give you a burst of dopamine, whether it's a new phone or an outfit you've had your eye on.

Taking a spontaneous vacation: Going on a short, spontaneous trip to an exciting location can create a rush of joy.

Watching a funny movie or binge-watching a series: Laughing at a comedy or getting lost in an engaging TV series can make you feel good in the moment.

Winning a small prize or achieving a minor victory: Whether it's winning a meat tray at the local RSL or beating your personal best in a game, these small victories provide a quick hit of pleasure.

Social media likes or online validation: Receiving positive feedback or 'likes' on social media posts can give you a quick boost of happiness too.

The key to experiencing hedonic happiness is to be truly *in the moment* – mindful of the joy these experiences bring as they happen. It's about appreciating these moments for what they are, without expecting them to create lasting fulfilment.

But while these quick bursts of joy can be fun and even necessary, the science of happiness is clear: true joy and wellbeing aren't just about chasing fleeting pleasures. They're deeply tied to eudaimonic happiness, the kind that comes from a sense of meaning, purpose and personal growth.

EUDAIMONIC HAPPINESS – FINDING MEANING AND PURPOSE

Eudaimonic happiness goes beyond these momentary pleasures. It's about living in alignment with your values, cultivating meaningful relationships, and engaging in activities that contribute to your personal development. This type of happiness leads to deeper satisfaction and a much longer-lasting sense of wellbeing. Here are some ways in which you can explore eudaimonic happiness:

Personal growth: Challenge yourself to learn new skills or take on projects that push your boundaries. Growth gives life a sense of progress and meaning.

Purposeful work: Find purpose in your work, whether that's through a career that aligns with your passions or by mentoring others and sharing your expertise.

Giving back: Volunteering or contributing to your community can foster a deeper sense of purpose. Helping others often brings a more lasting joy than personal achievements alone.

Nurturing relationships: Building and maintaining strong, meaningful relationships with family and friends is a really valuable factor in long-term happiness. These connections give life a sense of belonging and purpose.

While hedonic happiness offers you those delightful moments of pleasure, eudaimonic happiness brings a more profound sense of wellbeing that's tied to living a life that resonates with who you truly are. Balancing both types of happiness allows you to experience life's joys while also building a foundation for long-lasting fulfilment.

SOCIAL OR RELATIONAL HAPPINESS – THE POWER OF CONNECTION

There's a third layer to happiness that is attracting more and more attention from scientists studying longevity, happiness and the power of communities. It's known as social or relational happiness. This form of happiness is created when we have meaningful interactions, shared experiences, and a sense of belonging that comes from being part of a community in which you are valued and nurtured.

As humans, we are inherently social creatures, and there is a growing body of research that shows that strong social connections are one of the most important predictors of long-term happiness and wellbeing. The Harvard Study of Adult Development, one of the longest-running studies of its kind, has been tracking the physical and emotional wellbeing of hundreds of participants for more than 80 years.[31] Its findings are clear: good relationships are the single most important factor in determining both our overall life satisfaction and our longevity. In fact, the study found that people who are more socially connected to family, friends and their community are not only happier, they also live longer, with fewer physical and mental health problems – an important observation we can all learn from. In contrast, in the same studies, loneliness was linked to a decline in both mental and physical health and has been shown to be as harmful as smoking or excessive alcohol consumption.

This idea is further supported by research into the so-called Blue Zones, areas of the world where people live significantly longer and healthier lives.[32] Researchers like Dan Buettner have studied regions such as Okinawa in Japan and Sardinia in Italy where centenarians – people who live beyond 100 years – thrive. One of the common traits in these communities is the strength of their social ties. People in Blue Zones often live in close-knit communities, where coming together to socialise is an integral part of daily life. They enjoy shared meals, regular social gatherings, and strong connections that span multiple generations, and all these things contribute to a sense of purpose and belonging.

When we think about our social happiness, there are a few things we need to consider.

FOSTERING DEEPER, HIGHER-QUALITY RELATIONSHIPS

It's not the quantity of friends you have but the quality of your relationships that matters. It's important to have strong, trusting connections with family, close friends and/or a partner. These play a crucial role in how happy and resilient you feel. The Harvard study emphasised that people who felt they could count on others in tough times experienced greater life satisfaction, even in old age.

ENGAGING IN COMMUNITIES

Belonging to a community, whether through hobbies, social or interest groups, or religious or cultural activities, gives each of us a sense of purpose as well as a collective identity. In Blue Zone communities, elders often play important roles, helping to foster a sense of belonging for the wider family and community group, and this sees them maintaining their social networks well into old age.

PRACTISING EMPATHY AND ACTIVE LISTENING

Building stronger relationships means really tuning in to others and how they are feeling too. Practising empathy and being present in your conversations can deepen your bonds with others and make your relationships more meaningful. Studies show that strong emotional bonds, particularly those formed through understanding, care and empathy, are vital for maintaining long-term happiness.

SHARING EXPERIENCES

The joys of life really are multiplied when they are shared. Whether it's enjoying a meal with family, taking a walk with a friend, or working on a common project, sharing experiences with others really does strengthen your social ties and enhance your overall wellbeing. Blue Zones researchers found that the one key reason for the longevity of the residents in these areas is their tendency to prioritise socialising and communal activities as a regular part of life.

Incorporating social or relational happiness into your life doesn't mean you need to make grand gestures. Just have regular, meaningful connections with people that matter. It's about being intentional with your time, surrounding yourself with people who bring out the best in you, and fostering relationships that give you a sense of belonging and purpose. By doing so, you not only boost your happiness but also improve your overall health and longevity.

The real key to happiness, though, according to scientists, is balance: combining hedonic, eudaimonic, and social happiness, and recognising the role each of them plays in creating joy, meaning and a sense of belonging. When you actively cultivate all three, you create a foundation not just for fleeting happiness but a lasting sense of joy and fulfilment.

REDISCOVERING JOY IN WORK

We often tell ourselves that we need to leave work to find real joy in our lives. But for many, work plays a central role in their sense of meaning and purpose. If you're still actively working, it's worth considering how you can align your job with what truly brings you happiness and joy – if you haven't already. Are there opportunities to take on projects that excite you? Can you mentor younger colleagues or shift your focus to areas you're passionate about? Or perhaps, if you're feeling an inner death, you can seek out different ways to use the skills you find put you in 'the zone'.

Happiness science emphasises the importance of autonomy, mastery and purpose in work. If you're able to tweak your role to give you more control over how you spend your time, focus on the skills you enjoy using, and connect your work to a larger sense of purpose, you'll likely find more joy in it.

REMEMBER, FINDING JOY IS AN ONGOING JOURNEY

Finding joy isn't a one-time discovery but an ongoing practice. As you move through life, what brings you joy may change, and that's okay. The key is to stay curious, be open to new experiences, and reconnect with what feels meaningful to you at that point in your life. Science shows us that happiness isn't something we passively wait to have happen to us – it's something we cultivate actively, through our choices, relationships and mindset.

Lesson 14
Look beyond work to hobbies, pursuits and communities

WHEN YOU'RE LYING ON YOUR DEATHBED, YOU'LL NEVER SAY, 'I WISH I'D WORKED more.' But what will you wish you'd done more of? It's an important question to stop and think about in midlife.

On one of my recent epic retirement courses, a really poignant question was asked that I think many of us in midlife can relate to:

'Throughout our lives as parents, friends and workers, many of us give our time to others to help them achieve their goals. When we are no longer needed in these situations, we may have lost sight of our own dreams. Where do we even begin to search for our purpose or find and rekindle forgotten dreams?'

There are a few things most people choose to lean into as they gradually get more selective about the work they want to do:

- Spend more meaningful time with family and closest friends
- Work on projects that give a powerful sense of meaning and purpose
- Prioritise their health
- Devote more time to experiences
- Find some hobbies and pursuits
- Build up communities.

And yet many of us, as we approach midlife and our prime time years, are out of practice on some or all of these things.

If this is you, I want you to reopen yourself up to exploring. You don't have to dive headlong into them all. Take the time to try out different ways of enjoying life more and see what sticks.

It's amazing how uncomfortable people can feel when they stop and look at their current work–lifestyle balance in midlife and start exploring their sense of self all over again. So let me give you some simple, easy to follow instructions for getting started. I call this the midlife kickstart.

THE MIDLIFE-KICKSTART

1. I want you to get an A4 page and divide it into six columns. Then, at the top of each column, I want you to write these words:
   - Family and friends
   - Meaning
   - Health
   - Experiences
   - Hobbies and pursuits
   - Communities.
2. Now I want you to brainstorm 3–5 things you could do to activate each part of your life. There are no right answers, only *your* answers.
3. Now, with a red pen, circle one item on each list that will take the least time to do.
4. Then, with a blue pen, circle the one that you think you will enjoy the most.
5. And finally, identify the activity on each list you want to do most.
6. Now, make some plans to get them started.

   And remember, you don't have to commit forever. See the first phase as experimenting to see what you like doing, and what gives you a rewarding feeling.

HOBBIES, PURSUITS AND COMMUNITIES

Some of this talk about finding your sense of purpose outside of work can feel a bit abstract, so let's break it down to something practical and actionable. As we move into midlife, there are three key areas we can focus on to build a fulfilling life outside of work: hobbies, pursuits and communities. These aren't just nice-to-haves; they're essential for maintaining happiness, personal growth and a sense of connection.

HOBBIES AND PURSUITS

By the time we hit midlife, many of us have lost track of our hobbies, or forgotten how important they can be for our mental wellbeing. In a busy world, hobbies often take a back seat to work, family and life's responsibilities. But hobbies are incredibly valuable.

A hobby is something you do with your time to relax, have fun or simply unwind. Think of it as an activity that brings you joy, like painting, gardening, reading, or playing a musical instrument. It's about enjoying the process, without the pressure to excel or achieve anything more than personal satisfaction. Hobbies are vital for keeping stress levels down and allowing your mind to take a break from life's demands.

Now, let's take that idea a step further with pursuits. I like to think of pursuits as hobbies on steroids. They're more than just activities for fun – they're deeper, more ambitious efforts to grow, learn or accomplish something that matters to you. Pursuits are about pushing yourself further, setting goals and seeking personal fulfilment on a larger scale. They challenge you in ways that hobbies might not, offering a sense of direction and purpose. Fundamental to a pursuit is the idea of investing in growing your knowledge in something and becoming better at it.

For example, gardening might be a relaxing hobby, but turning your garden into a thriving vegetable patch, learning sustainable practices, and even selling your produce at a local market – that's a pursuit. Playing the guitar in your living room for enjoyment is a hobby; practising regularly, composing music and perhaps performing at a local event transforms it into a pursuit.

While hobbies help you unwind, pursuits push you toward growth and mastery. They give you something bigger to strive for – a project, a challenge or a passion that ignites your curiosity and keeps you moving forward.

REDISCOVERING HOBBIES IN MIDLIFE

For many, rediscovering hobbies can feel like reconnecting with something you lost along the way. The busy pace of life often crowds out these smaller joys, but they're essential for your wellbeing. If you're not sure where to start, ask yourself what used to make you happy before life got too busy. Did you enjoy sketching, fishing, cooking or collecting? These are the kinds of activities that can still bring you joy, especially if you carve out time for them again.

You can also explore new hobbies. Maybe you've always wanted to learn photography or ceramics, or take up hiking. The beauty of hobbies is that there's no pressure to perform or be the best; they're for your enjoyment and relaxation, nothing more.

FINDING PURSUITS

Pursuits, on the other hand, are those activities that demand more focus and ambition. They're hobbies taken to the next level, where you set goals and push yourself to grow in a meaningful way. Pursuits often give you a sense of purpose because they're about progress, achievement and fulfilment.

For example, maybe you've always loved writing, but instead of keeping a private journal, you decide to start working on a novel, join a writing group or take a creative writing class. You've moved from a casual hobby to a pursuit that challenges and stretches you.

The key with pursuits is that they provide a sense of growth. They ask more of you and often involve learning something new or working toward a specific goal. You can think of pursuits as projects or passions that require dedication and effort, but offer deep satisfaction in return.

FINDING COMMUNITY

Community is really the third leg of the stool when it comes to happiness and fulfilment. You can fill your days with hobbies, but without a sense of connection, something will always feel like it's missing. The best way to build those connections is often through your pursuits.

Communities provide support, shared interests and a sense of belonging. Most members are active participants, meaning they share your passion and commitment, which leads to genuine connections and great conversations.

We're wired for connection, and research like the Harvard Study of Adult Development and that done on Blue Zones show that people with strong social ties are not only happier, they also live longer, healthier lives. Whether it's a local book club, running group or community garden, being part of something bigger than yourself fulfils that deep human need for connection.

If you're transitioning out of work, don't let your social life fade. Be proactive – join groups that align with your passions or reconnect with old friends. These communities offer not just companionship but also help support your mental and emotional wellbeing.

Looking for inspiration? Here are some examples of how hobbies can grow into pursuits and communities.

Running – Hit trails or streets solo for a hobby. Or pursue a run club, triathlons or marathon running locally or all over the world.	**Tennis** – Play matches with friends, or as a pursuit, join a local club and play competitions.
Cycling – Take long solo rides for a hobby, or pursue in a cycle group, charity rides or expedition cycling trips.	**Golf** – Hit the course with a group of friends, or join a club and play routinely, and perhaps even put your name down for tournaments.
Painting – Express creativity in your own space for a hobby. Or take classes and look for ways to build your artistic talents as a pursuit.	**Cooking classes** – Learn new recipes and cook for friends, or, as a pursuit, take cooking classes to become a master baker or specialist in a type of cooking you love.
Meditation – Find peace and focus by yourself as a hobby, or go on meditation retreats, seek out new practices from gurus, or even travel overseas to learn in other cultures.	**Handywork and renovation** – Enjoy the handiwork around the house, or buy a 'renovator's dream' property, do it up and either enjoy it or sell it for a profit as a pursuit.

Photography – Capture landscapes or urban shots alone as a hobby, or study photography and join a photography club – make it a pursuit.	**Book clubs** – Chat with others about the latest reads, or lead the way with your own group.
Crosswords – Challenge your mind with puzzles, or learn about cryptic crossword processes and challenge yourself with more and more difficult ones.	**Sailing lessons** – Try sailing with a twilight sail at your local club, usually offered weekly. Or pursue it by taking sailing lessons and joining a local sailing club.
Workouts – Get fit at your own pace, or join a gym, group fitness classes, or see a personal trainer to make it a pursuit.	**Crafting** – Take up crochet, knitting, scrapbooking and other handy crafts. Or pursue crafts in a club with others who teach and help you improve your skills.
Journalling – Reflect and write personal thoughts as a hobby. Or consider publishing your journals as a blog or as opinion articles to take it to the next level.	**Build tracks and play with model trains** – There are clubs of passionate train lovers you can visit or join. You can also invest in your trains and build a peer community.
Fishing – Enjoy the calm of solo fishing trips. Or make it a pursuit by joining a club or finding a group of friends who want to fish regularly and improve their catch.	**Learn a new language** – Take up Duolingo lessons, or pursue it further by joining a language school and attending classes to allow you to find a peer group.
Yoga or Pilates classes – Practice mindfulness in a group setting. Or, as a pursuit, seek out advanced levels of yoga and Pilates, or even learn to teach it.	**Music** – Learn an instrument or sing regularly, or as a pursuit, take lessons, join a band or choir, and perform for audiences.

Lesson 15
Recognise transitions and embrace the journey they offer

Most of us have faced significant life changes, whether it's a divorce, redundancy, serious illness, moving out of the family home, or the loss of a loved one. These events bring abrupt endings to things that were once meaningful, and the more attached we were, or the less prepared we felt, the more deeply the impact hits us. This often leaves us feeling unsettled for two reasons:

1. **Change makes us uncomfortable**: Humans are creatures of habit, and change throws us into unfamiliar territory, which naturally causes discomfort.
2. **Loss creates a void**: When something we value is suddenly gone, it leaves a gap in our lives, and most of us struggle with the uncertainty of how, or if, we can fill it again.

We feel an emotional turmoil from sudden loss, and that is intensified by the need to adapt, often before we feel ready to. Recognising that these feelings are normal is the first step in moving forward.

THE BRIDGES TRANSITION MODEL

There's a great set of theories about transitions in life that can act as a template for navigating change, both emotionally and practically. The concept of transitioning was coined by social scientist and author

William Bridges in the 1980s, and to this day it is used to explain the way we cope, adapt and grow when faced with change.[33] His theories underpin common change-management practices in business, as well as guiding us during major upheavals in our personal lives. They're a good way to turn feelings and emotions into a more logical process we can understand and somewhat predict.

Bridges' theory says we all go through transitions – increasingly more noticeable ones in mid and later life – and that the experience of a transition can be mapped into three parts.

1. THE ENDING

This is the initial stage, where you're letting go of something familiar, whether it's a job, a relationship or a way of life. Even if the change is positive or necessary, the ending often comes with feelings of loss, uncertainty or resistance. It's a time of acknowledging that a chapter is closing and learning to detach from the old ways. Recognising where you are at this stage is important. You need to be able to process the emotions that come with endings before you can prepare for what's next. And until you've properly accepted the ending, you'll probably find it hard to move into the next phase.

2. THE MIDDLE ZONE

The second phase is the middle zone, sometimes also called the 'neutral zone', the in-between phase where you've left the old behind but haven't yet fully embraced the new. It's often a time of confusion, discomfort and uncertainty as things feel unsettled and unclear. But it's also a stage of reflection and creativity. In the middle zone, you're exploring new ideas, testing possibilities and slowly shaping the next steps. When you're in it, things can feel chaotic, and you can feel quite lost, eager to move forward but unable to make sense of it. Despite this, it's an essential time for growth and transformation.

3. THE NEW BEGINNINGS

The final stage of transition is where you start to emerge into a new reality. This is when you begin to embrace a new identity, direction, relationship or way of life. There's a sense of renewal, motivation and energy as you move forward with fresh goals and purpose. The new beginning comes from successfully navigating the earlier stages, and it brings a sense of clarity about where you're headed and what's important to you.

When we look at these in relation to our Prime Time, we can find they apply to life in a number of ways.

Our Prime Time can be a series of transitions, as we consciously create endings in our lives so that we can choose new directions and make new beginnings. We might find ourselves leaving a corporate role to give ourselves space to start a business, take up further study or make more time for passion projects.

Just as commonly, we can find ourselves grappling with endings that happen to us, outside our control, causing us to rethink and reshape our lives. Whether it's the breakdown of a marriage, the death of a loved one, being laid off, giving up work to become a carer for a loved one, or the ending of a business, each can leave you wondering about what comes next, with trepidation.

Consider Linda's experience. She was a 54-year-old marketing executive who was living what she thought was a pretty stable life. She had a successful career, a comfortable home and two grown children who had moved out. But when her company went through a major restructure, Linda was made redundant after 25 years in the same industry. It hit her hard. Suddenly, the two roles that had defined much of her adult life were gone, and with it, her sense of purpose and identity.

At first, Linda resisted the idea that this was an 'ending'. She tried to brush it off, telling herself that she'd just find another job and get back on track in the same industry pretty easily. But as weeks turned into months, Linda found herself stuck in the first stage of transition. She was grieving the loss of her professional identity and struggling to detach from what had once been so familiar. Every rejection of a job application deepened her sense of loss. But she didn't want to change – she wanted to find a similar role in a similar space.

During this time, Linda started to recognise that the end of her job was more than just losing work – it was the beginning of a bigger life shift. She realised she was entering a transition, even if she didn't feel ready. It was uncomfortable, but knowing this was a normal part of change helped her start to accept the process.

After months of feeling unsettled, Linda entered the 'neutral zone', where you've let go of the old but haven't quite found the new. It was a confusing time. She had no clear direction, but with some encouragement from a career coach, Linda allowed herself the space to explore. She tried freelance work, took a short course on interior design, and even rekindled her love of painting – something she hadn't done since her 20s.

In the middle zone, she really did feel like she was spinning her wheels sometimes, unsure of what the future held. But slowly, as she experimented and reflected, she began to see new possibilities emerging. She realised she didn't want to return to corporate life. Instead, she found herself drawn to using her marketing skills in a way that aligned with her creative interests and her values.

Finally, after about a year of feeling lost and uncertain, Linda reached what Bridges describes as 'the new beginnings'. She embraced her new identity as a freelance consultant and started helping small businesses with branding and marketing while also carving out time for her artistic pursuits, building a portfolio life. This new chapter brought a sense of excitement and energy that she hadn't expected, along with clarity about the life she wanted to lead moving forward.

Linda's journey is a perfect example of how transitions, though painful and uncomfortable at times, *can* lead to growth and new beginnings. Her story reminds us that our Prime Time can be filled with a series of transitions – some we choose, and others that are thrust upon us. What matters is recognising where we are in the process and embracing the journey, even when it feels uncertain.

THINK ABOUT HOW YOU HANDLE TRANSITIONS

Take a moment to reflect on how you've navigated previous transitions in your life. Can you pinpoint moments of significant upheaval where you had to face an ending, uncover new opportunities and eventually commit to a fresh direction? Consider how you embraced these changes and what they taught you along the way, and how you might do it next time.

- How have I navigated significant life transitions in the past?
- What challenges did I face during those times, and how did I overcome them?
- What lessons did I learn from those transitions that I can apply now?
- Were there any unexpected positive outcomes or instances of growth that resulted from past changes?
- What transitions or changes do I anticipate in the near future, either by choice or circumstance?
- How can I prepare emotionally, mentally and practically for those upcoming changes?
- What values or priorities do I want to guide me as I move into future transitions?

Lesson 16
Remind yourself that curiosity, learning and flexibility are crucial

DAVID AND LOUISE, TWO EXPERIENCED BANKERS IN THEIR EARLY 50S, WORKED IN the same department of a large financial institution. Both had been with the bank for decades, but when the industry began adopting new fintech innovations, like blockchain, AI-driven customer service and automated operational systems, their responses couldn't have been more different.

David had built his career the traditional way: face-to-face client relationships, manual processes, and relying on his deep understanding of the old systems and interpersonal connections. When the bank started rolling out new technology, David resisted. He avoided learning about advanced digital banking platforms, ignored the shift toward data analytics, and scoffed at the rise of AI in customer service. 'This tech stuff is just a phase. It'll fail and then we can get back to doing it the right way,' he'd say, confident that his tried-and-true methods would continue to serve him well. When the bank pushed for more employees to adopt these new tools, David dug in his heels, refusing politely to adjust to the new workflows or to be curious about the skills he might need as the business changed.

Eventually, the bank underwent a digital transformation, prioritising tech-savvy employees who could navigate the new fintech landscape. David, who had avoided upskilling, was laid off during a round of redundancies. His refusal to embrace change and adopt new technology left him on the outside, despite his years of experience and his loyalty.

Louise had started in banking around the same time as David and had a similarly strong foundation in traditional banking and customer service. But when the digital revolution came to their industry, she saw it as an opportunity rather than a threat. Louise eagerly took every training session the bank offered, learning about AI, data analytics and even blockchain applications. She also explored fintech courses in her spare time, recognising that the future of banking lay in technology, and got involved in an emerging practice groups.

Her willingness to embrace learning and adapt to the changes positioned Louise as a leader in the digital transformation within her department. When others struggled to adjust, she was promoted to a senior role, overseeing the bank's shift toward integrating tech with traditional services. Louise's openness to change kept her career thriving while others were left behind.

We all know someone like David and someone like Louise. They might be in a different industry, or even in a different phase of life. But their experiences are just one example of how resistance to change, lack of curiosity and inflexibility in life can have serious consequences for the way we get to participate in the future.

David's story is one of missed opportunities – not because he wasn't skilled or experienced, but because he clung to the past and failed to stay relevant. Louise, by contrast, saw the changes as a chance to grow, and that mindset opened up new doors for her.

This isn't just a lesson for the workplace; it extends far beyond that. Think about the people you enjoy spending time with. Are they the ones stuck in old ways, resistant to new experiences and ideas? Or are they the ones who embrace learning, are curious about life and are open to change? The people who remain curious, flexible and willing to learn are often the ones who stay dynamic, engaged and fun to be around, whether they're your colleagues, friends or family members.

In our fast-paced world, adaptability is not just a professional asset, it's a personal one too. If we stop learning and growing, we can quickly become out of touch, not only in our careers but also in how we relate to others and play our role in society.

Ultimately, the world is evolving, and so must we – inside and outside the workplace.

I think there are three fundamental values we need to approach midlife with if we want to get the most out of it. These are things that if we lived 50 years earlier might not have been a priority for us. But remember, those templates of life are broken. The values are:
1. Lifelong learning
2. Curiosity and courage
3. Structure and flexibility.

1. LIFELONG LEARNING

It frustrates me when I hear people in midlife saying, 'I'm too old to go back and learn new things,' or, 'I don't want to learn anymore. I know enough. I'm ready to get off the wheel'. I just want to give them a big hug and say, 'But you've got so much life ahead of you! If you stop learning now, what will your world become?'

We've got to keep finding ways to learn and grow throughout our lives. Sure, what we're learning and how we grow may change over time, and our interests might shift too. But the act of learning is key. It's not just about picking up new skills for work; it's also about evolving mentally, emotionally and even spiritually. It's about developing our interests and passions, staying curious about the world.

Whether it's taking up a new hobby, diving deeper into a pursuit you love, travelling to places where you learn along the way, or simply reading more widely, lifelong learning expands our minds. It makes us more empathetic, more interesting, and more engaged with the world around us. It gives us things to talk about, to think about, to enjoy. Honestly, I can't imagine life without it.

When we toss out the outdated templates that suggest we stop learning and begin to decline in the second half of life, it's time to reconsider our attitude toward learning. For many, learning in the first half of life is seen as formal, structured through school, university or vocational training, all with a focus on building skills and knowledge to improve career prospects.

But as people approach what they perceive to be the end of their career, they often relax and, in many cases, stop learning altogether. They forget or fail to recognise that life is long, and the latter years of your working life can be filled with renewed energy, creativity and initiative – if you choose to embrace it. More importantly, the years after you finish working are also significant, and without continued learning or stimulation, they can easily become stagnant or even dull.

The question is, what will you learn about, and where will you invest your intellectual energy? In the second half of life, you have an incredible range of choices. I like to break it down into three main areas:

1. **Formal education**: Don't think formal education is only for the young. Many people return to university or enrol in formal qualifications later in life, pursuing subjects they've always been interested in but never had the time to study. And universities are interested in building whole-of-life education. In fact, some of the world's biggest universities have launched some really interesting lifelong learning platforms worth exploring.
2. **Courses and personal development**: Whether it's a short course, a workshop or professional training, investing in your personal development can open new doors and ignite new passions. This could include anything from public speaking to creative writing, financial management, learning a new language, board-level management skills or small business skills.
3. **Prime time pursuits**: These are those activities that go beyond hobbies that we learned about in the last section. Prime time pursuits are about deepening your knowledge and skills in something that truly excites you. Whether it's learning a language, becoming a master in gardening, or diving into

music, financial literacy, art or languages, the goal is to invest in your own personal growth because you want to, and because it makes you feel good.

Lifelong learning is about keeping your curiosity alive, staying mentally engaged and continually challenging yourself. The second half of life presents the opportunity to learn what truly interests you – not for career advancement, but for personal growth and joy.

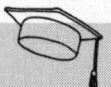

LIFELONG LEARNING OPTIONS ARE BROADER THAN YOU MIGHT THINK

Short-course university programs: Some universities have developed dedicated short-course programs for lifelong learners, allowing you to study non-degree courses that pique your interest without the pressure of exams or grading. Institutions around the world, from Australia to the UK and the US, offer these options online, so the possibilities are virtually endless. Some rather cool examples include:

- Oxford University – Creative Writing Summer School, and Philosophy and Ethics
- Harvard University – Harvard Extension School – Introduction to Data Science, and Modern Masterpieces of World Literature
- University of Sydney – Centre for Continuing Education – History of the World in 100 Objects, and Introduction to Psychology
- Stanford University – Stanford Online – The Science of Well-Being, and Introduction to Innovation and Entrepreneurship
- Monash University – FutureLearn – Mindfulness for Wellbeing and Peak Performance, and Food as Medicine.

Workshops and online courses: Platforms like Udemy, Coursera and LinkedIn Learning offer a range of courses on everything from creative writing to coding to emotional intelligence. These courses are usually more practical and hands-on, helping you immediately apply what you learn. And they're usually quite affordable. You could also seek out speciality courses in your local community or interest area.

Self-improvement and professional growth programs: When I talk about personal development, I include doing workshops, seminars or programs that are designed to help you grow – professionally and personally. This could mean attending a leadership workshop, learning to improve your public-speaking skills, or joining a workshop on finding fulfilment in your 50s.

Health and wellbeing: Courses on mindfulness, nutrition and fitness also fall under personal development, helping you stay physically and mentally healthy as you navigate your Prime Time. These can help you live a longer, better-quality life.

Financial confidence: Knowing your retirement is ahead of you, understanding the financial frameworks you should have in place and understanding how money works in that phase are important. Consider courses and workshops that can help you.

University programs: Of course, there's also the option to go back to university and pursue a degree, postgraduate qualification or professional certification. Universities offer programs specifically for mature students, with flexible learning schedules and online options.

2. CURIOSITY AND COURAGE

Curiosity might seem like an abstract idea, but it's a real, practical driver of how we learn, grow and engage with the world. When we're curious, we open ourselves up to new ideas, perspectives and possibilities. It's what gets us asking questions, exploring different paths, and starting conversations that challenge what we know. But curiosity isn't just about thinking – it's the first step toward doing. It's what pushes us to try something new, to step outside our comfort zones and explore fresh opportunities.

CURIOSITY: THE STARTING POINT FOR ACTION

Curiosity works by activating our brain's reward system. When we're interested in something, we get a dopamine hit, making us feel good and motivating us to keep exploring. This sense of reward keeps us asking questions and diving deeper into things that catch our attention. Plus, because curiosity engages the hippocampus, the part of the brain responsible for memory, we're more likely to remember and apply what we learn when we're genuinely curious.

People often ask me how you build curiosity. Well, it's a progressive process with two key steps:

1. Start small: Asking simple questions about things you normally wouldn't. Dive into a new topic that piques your interest, no matter how random it seems, and see what captures your attention and makes you want to go deeper.
2. Look more widely: Try reading about unfamiliar subjects or talking to people with different perspectives and sparking conversations about things you wouldn't always find yourself talking about. This will keep your curiosity active and open new pathways of learning.

Once curiosity sparks, it naturally builds momentum. The more we explore, the more motivated we become to keep going, creating a cycle of learning and growth. See if you can recognise how the dopamine powers you and your interests once curiosity strikes.

COURAGE: TURNING IDEAS INTO ACTION

While curiosity gets us thinking, courage is what gets us doing. Courage isn't about being fearless. Rather, it's about taking action in the face of fear. It's what helps us step forward, even when we're unsure or nervous.

In your brain, the amygdala processes fear, sending out signals when something feels risky. But courage activates the prefrontal cortex, allowing you to assess situations rationally and push through those fear signals. Over time, the more you practise courage, the easier it becomes to step outside your comfort zone. This is where neuroplasticity comes into play – the brain's ability to rewire itself. By continually acting courageously, you train your brain to become less fearful of the unknown.

SOME SIMPLE WAYS TO WORK ON YOUR COURAGE

- **Take small steps**: Start with manageable risks. Whether it's trying something new or speaking up in a meeting, each small act of courage builds confidence.
- **Visualise what success looks like**: Imagine what it looks like when you succeed. Learn to picture the positive outcomes you want to have to lower your anxiety. When you focus on potential rewards instead of fears, it becomes easier to act.
- **Be kind to yourself**: Courage isn't about being perfect but about trying. Even if things don't go as planned, celebrate that you took the step forward, learned from the experience and were able to take those learnings forward into your next decisions.

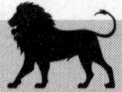

FEAR, COURAGE AND THE BRAIN'S FIGHT-OR-FLIGHT RESPONSE

In the days of our primitive ancestors, the brain's fight-or-flight response was crucial for survival. Imagine a caveman confronted by a dangerous predator, like a sabre-toothed tiger. The brain's amygdala would kick in immediately, triggering the fight-or-flight response to prepare the body to either defend itself or run. The prefrontal cortex would assess the situation logically, helping the caveman decide whether to fight, flee or find another solution.

Fast forward to today, and while we no longer face sabre-toothed tigers, our brains still react the same way to perceived threats. The amygdala can trigger fear in situations like career

> changes, financial uncertainty or starting something new. The feeling of fear may make you want to retreat or avoid taking action, just like running from a predator.
>
> But that's where your prefrontal cortex comes into play. It helps you assess the situation rationally, considering your options and allowing you to overcome the initial fear response. Courage isn't about eliminating fear; it's about allowing the prefrontal cortex to take the lead, so you can make decisions that move you forward despite feeling nervous or uncertain.

When you combine curiosity and courage, you create a powerful duo. Curiosity opens the door by sparking ideas and leading you toward new possibilities. Courage gets you through that door, helping you take those ideas and turn them into real action. Together, they allow you to break out of routines, try new things, and grow in ways you might not have imagined.

3. STRUCTURE AND FLEXIBILITY

As we move into midlife, a lot of the things that used to give our days structure, like work schedules or raising kids, start to fade. That can leave you feeling a bit aimless. But there's actually some solid science behind why building a new structure, while keeping flexible, is important to staying engaged and feeling good.

WHY YOUR BRAIN NEEDS STRUCTURE

Our brains love routine and predictability, especially when there's change happening around us. The part of your brain that handles decision-making and planning – the prefrontal cortex – relies on structure to keep things running smoothly. Without it, you can end up feeling mentally overloaded because your brain is constantly trying to figure out what's next. Structure gives your brain a clear roadmap, which means less stress and fewer decisions to make on the fly.

For example, having a routine like regular exercise, a weekly catch-up with friends or a financial plan keeps you grounded and feeling in control. Studies have shown that people with a bit of structure in their lives tend to feel less anxious and more focused. It's like giving your brain some breathing room so you're not always scrambling.

WHY FLEXIBILITY IS JUST AS IMPORTANT

At the same time, you've got to stay flexible. Life throws curveballs, whether it's health issues, changes in relationships or shifts in your financial situation. Being flexible is all about keeping your brain adaptable, which is something it's wired for.

Your brain's ability to adapt is thanks to neuroplasticity, which means it can rewire itself when new challenges come up. Staying open to changes and continuing to stimulate your brain, whether that's adjusting your plans, trying something completely new or simply exercising it, helps keep your brain sharp. Research shows that people who work on their neuroplasticity tend to handle stress better and are more resilient when life doesn't go to plan.[34]

FINDING THE BALANCE

The trick is finding a balance between structure and flexibility. Too much structure, and you might feel trapped in a routine that doesn't allow for spontaneity or new opportunities. Too much flexibility, and you can end up feeling lost or unproductive.

So build enough structure to keep you on track, whether that's sticking to a budget, setting health goals or making time for hobbies. But leave space to adjust when life shifts. Maybe your fitness plan needs tweaking because of a new health issue, or your financial goals shift as priorities change. Flexibility lets you adapt without losing sight of what's important.

Practical ways to balance structure and flexibility include the following:
- **Set daily or weekly goals**: Even in midlife, having goals for your week (exercise, social connections, financial tasks) gives you a sense of purpose and keeps your routine grounded.
- **Create a loose routine**: Structure your days with key activities but allow for flexibility. For example, schedule exercise or

self-care, but leave afternoons open for spontaneous plans or downtime.
- **Plan for adjustments**: Recognise that life changes, and so your structure should too. Check in monthly to see if your routines and goals need tweaking based on your current priorities.
- **Embrace new opportunities**: Don't get too stuck on 'the plan'. If a new opportunity or challenge arises, assess how it fits into your life. Be willing to adapt while still keeping your main goals in focus.
- **Keep experimenting**: In this phase, it's about experimenting with new ways to structure your life. Try new hobbies and pursuits, ways to stay active, or projects that excite you. Stay curious, and don't be afraid to adjust your structure as you go.

Activity 1
YOUR WORK AND YOUR PURPOSE

With all that theory behind us, it's time to get practical about assessing whether you are getting enough of a sense of purpose from what you do at work, or whether you need change. I have a simple process you can work through. You just need to set aside 20–30 minutes in a quiet space where you can focus and reflect.

STEP 1: RATE YOUR CURRENT JOB SATISFACTION
On a scale of 1 to 10 (1 being completely unsatisfied and 10 being completely fulfilled), rate your current level of job satisfaction. Don't overthink it – just write down the first number that comes to mind.

STEP 2: REFLECT ON THE FOLLOWING QUESTIONS
Write down your answers to these questions on a piece of paper:
- What aspects of my work do I enjoy most?
- Are there parts of my job that bring me a sense of purpose or joy?
- Do I feel appreciated and valued in my current role?
- Am I learning and growing in this position, or do I feel stagnant?
- How does my job align with my values and long-term goals?

STEP 3: IDENTIFY SIGNS OF CHANGE
Now let's think about whether your work might need a change:

Think about your energy levels: Do you feel energised or drained at the end of most workdays? Constantly feeling drained could be a sign of burnout or misalignment.

Think about your sense of passion versus your sense of obligation: Are you working because you're passionate about what you do or simply out of obligation? If it's more of an obligation, think about what might reignite your enthusiasm.

Contemplate your sense of challenge and growth: Does your job challenge you in a meaningful way, or do you feel like you're coasting? Lack of growth can indicate it's time to look for new opportunities.

Think about how your job connects you to your sense of purpose: Does your job connect with something meaningful to you? If your work feels detached from your personal purpose, it might be time to realign your career with your values.

STEP 4: DECIDE ON THE ACTIONS YOU WANT TO TAKE

Look back over your reflections and make a decision on whether your current job is fulfilling you, or if you need to make some changes. Consider the following actions:

- **If you're satisfied**: Celebrate what's working and consider how you can continue to grow in this role.
- **If change is needed**: Identify one small step you can take toward finding more joy and purpose in your work. This could involve upskilling, looking for a new role, or having a conversation with your manager about ways to make your current job more fulfilling.

STEP 5: PUT A NOTE IN YOUR DIARY

Set a reminder in your diary to revisit your reflections in a month. Sometimes when you look back, you can see how reflecting has, over time, shifted your feelings, and whether taking small actions, or even just noticing your sense of purpose, has improved your job satisfaction at all.

Activity 2
RECLAIMING AND REFRAMING YOUR IDENTITY

As we enter our Prime Time, our identity naturally evolves. It's a time to reflect on who we are now, re-evaluate our goals and values, and choose learning goals and pursuits that align with our current passions and interests. This activity will guide you through practical steps to reframe (or reclaim) your identity, embracing curiosity and lifelong learning as key tools for growth.

It's easy to get caught up in the roles we've played over the years: a parent, a worker, a professional, a partner. Now it's time to step back and reflect on *who you are today* – just you. Ask yourself the following questions.

WHO AM I NOW, OUTSIDE OF THE ROLES I'VE PLAYED?
Write down words or phrases that come to mind.

_____

_____

_____

HAVE YOUR PASSIONS, INTERESTS OR EVEN DISLIKES CHANGED OVER TIME?
Embrace the idea that who you are is fluid and can evolve as you move through your Prime Time.

_____

_____

_____

Activity 3

RE-EVALUATE YOUR GOALS AND VALUES, AND RECOGNISE IT'S TIME TO GROW

Your goals and values may have shifted fundamentally from what they were in your 30s or 40s, and that's perfectly fine. This stage of life is about realigning your pursuits with what's important to you now.

Here's another exercise to help you explore the shift:
1. Get a piece of paper.
2. Create two columns. In one, list your core values (for example, integrity, creativity, family, freedom, adventure, learning).
   In the other, list your current goals, the things you want to achieve in your life. Do they align? If not, think about how you can adjust your goals to better reflect your values.

A good tip: Values like time, autonomy or experiences may take priority in Prime Time, so ensure your goals reflect these shifts.

Core values	Goals

Activity 4
CHOOSING AND BUILDING PRIME TIME PURSUITS THAT ALIGN WITH YOUR VALUES AND INTERESTS

Now that you've re-evaluated your values, it's time to build a life that aligns with them. Prime time pursuits can range from career changes and hobbies to community involvement and personal growth.

- Get another piece of paper, divide it into two columns, and mark the first 'Ideas' and the second 'Actions'.
- Brainstorm 3–5 activities or pursuits that excite you and align with your values. Ask yourself this question: 'What do I want to explore, achieve or experience in the next few years?'
- Now complete the action column with the first action you can take to self-start. Thing about taking a small step toward one of these pursuits, whether it's enrolling in a course, joining a new group, or simply dedicating time each week to a passion project.

Ideas	Actions

Activity 5
CURIOSITY AND LIFELONG LEARNING ARE CRITICAL

One of the best ways to stay engaged and fulfilled in Prime Time is through lifelong learning. Curiosity opens doors, introduces you to new ideas and keeps your mind active.

In this exercise, I want to challenge you to learn something new each month. It could be a skill, a hobby, or even a small subject area you've always been curious about.

- I want you to identify the first thing you are going to learn in the first month.
- Then set a diary alert for one month's time and explore and reflect on your learning process.
- How does learning something new make you feel?
- Does it reignite a sense of wonder or accomplishment?
- Now think about making a monthly learning objective. What will you learn next?

Part 4
HEALTH

THERE ARE PLENTY OF REASONS – PHYSICAL, EMOTIONAL AND MENTAL – WHY prioritising our health during midlife is essential. For some, it's about wanting to live long, energetic lives and knowing that diet, exercise and good health practices are the keys to making that happen. Others are motivated by the need to manage health issues that are starting to surface, recognising that they feel better when they look after their health.

The main reason I prioritise my own health is because, on average, people spend 6–10 years at the end of their lives in poor health. And science now shows that we *do* have the power to shift this toward the lower end of that range. By making proactive choices, we can reduce the time we spend in poor health and enjoy a longer, healthier Prime Time and Epic Retirement.

We're living in a time when the science and medicine around age-related diseases is rapidly evolving. It's commonly referred to as the science of modern ageing, and not just because of the crazy billionaires looking for attention by reversing their biological age – that stuff is nuts. I want you to understand the proactive choices we can all make now, daily and for free, that will enhance both our longevity and our quality of life, and to start taking them seriously.

I keep saying to myself, *I choose to do the things that will make future me happy with me.* I know the choices I make today with food, exercise and mental health will affect the quality of my life tomorrow.

Since writing *How to Have an Epic Retirement* and launching the *Prime Time* podcast, I've been fortunate to be able to speak with some of the leading scientists and medical experts in the space of longevity and health. Alongside this, I've read so many papers exploring how we can take better charge of our health from midlife onward. Of course, while these are universally recognised lessons, please consult your own medical practitioner for any individual health or medical advice.

Having done this research, I want us to focus in our Prime Time on just three big areas, because I think we should keep things as easy to act on as possible:

1. Make health your top priority
2. Learn how to age better according to science
3. Become literate in reading your biometrics and take your prevention testing seriously.

They're all important. In fact, they could be the keys to living a good second half of life. Because all lives, long or short, suck if they're spent in poor health.

Lesson 17
Make your health your top priority

It honestly boggles my mind that so much of the focus for midlife planning and goal setting is financial. Don't get me wrong – money matters. But here's the truth: you can live a fulfilling life without a lot of money, but you absolutely cannot live a fulfilling life without your body and mind being in good shape.

As you move into the second half of life, health needs to be right at the top of your list, because it's not the same as it was in your 20s or 30s. In midlife, you're tackling a whole new set of challenges, ones that can't be 'fixed' as easily, or sometimes not at all, if you wait until they've become real problems. This isn't about scare tactics. It's about being realistic about how much your body changes over time, and how those changes need a proactive approach, not a reactive one.

WHY HEALTH NEEDS TO TAKE CENTRE STAGE IN MIDLIFE

In your 20s or even 40s, your body often bounces back from stress, lack of sleep or poor lifestyle choices. But in midlife, the stakes are higher. Health issues like heart disease, diabetes and cognitive decline start to creep up on people. They don't just 'happen' overnight but develop over time, and often, by the time we notice them, we're already dealing with the long-term impacts.

We're also facing changes we can't avoid: muscle loss, decreased bone density and slower metabolism. These are natural parts of ageing, but how we handle them makes all the difference. What we can do is take proactive steps to ensure these natural processes don't have to stop us from living full, active lives.

THINKING ABOUT OUR HEALTHSPAN: WHY IT MATTERS

One of the big realities we're facing is our increasing longevity. We're living longer, healthier lives than ever before. Alongside this we need to recognise that, on the whole, women tend to live longer than men – in Australia, the US and many other countries, women are living about six years longer on average. But here's the catch: men tend to have better healthspans – the number of years we live in good health. That means men often live more of their lives in good health, even though they might die younger. Essentially, men and women may have a similar number of good-quality years, even if women live longer.

If you're part of a couple, you can expect to add up to three years to your lifespan. There's something about sharing life with someone that boosts longevity, perhaps the support, the shared activities or simply the companionship.

Here's the tough reality: many women spend the final years of their lives alone, often dealing with chronic and debilitating illnesses after their male partners have passed away.

None of these outcomes are set in stone, but they're worth considering as we pass through midlife and into our second half of life, because the things we do today and in fact every day can make a difference each step of the way. The good news is that modern science is increasingly showing us ways to improve our healthspan. By being proactive about our physical and mental health, we can not only live better during our midlife and retirement years, we can also slow down the ageing process in ways that weren't possible for previous generations.

THE BIG HEALTH CHANGES OF MIDLIFE

As we head into midlife, there's a lot of new stuff going on, physically and mentally, for both men and women. Our metabolism starts to slow down, women's and men's hormone levels fluctuate, and it becomes more important than ever to adjust our lifestyle to stay healthy to avoid the onset of chronic diseases, which typically start to raise their heads at this time. So let's take a closer look at the big four – the massive changes of midlife that people find most challenging to adapt to:

- Our metabolism changes
- Our hormones shift
- Our health risks rise
- And we all need to take proactive steps toward living healthier for longer.

Let's take some time to understand each of these, and learn how we should change our priorities.

OUR METABOLISM CHANGES

One of the most noticeable shifts during midlife is a slower metabolism, for both men and women. This natural decline means your body doesn't burn calories as efficiently as it used to, which can lead to weight gain even if your diet and activity level haven't changed. This shift is partly due to a decrease in muscle mass, which typically occurs as we age. Muscle tissue burns more calories at rest than fat tissue, so as muscle mass decreases, so does your resting metabolic rate.

There are a few ways in which we can attempt to counteract this shift.

Increase your protein intake

Increasing your protein intake helps maintain and even build muscle mass, which is crucial for keeping your metabolism active. Think lean meats, fish, eggs, legumes and dairy.

Lift your exercise levels

Incorporate aerobic exercises, like walking or cycling, and strength training into your routine. Strength training in particular helps preserve muscle mass and boosts your metabolic rate.

Re-balance your diet
Focus on a diet rich in nutrient-dense foods. Whole grains, fruits, vegetables and lean proteins should form the foundation of your meals. Avoid overly processed foods and sugars, which can contribute to fat storage and metabolic slowdown.

Eat smaller, more frequent meals
Eating smaller, more frequent meals can help keep your metabolism engaged throughout the day.

Consider fasting
Fasting can help improve your metabolic flexibility by encouraging your body to burn stored fat for energy during fasting periods. This can be particularly helpful in preventing midlife weight gain.

Don't forget to drink water
Water plays a critical role in maintaining your metabolic rate. Dehydration can slow down your metabolism, so make sure to drink plenty of water throughout the day.

OUR HORMONES SHIFT
Hormones are the body's chemical messengers. They play a critical role in regulating various functions, from metabolism to mood. As we enter midlife, the hormones flowing through our body change significantly, and this can affect both men and women in unique ways. A whole raft of unappealing and unexplained symptoms can start to rear their heads. It's important to be kind to yourself about the changes going on in your body during this phase of your life. And it might help to know that what you're going through is common and quite normal – and thankfully, now medically recognised and treated.

Menopause and women's health
Women get the worst of it. Somewhere between the ages of 45 and 55 they run headlong into menopause. Menopause is medically defined as the day that occurs one year after a woman has had

her last period ever, but the term is commonly used for the whole period of life when hormonal changes occur. The hormonal changes can start years before, in a phase called perimenopause, when oestrogen and progesterone levels start to drop, and symptoms start to appear that can be quite confronting. There are more than 30 symptoms that are known to be caused directly by these changes in our hormones and the process of menopause, none of which are pleasant and many of which can have an impact on your happiness and your relationships. Just some of the more common changes include hot flashes, night sweats, irregular periods, vaginal dryness, mood swings, irritability, anxiety, depression, fatigue, sleep disturbances (insomnia), weight gain, slowed metabolism, thinning hair and dry skin.

Be cognisant of these and the many other symptoms of menopause, and know that doctors can tackle them in one of two ways. They can either address the whole lot using hormone replacement therapy (HRT), or they can address the discomfort of each symptom one by one if you are unsuited to HRT.

The good news is that menopause and menopause treatments are going through a renaissance. HRT remains the most common treatment, and while it has had a complex history, advancements have led to a more nuanced and personalised approach to managing menopause.

HRT is designed to alleviate menopause symptoms by replacing hormones that decline during menopause, such as oestrogen and progesterone. It can be effective in managing hot flashes, night sweats, vaginal dryness, low libido and mood swings, among many other symptoms. Modern HRT options offer a variety of formulations, including oestrogen-only therapy for women who have had a hysterectomy, and combined therapies for those who haven't. These treatments come in various forms, including creams, and stick-on patches that release hormones through the skin.

The idea of using HRT still carries some stigma among older generations. But as a midlifer, you might want to do your own research and become your own advocate around the menopause conversation.

Andropause and men's health

While men don't experience a sudden hormonal shift like menopause, they do undergo a gradual decline in testosterone levels, often referred to as andropause. This process typically begins around the age of 40 and can lead to various subtle changes over time.

One of the first effects is often a change in muscle tone and an increase in body fat. Testosterone plays a crucial role in maintaining muscle mass and strength, so as levels decrease, men may find it harder to retain muscle and might notice more fat accumulation, particularly around the abdomen. This can be frustrating, especially if your diet or activity level hasn't changed.

Do the following to counteract these shifts, in consultation with your medical practitioner:

Strength training: Several scientific studies show that resistance training is particularly effective in elevating testosterone levels in men, especially when it targets large muscle groups in the lower body. Exercises like squats, deadlifts and power cleans are proven to have the most substantial impact on testosterone production. This is because activating larger muscle groups causes a greater hormonal response, boosting not only testosterone but also other anabolic hormones that help maintain muscle mass and overall strength as men age.[35] It's also important to point out that muscle mass is metabolically active, meaning it burns more calories – even at rest.

Prioritise protein: A diet rich in lean proteins (like fish, eggs and legumes) is crucial for maintaining your muscle mass, especially as your testosterone levels decline with age. Adequate protein intake supports your muscle repair and growth, which is critical for counteracting any age-related muscle loss (sarcopenia) that might be starting to set in. Importantly, research shows that consuming enough protein not only helps maintain your muscle mass but also positively influences your testosterone production,[36] making it a key dietary focus for men in midlife looking to sustain and improve both their muscle health and hormone levels.

Another common symptom of lower testosterone is fatigue and reduced stamina. You might find that activities you used to power through now leave you feeling drained. Your energy levels can be maintained or improved with a combination of regular exercise, getting enough sleep and eating a balanced diet. Supplements like vitamin D and magnesium, which support testosterone production, might also be worth considering, but always check with your doctor first.

It's important to point out that testosterone decline is a natural part of ageing and can also affect libido and sexual function. While these changes can feel uncomfortable to talk about, recognising that they are normal can help you address them more openly with your partner and your doctor. Testosterone replacement therapy is an option for some men, but it's not usually the first step. Lifestyle changes can make a significant difference and are the best place to start.

OUR HEALTH RISKS RISE

As we enter midlife, our health risk levels naturally begin to increase. This phase, which typically occurs between ages 45 and 65, brings with it the first interactions most people have with chronic disease. Understanding these risks and taking proactive steps to mitigate them can make a significant difference in maintaining your overall wellbeing. The leading causes of death among over-50s in the Western world are, in order, heart disease, cancer, chronic respiratory disease (COPD), stroke, dementia and diabetes, all chronic diseases linked to the central disease of ageing. Following are the things we need to concern ourselves with.

Cardiovascular health

Midlife is a critical period for cardiovascular health. Blood pressure tends to rise with age, partly due to increased stiffness in the arteries. Cholesterol levels may also become less balanced, with LDL (bad cholesterol) potentially increasing while HDL (good cholesterol) decreases. These factors contribute to a higher risk of heart disease and stroke. Regular cardiovascular exercise, a heart-healthy diet and routine check-ups can help manage these risks. Monitoring blood pressure and cholesterol levels regularly is crucial for early detection and management.

Metabolic changes

Metabolism naturally slows down with age, making it easier to gain weight even if your diet and activity level remain unchanged. Weight gain and poor diet can lead to an increased risk of type 2 diabetes and other metabolic disorders known to be some of the leading causes of death. Of course, the best way to mitigate this risk is with a balanced diet rich in whole foods and regular physical activity, alongside monitoring blood sugar levels if you're at risk. Weight management is also really important, as excess weight is a significant risk factor for metabolic diseases.

Bone health

Bone density tends to decrease with age, particularly for women after menopause due to declining oestrogen levels. This increase in risk can lead to osteoporosis, making bones more susceptible to fractures. Weight-bearing exercise, adequate intake of calcium and vitamin D, and more regular bone-density scans can help you stay strong as you age, particularly if osteoporosis is a risk factor for you.

Cancer risks

The risk of developing cancers, like breast, prostate and colorectal cancer, rises with age. Regular screenings are vital for early detection. For women, mammograms and pelvic exams are essential; for men, prostate-specific antigen (PSA) tests and digital rectal exams can help monitor prostate health. Colonoscopies are recommended for both men and women to screen for colorectal cancer. Adhering to recommended screening schedules can significantly improve outcomes through early intervention.

Mental and cognitive health concerns

Midlife can also bring challenges to mental health. We can find ourselves under increased stress, juggling family responsibilities for both our parents and our children, and trying to navigate our own life transitions, and each of these can contribute to anxiety and depression. The experts say we should all get better at stress-management techniques, work harder to stay connected with our loved ones, and not be shy about getting medical help to support our mental wellbeing during this phase of life. Doing it tough is nothing to be embarrassed about. You should also be alert to changes in your cognitive health, as early signs of cognitive decline or memory issues can sometimes appear in midlife, as well as struggling with issues often related to menopause.

Joint and muscular health

Joint pain and muscle stiffness are really common from our mid to late 40s onward. You might start to see instances of arthritis appear in your joints, particularly in the winter. Regular physical activity, maintaining a healthy weight, and incorporating flexibility and strengthening exercises can help with your joint health, ideally reducing the risk of developing arthritis. Or, if you end up managing it, taking a proactive approach to anti-inflammatory eating has also been shown to help some people.

Eyesight and hearing

Vision and hearing changes are both more noticeable in midlife. Regular eye exams can help you maintain quality of vision and detect issues like presbyopia or early signs of age-related macular degeneration. Hearing tests are essential, not just to maintain your quality of life, but also because hearing loss has been directly connected by neuropsychologists to the risk of dementia. Don't put this off.

Gut and digestive concerns

Gut health issues, allergies and other gastrointestinal disorders can become more common in midlife. And they shouldn't be ignored. Our gut health has been directly linked to our mental and cognitive health. So pay attention to symptoms such as persistent heartburn, changes in bowel habits and abdominal pain, and understand more about how you can improve your gut health with pre-biotics, probiotics and an appropriate amount of fibre in your diet.

TAKE PROACTIVE STEPS TOWARD LIVING HEALTHIER FOR LONGER

What if you could get a sneak peek into how your body is performing and catch potential issues before they become serious? Thanks to advances in technology and health screening, this has never been easier or more possible. Today, you can do two important things to stave off chronic disease that might shorten your healthspan – become literate in reading your biometrics and take your prevention testing seriously.

MONITOR YOUR BIOMETRICS

More and more midlifers are learning to keep tabs on their health in the comfort of their own home using a range of innovative tools that were once beyond reach. You can use this information to make changes to your behaviour, diet, or to seek medical interventions.

Wearable devices such as Apple Watches, Fitbits and Oura Rings are leading the way in measuring our biometrics. These gadgets can keep track of vital signs such as heart rate, sleep patterns and physical activity levels. They keep you informed about your heart health, alert you to irregularities, and provide data that helps you understand how well you're managing stress and exercise. For instance, a smartwatch can notify you if your heart rate is unusually high or low, prompting you to take action before it becomes a problem.

But wearables are just the beginning. At-home tests and monitoring devices are now available to track everything from blood pressure and glucose levels to cholesterol and hormone levels, and they are really easy to use. These tools are incredibly user-friendly and can deliver real-time feedback on critical health metrics. Imagine being able to check your blood sugar levels after a meal, so that if you notice spikes after eating certain food types, like simple carbohydrates or sugary fruits, you can tweak your diet. Or use a blood pressure cuff that syncs with your smartphone (or acts alone) to alert you to hypertension concerns. Or monitor your cholesterol to gain insights into your lipid profile without visiting a doctor or pharmacy. Well, these are now readily available to all of us.

In the era of what health experts are calling Medicine 3.0, where general practitioners often struggle to keep up with the volume of patients, it makes even more sense to take charge of your own health monitoring.

Let's look at some of the big health issues today and how you can monitor them simply by watching your biometrics.

HEART HEALTH

High blood pressure and irregular heart rhythms can be early warning signs of cardiovascular issues. Keeping track of your heart rate and blood pressure regularly can help you spot changes early and take action if needed.

What to measure:
- **Blood pressure:** Blood pressure is recorded as two numbers; for example, 120/80 mmHg. The first number (systolic) measures the pressure in your arteries when your heart beats, while the second number (diastolic) measures the pressure between beats. Normal blood pressure is around 120/80 mmHg. Elevated or high blood pressure can indicate an increased risk of heart disease and stroke.
- **Heart rate:** Your heart rate, measured in beats per minute (bpm), reflects how often your heart beats while at rest. A normal resting heart rate for most adults ranges from 60 to 100 bpm. Persistent abnormalities can signal heart issues or stress.

How to monitor: Smartwatches and fitness trackers can continuously monitor heart rate, alerting you to irregularities, and at-home blood pressure monitors allow you to check your pressure regularly and monitor for changes that require attention.

BLOOD SUGAR LEVELS

Monitoring blood sugar is important for detecting early signs of diabetes, managing insulin levels and reducing the risk of chronic inflammation linked to poor glucose control. Keeping an eye on your levels can help you make adjustments before issues escalate.

What to measure:
- **Fasting blood glucose**: This test measures blood sugar levels after fasting overnight. Normal fasting blood glucose levels should be between 4.0 and 5.5 mmol/L. High levels could indicate pre-diabetes or diabetes.
- **Postprandial blood glucose**: Measure two hours after eating. Normal levels should be less than 7.8 mmol/L. Elevated levels can help diagnose diabetes and necessitate glucose management.

How to monitor: Glucometers can be used ad-hoc to test your blood sugars, or increasingly people are choosing to wear continuous glucose monitors (CGMs) for real-time glucose readings driven by a sensor placed under the skin.

CHOLESTEROL LEVELS

High cholesterol is a major risk factor for heart disease, but keeping track of your levels can help you take control of your cardiovascular health. Regular monitoring allows you to make dietary and lifestyle adjustments before issues escalate.

What to measure:
- **Total cholesterol**: Total cholesterol should be less than 5.0 mmol/L. High levels can increase your risk of heart disease.
- **LDL (bad) cholesterol**: Ideally, LDL cholesterol should be below 3.0 mmol/L. Elevated levels are linked to a higher risk of arterial plaque build-up.
- **HDL (good) cholesterol**: HDL cholesterol should be above 1.0 mmol/L for men and 1.3 mmol/L for women. Higher levels are beneficial as HDL helps remove LDL cholesterol from the bloodstream.

- **Triglycerides**: Normal levels should be less than 1.7 mmol/L. Elevated triglycerides can contribute to heart disease and metabolic syndrome.

How to monitor: At-home testing kits that use finger-prick blood samples to measure cholesterol levels. Some kits provide a full lipid profile, helping you track and manage your cholesterol.

BONE DENSITY

Osteoporosis is a big concern as we age. While home testing for bone density is more complex, wearable devices and apps can track physical activity and alert you to changes in your strength and balance, which can be early indicators of bone health issues.

What to measure: Bone mineral density (BMD), measured in grams per square centimetre, identifies the minerals packed into a specific area of bone tissue. Doctors use a T-score to compare your bone density to the average peak bone density of a healthy young adult of the same sex. A T-score of –1.0 or higher is normal, –1.0 to –2.5 indicates osteopenia (bone loss), and a T-score below –2.5 indicates osteoporosis.

How to monitor: DEXA scans from your doctor or a scan provider offer a detailed measurement of bone density. Regular scans help monitor bone health, especially if you have risk factors for osteoporosis.

WEIGHT MANAGEMENT

Keeping tabs on your weight is crucial for maintaining overall health and wellbeing. It's not just about the number on the scale; it's about understanding your body composition and how it changes over time. Smart scales can offer more detailed insights than traditional scales, providing data on muscle mass, fat percentage and body composition, which can guide your diet and exercise choices.

What to measure:
- **Weight**: Regular monitoring helps you track weight changes and manage your overall health effectively. Aim to weigh yourself at the same time each day or week for consistency.

- **Body composition**: Beyond weight, smart scales can measure muscle mass, fat percentage and body mass index (BMI). BMI is calculated using your weight and height, with a normal range being between 18.5 and 24.9.
- **Waist circumference**: Measuring waist circumference helps identify excess abdominal fat, with higher health risks for men of European descent with a circumference of more than 94 cm, men of Asian descent of more than 90 cm, and women of all ethnicities of more than 80 cm.

How to monitor: Consider the use of smart scales that measure muscle mass and body fat percentage; and use a tape measure to track waist circumference, just above the hip bones.

SLEEP PATTERNS

Poor sleep can impact energy levels, cognitive function and overall health. Tracking your sleep can help identify patterns and improve sleep quality over time.

What to measure:
- **Sleep duration**: The number of hours you sleep each night.
- **Sleep quality**: Includes the amount of time spent in deep sleep and REM sleep.

How to monitor: Use wearables to track your sleep patterns and get insights into sleep stages and quality. If you need more insights, sleep apps can be purchased that record additional information.

PREVENTION TESTING

None of us want to deal with the rough stuff in our later years, like cancer, heart disease or diabetes, or have them cut our time short. That's where prevention testing comes in. Over the years, our longevity has improved because we're getting better at catching and treating these conditions early. Scientists and medical professionals now recommend we have a barrage of tests, semi-regularly, to reduce our risks. Consider these tests your early warning system, helping you spot potential issues before they become major problems. It's all about catching things early so you can deal with them promptly and keep enjoying life to the fullest.

Here are the tests you should be having from somewhere in your late 40s onward. As always, consult with your GP to discuss your individual health concerns and any underlying issues.

Blood tests

Blood tests can check cholesterol levels, blood sugar (for diabetes), kidney and liver function, vitamin and mineral deficiencies, and general health markers.

Starting age: Regularly from age 50.

Frequency: Annually or as recommended by your GP, depending on your health and risk factors.

Mammograms (for women)

Mammograms check for early signs of breast cancer.

Starting age: 50.

Frequency: Every two years.

Colonoscopies

Colonoscopies check for early signs of colorectal cancer and polyps.

Starting age: 50.

Frequency: Every five years, or as recommended based on initial findings or family history.

At-home bowel cancer screening

At-home bowel cancer screening is an important check for early signs of colorectal cancer and polyps that you can do yourself. In Australia, it will arrive in the post when you turn 45, and every two years after that. In other countries, you'll have to get tested by a doctor.

Starting age: 45.

Frequency: Every two years, or as recommended based on initial findings or family history.

Hearing tests

Hearing tests are not mandatory, but it's worthwhile to check for a deterioration in hearing or hearing loss.

Starting age: From age 50, especially if you notice any hearing changes.

Frequency: Annually, or as needed based on symptoms or recommendations from your healthcare provider. In most countries, there is no requirement to ever get a hearing test, but hearing is an issue known to contribute to dementia, so don't be a dummy and put it off.

Bone-density scans

As discussed earlier, bone-density scans check for osteoporosis and bone-density loss.

Starting age: Discuss with your GP. Women's scans are more common from age 65 and men from age 70, or earlier if risk factors are present.

Frequency: Every two years, or as advised by your GP based on your bone health and risk factors.

Prostate checks (for men)

Prostate cancer checks are usually done as both a PSA blood test and a digital test, to assess prostate health and look for symptoms of prostate cancer.

Starting age: Discuss with your GP from age 50.

Frequency: Varies based on individual risk factors and discussions with your GP. Regular checks are generally advised, every year or as recommended.

Skin checks

Skin checks should be done by a doctor using a dermoscope, looking for skin cancers including melanoma.

Starting age: Commonly from age 50, but talk to your GP about your individual situation.

Frequency: Annually, or more frequently if you have a history of skin cancer or have had significant sun exposure.

Eye exams
Eye exams check for vision loss and also for age-related eye conditions like macular degeneration, glaucoma and cataracts.
Starting age: From age 50.
Frequency: Every two years, or as recommended based on your eye health and risk factors, increasing to every year from 65.

MANAGING YOUR MENTAL AND COGNITIVE HEALTH
Finally, it would be remiss of me not to talk about mental and cognitive health, as they are such a significant part of living a long and healthy life. We need to recognise that our mental health and our cognitive capability are very tightly woven in with other physical and hormonal changes in our lives, especially through the middle years, when we are often damaging our bodies simply by neglecting to do the things we should be doing to look after ourselves. So if we are looking after our bodies with regular exercise, healthy eating and an eye to prevention, then we're off to a great start. But it's also important to take the time to look within, to what we need emotionally, and for good mental health; and more practically, to maintain and support our cognitive health.

Midlife brings challenges such as trauma and grief, which can lead to anxiety and depression – common ways that mental health issues arise. Gen Xers and boomers often don't talk about these symptoms – but they should. Persistent sadness, loss of interest, fatigue and difficulty concentrating are signs something isn't right. So are irritability, sleep changes, appetite fluctuations, and even physical symptoms like headaches. Feelings of worthlessness, guilt and social withdrawal should also be addressed.

Recognising these symptoms is key as is being proactive about seeking help from your doctor for support, medication and counselling.

And finally, maintaining a focus on our cognitive health is vital as we age. It's not just about preventing decline and dementia, but fostering a vibrant mind that keeps learning and growing. A resilient emotional state and a positive approach to overall health are essential.

DEMENTIA PREVENTION: WHAT YOU NEED TO KNOW

The latest report from The Lancet Commission highlights that dementia is not an inevitable part of ageing – it can be prevented. By addressing key risk factors like hearing loss, high blood pressure, smoking, obesity, depression, physical inactivity, diabetes and social isolation, we can significantly reduce our risk of developing dementia.[37]

Recently, two more critical factors have been added to this list: untreated vision loss and high LDL cholesterol. For those under 65, even a 1 mmol/L increase in LDL cholesterol can raise the risk of all-cause dementia by 8 per cent, according to a large study involving over a million participants.[38]

By taking proactive steps to manage these risk factors, we can protect our cognitive health and reduce the likelihood of developing dementia as we age.

REMEMBER WHY YOU'RE DOING IT

Everyone who stays proactive about their health has a personal motivation. Maybe it's the desire to avoid the frailty you saw in your parents. Maybe it's about staying strong and in control of your body. Or perhaps it's the boost in energy, the dopamine hits, and the overall sense of wellbeing you get when you're looking after yourself.

There are plenty of things you can aim to improve. Consider the following for inspiration:
- Lengthening your healthspan
- Building and maintaining muscle mass
- Strengthening your body
- Improving your balance
- Enhancing cardiovascular health

- Reducing the risk of chronic disease
- Feeling more energetic
- Looking and feeling good.

Take a moment to reflect on your 'why'. What's going to get you out of bed in the morning, into your workout gear, measuring and monitoring your health, and making healthier choices throughout the day? Whether it's to stay strong for your family or to enjoy a long, independent life with a better healthspan, having a clear motivation will help keep you on track.

And remember that you're choosing your own adventure in midlife, taking the proactive steps today that your future self will thank you for. No-one should have to nag you about looking after your health. This is something you'll benefit from directly. So take positive action, because it's not just good for you – it's essential.

Lesson 18
Learn how to age better according to science

THE SCIENCE OF MODERN AGEING IS ADVANCING AT AN EXTRAORDINARY PACE, YET IF you haven't been following the breakthroughs in science and medicine, you might have missed just how far we've come – and, more importantly, how you can use these discoveries to live a longer, healthier life.

In the last 20 years, scientists have connected many dots about what causes our bodies to age. They've discovered that ageing is more than just the passing of time and the wrinkling of skin and deterioration of our muscles and bones. It's deeply connected to the major diseases that become more prevalent as we grow older: heart disease, dementia, diabetes and cancer. According to recent scientific discoveries, these aren't just separate conditions that pop up independently. They're all connected to a bigger, more central issue that most people don't even think of as a disease: ageing itself.[39]

This idea, that ageing could be considered a disease, is a newer concept in the scientific community. Traditionally, ageing has been viewed as a natural, inevitable process. But with modern research, some scientists are now suggesting that ageing could be treated as a condition that drives and underpins many chronic diseases. This perspective isn't universally accepted yet, but it's gaining traction, particularly as we learn more about the cellular and genetic mechanisms at play.

The science shows that our cells' DNA gets damaged over time due to a mix of everyday wear and tear, exposure to things like UV rays and pollution, and lifestyle choices like diet and smoking. This damage messes with how cells do their jobs. Some cells eventually stop dividing and enter a state called cellular senescence, where they stop working properly and become less effective at fighting off toxins and disease. And this leads to age-related diseases taking hold.

What's really exciting, and could change how we age, is that scientists now see ageing as something we might be able to treat by tackling the problem of cellular senescence.[40] Modern science is uncovering ways to slow down this cellular breakdown, which could help keep our bodies and minds from deteriorating as quickly as they have in past generations.[41]

Some studies point to simple everyday habits that can make a big difference, while others suggest that medical breakthroughs could be on the horizon, though they might take 10–20+ years to become available. It's clear in the research that the sooner we start making positive behavioural changes in our lives, the sooner we can enjoy the benefits of longer healthspans.[42] And as people in midlife, we're in a great position to take advantage of these lessons.

I DON'T FEEL OLD ENOUGH TO TALK ABOUT AGEING BETTER

If the Prime Time of our lives falls between 47 and 75 – give or take, depending on when we had our kids and when we start to feel a bit freer from those responsibilities – and our life expectancy, especially for those who are wealthier and more proactive about their health, is edging further into our 90s, getting closer and closer to 100, then it's time to think about when we should have that conversation with ourselves about ageing better. It's hard to talk about ageing to someone who is 47 or 50. The conversation doesn't really feel relevant, because all too often we use that word to refer to the stages of life when we are frail, or beauty therapies that try to make us look younger than we are, both of which are irrelevant when we want to talk about true healthy ageing.

But ageing well starts very much in your midlife, hopefully at a time when you do not feel 'old'.

Old, by my definition, is the last 10 years of our life. For many of today's proactive Prime Timers, with luck on our side, that means we won't be old until our early, mid or late 80s. And, as we work our way through the years before this, we don't want our physical, cognitive or emotional health to take a dive and pull us into ageing prematurely. This section focuses on the things we can do to prevent that.

You don't have to feel old to start wanting to age better, improving your heathspan and your quality of life. And it doesn't have to be about how you look. Sure, looking good can help you feel good about yourself, but in my opinion it is far more important to focus on your physical and cognitive health and the quality of the life you want. You'll no doubt reap plenty of benefits in terms of how you look from taking care of yourself better, even if you don't focus on looks alone.

So what does the science of modern ageing say about slowing down, or even reversing the ageing process? According to leading researchers, the key lies in targeting the biological mechanisms that drive ageing. Here are some of the most promising strategies.

RESTRICTING CALORIES AND FASTING

Eating less and keeping your blood sugar consistent through fasting are two simple yet powerful strategies that are gaining attention in the science of ageing. These approaches have shown promising effects on both how long we live and how healthy we stay as we age.[43]

CALORIE RESTRICTION
Calorie restriction is all about eating fewer calories each day – about 20–40 per cent less – without starving yourself. Studies, especially

of animals like mice and rhesus monkeys, have found that this can help you live longer and it reduces the risk of diseases like cancer, heart problems and brain disorders.[44] The magic happens because eating less activates certain 'longevity genes' in our bodies known as sirtuins, which help repair DNA, reduce inflammation and boost energy production in our cells.[45] When these genes are active, our cells stay healthier for longer, which slows down the ageing process.

INTERMITTENT FASTING

Intermittent fasting is a way of managing our diet that sees us cycling between eating and fasting periods. Some of the most well-known methods include the 16:8 plan, where you fast for 16 hours and eat within an eight-hour window, or the 5:2 diet, where you eat normally for five days and cut calories significantly for two days. Fasting pushes your body to switch from burning sugar for energy to burning fat, which produces ketones. These ketones help clean out damaged cells and create new, healthy ones. It's a process known as autophagy, and something scientists have identified as one of the key ways to counteract cellular senescence. This clean-up is crucial for keeping your cells in top shape, which could help you live longer and stay healthier.[46]

Fasting has also been shown to boost our brain health by increasing a protein called BDNF, which supports brain function, and lowering levels of a hormone called IGF-1, which, when too high, is linked to ageing and cancer.[47]

WHY BOTH CALORIE RESTRICTION AND FASTING WORK

Calorie restriction and intermittent fasting share similar benefits. They activate stress-response pathways in your cells that help your body resist the effects of ageing and disease. By eating less and giving your body regular breaks from food, you could be turning on these protective mechanisms, which might keep your cells healthier, delay age-related diseases, and extend the years you spend in good health.

The bottom line is that these dietary strategies do more than just help manage weight. They may actually slow down the biological clock, keeping you feeling younger and more vibrant as you age.

BOOSTING NAD LEVELS

NAD+ (nicotinamide adenine dinucleotide) is a molecule that plays a key role in keeping our cells energised and functioning well.[48] As we age, our NAD+ levels naturally decline, which can lead to signs of ageing like weaker muscles, slower thinking and longer recovery times.

The good news is that there are natural ways to help maintain or even boost your NAD+ levels. Regular exercise and intermittent fasting are two of the most effective methods. When you exercise, your body kickstarts processes that help preserve NAD+, keeping your cells healthier and more resilient. Intermittent fasting can also help boost NAD+ by promoting cellular repair and improving overall cell function.[49]

You might also see supplements like NMN (nicotinamide mononucleotide) and NR (nicotinamide riboside) gaining in popularity as potential boosters of NAD+ levels. These supplements are converted into NAD+ in the body and have shown promising results in animal studies, such as improved muscle strength, better endurance and even extended lifespans. However, it's important to point out that the effectiveness of these supplements in humans is still unproven. While the early research is encouraging, we don't yet have enough evidence to say they definitely work or to fully understand any potential risks.

EXERCISE AND HORMESIS

Regular exercise, especially high-intensity interval training (HIIT), is one of the best things you can do for your health as you age. HIIT involves short bursts of intense exercise followed by rest or lower-intensity periods.[50] This kind of workout helps your body in several ways:

- **It boosts mitochondrial function**: Mitochondria are like the powerhouses of your cells, providing them with energy. Regular exercise helps these powerhouses work better, giving you more energy and keeping your cells functioning well.[51]

- **It promotes autophagy**: This is that fancy term for the process where your body cleans out damaged or old cells suffering from cellular senescence and regenerates new, healthy ones. Think of it as a spring clean for your cells. This natural clean-up helps keep you feeling younger and more energetic.
- **It drives hormesis**: Exercise also takes advantage of a concept called hormesis. This means that a small amount of stress, such as the stress from working out, actually makes your body stronger. Just like lifting weights helps to build muscle, the small stress from exercise encourages your cells to become more resilient and efficient. It's a way of using mild stress to strengthen your body and improve overall health, and it's been scientifically proven to directly impact longevity in mice and mammals, and indirectly in humans.

The cool thing about exercise is that it's a natural way to slow down the ageing process. By making exercise a regular part of your life, you're not just staying fit, you're also helping your body fight off the effects of ageing. Remember, though, it's always advisable to have a health check with your GP before embarking on any new exercise program.

THE POWER OF EXERCISE

As we enter midlife, and undertake exercise in the second half of our lives, it's worthwhile understanding the different roles that different types of exercise can play in managing your heart, health, mood, balance, weight, flexibility and strength.

Boosting cardiovascular health

First up, regular cardiovascular exercise is fantastic for your heart. Engaging in physical activity helps keep your cardiovascular system in top shape by lowering blood pressure, improving blood flow and reducing the risk of heart disease. When you get your heart pumping, you're not only helping your body use oxygen more efficiently but also actively reducing the risk of stroke and heart attack by promoting better blood circulation. It's like giving your heart a workout, making it stronger and more resilient.

The World Health Organization (WHO) recommends 150 minutes of moderate-intensity cardiovascular exercise per week for adults aged 18 and over, including those over 65. Moderate intensity means you're working hard enough that you'd be puffed and find it challenging to have a conversation with someone walking beside you. While this is considered the minimum, incorporating more cardiovascular exercise into your routine can provide even greater health benefits.

HIGH-INTENSITY INTERVAL TRAINING: A GAME-CHANGER FOR FITNESS AND BRAIN HEALTH

HIIT is a workout approach that alternates between short bursts of intense exercise and periods of lower-intensity recovery or rest. This method has become popular due to its efficiency and effectiveness, delivering significant benefits in a shorter amount of time compared to traditional exercise routines.

During a HIIT workout, you might perform an exercise like uphill walking, sprinting, cycling or bodyweight exercises at maximum effort for 20–30 seconds, followed by a brief period of slower activity or rest. This cycle is repeated several times. The intensity of the exercise pushes your cardiovascular system to its limits, which enhances overall fitness and increases calorie burn long after the workout is over, a phenomenon known as the afterburn effect.

But HIIT isn't just about improving cardiovascular health. Recent research has shown that it can also have profound effects on brain health. By challenging the body with high-intensity bursts, HIIT helps improve metabolic function, increase muscle mass and enhance endurance. This intense form of exercise has also been linked to better cognitive function, particularly in older adults, by promoting neuroplasticity and improving brain connectivity.[52]

A recent study by the Brain Institute at the University of Queensland explored how different types of exercise affect cognitive health, focusing on the hippocampus, a brain area essential for memory and learning.[53] The researchers recruited 151 healthy older adults, aged 65–85, and divided them into three groups: one group did low-intensity exercises, another did medium-intensity exercises, and the third group engaged in HIIT on an inclined treadmill at a cardiovascular intensity of 85–90 per cent. Each group completed 72 supervised sessions over six months.

The results were impressive. While all groups remained active, the HIIT group showed significant improvements to their memory and learning abilities, reduced age-related brain shrinkage, and enhanced brain connectivity. Remarkably, these benefits persisted for at least five years, highlighting that HIIT not only boosts cognitive function but also provides lasting brain health protection.

Strengthening muscles and bones

Next, let's talk about muscles and bones. As we age, we naturally lose muscle mass and bone density, which can lead to frailty and an increased risk of fractures much earlier in life than we'd like. But exercise, especially strength training, can help counteract this. Lifting weights, using resistance bands and even doing bodyweight exercises like squats and push-ups, can build muscle and strengthen bones. This isn't just about looking good; it's about maintaining functional strength and preventing falls. For those of us in our late 40s, 50s and 60s, it's especially important to focus on maintaining muscle mass and bone density.

WHO guidelines say we should aim for at least two days a week of strength training exercises. And try to focus on all the major muscle groups: legs, arms, back and core. Exercises like squats, lunges, push-ups and rows are simple to do at home, without inconvenience. You can get yourself a mat and some hand weights at varying levels and really start to take your strength more seriously.

Stimulating bone growth with weight-bearing exercises

Weight-bearing exercises are essential for maintaining and improving bone density as we age. It's an area that is particularly of concern for post-menopausal women, who find their bone density can really start to drop at an astounding pace in their 50s, 60s, 70s and 80s, and men also suffer age-related bone density decline.[54] Weight-bearing exercises require you to support your body weight against gravity, which helps to stimulate bone growth and strengthen the bones. They have been shown to have a significant positive impact on our risk of osteoporosis and fractures.

The types of weight-bearing exercise to consider doing can be divided into two different categories:

1. **Weight-bearing aerobic exercises**: usually impact activities where arms, feet and legs are bearing the weight (i.e., walking, stair climbing, jogging, volleyball, tennis and similar sports, tai chi and dancing).
2. **Strength and/or resistance exercises**: where the joints are moving against some kind of resistance, like free weights, machines, bands or simply body weight.

There is no scientific agreement on the amount of weight-bearing exercise we should include in our week, but evidence shows that combining both of these types can have a significant effect on bone density.

Maintaining balance and flexibility

Maintaining good balance and flexibility is crucial as you get older, and it's something you can actively work on from midlife so that it becomes ingrained. According to the WHO guidelines, balance becomes a concern once we reach the age of 65, which is when it's suggested that people incorporate three sessions designed to improve our balance each week. But I think we should start earlier.

Activities like yoga, Pilates and tai chi are excellent choices, as they focus on controlled movements and flexibility, which help you stay steady on your feet. Simple balance exercises, such as standing on one leg or walking heel to toe, are also effective and easy to do at home.

Strengthening your core also plays a pivotal role in improving your balance. Exercises like seated leg lifts and gentle twists can help to build up the muscles that support your stability. Regular stretching can enhance your flexibility, reducing stiffness and helping you move more fluidly, something everyone wants in the second half of life.

BUILD A PROGRAM YOU ENJOY

One of the really important aspects of exercising in midlife is finding a variety of activities that you genuinely enjoy and building some structure and organisation around them. Consistency is key, but mixing up your routine is also valuable. Variety not only keeps things interesting but also helps prevent injuries from overuse and ensures that different muscle groups are worked. It's less about pushing yourself to the limit and more about maintaining a balanced and steady approach. Enhancing and preserving cardiovascular health, muscle and bone strength and balance and flexibility requires regular, varied exercise rather than just focusing on high-intensity or cardio exercise alone.

If you're new to strength training, start with lighter weights and fewer repetitions. Gradually increase the weight and intensity as you build strength and confidence. It could be worth working with a fitness trainer or an exercise physiologist who can tailor a strength-training program to your needs and ensure you're using proper form, to prevent injury.

GOOD NUTRITION

As we move through our prime time years, our metabolism naturally slows, and inflammation often becomes more frequent, sometimes triggered by the foods we eat. Suddenly, what we put in our mouths matters a lot more. It's no longer just about satisfying hunger. Instead, it's also about providing the right nutrients to keep our body functioning smoothly and preventing inflammation that accelerates ageing and increases the risk of chronic diseases. Nutrition is the fuel that keeps our cells healthy and energetic, while poor dietary choices can lead to cellular damage.

Let's look at nutrition from three main angles:
1. Anti-inflammatory eating
2. Embracing the Mediterranean diet
3. Contemplating your protein.

ANTI-INFLAMMATORY EATING

As we grow older, chronic inflammation becomes a much more significant concern, contributing to many common age-related health issues that usually start to pop up for the first time in midlife, like hypertension or high blood pressure, blood sugar issues, and the aches and pains of arthritis. What most people don't realise is that persistent, low-grade inflammation can subtly damage cells and tissues, leading to a range of health problems that simply worsen over time. But there is something that you can do that has been tried and tested by many: adopt an anti-inflammatory diet.

Inflammation is the body's natural response to injury or infection, part of the immune system's protective mechanism. And when your body is unhappy for an extended period, the inflammation can become chronic. Then it can start harming healthy cells and tissues. Diet plays a significant role in driving chronic inflammation up and down, so focusing on the right foods and the right practices can be rewarding.

There's a whole raft of evidence that shows certain types of foods can increase inflammation and contribute to chronic health conditions. The four main categories to be wary of are as follows:

1. Processed foods

Processed foods often contain unhealthy fats, sugars and additives that can disrupt your body's balance and fuel inflammation. These ingredients can exacerbate chronic inflammation and contribute to various health issues. A quick way to identify processed foods is to check the ingredient list on the label. If you see more than six ingredients, especially ones with complex chemical names or ones that sound more like lab experiments than food, it's best to avoid them. Opt for products with short ingredient lists and names you can easily recognise. This often means the food is less processed and more nutritious.

2. Sugary snacks and drinks

Excessive sugar intake is a major culprit in raising blood glucose levels and increasing inflammation in the body. This isn't just about obvious sweets, cakes and pastries; it includes sugary drinks like soft drink and fruit juices, and starchy carbohydrates like white bread, pasta and certain cereals. Each can cause rapid spikes in blood sugar, leading to inflammation and potentially long-term health issues.

To keep inflammation in check and maintain stable blood sugar levels, aim to limit your intake of these sugary and starchy foods. Instead, opt for whole foods and naturally sweet options. Fresh fruit, while it still contains sugar, provides essential nutrients and fibre that help manage blood sugar more effectively. Whole grains like quinoa, brown rice and oats are better choices than refined carbohydrates because they have a lower glycaemic index and provide steady energy without the sugar crash.

When tempted, replace sweet drinks with water, herbal teas, or sparkling water with a splash of lemon or lime. If you're craving something sweet, try making a smoothie with unsweetened yoghurt, fresh fruit and a handful of spinach or kale for a good stash of nutrients.

3. Saturated and trans fats

Unhealthy fats, like trans fats and excessive saturated fats, can significantly impact your health. Trans fats are artificial fats found in fried foods, some baked goods and processed snacks. They're created through hydrogenation, which makes oils solid and extends shelf life but also increases bad LDL cholesterol while lowering good HDL cholesterol. This imbalance raises the risk of heart disease and promotes inflammation. Look out for 'partially hydrogenated oils' on ingredient lists and choose foods made with healthier fats like olive or avocado oil.

Saturated fats, found in fatty meats, dairy products and some plant oils, can also elevate LDL cholesterol levels, contributing to heart disease and inflammation. To reduce your intake, choose lean meats, low-fat dairy and healthier cooking oils. Reading labels and opting for whole, minimally processed foods can help you avoid these harmful fats and support better overall health.

4. Nightshade vegetables

Nightshade vegetables, which include tomatoes, capsicums, eggplants and potatoes, contain compounds such as solanine and alkaloids that some people believe can contribute to inflammation and joint pain. While not everyone is sensitive to nightshades, if you notice that these foods seem to worsen your symptoms, consider reducing or eliminating them from your diet to see if it makes a difference.

Anti-inflammatory foods

On the flip side, many foods are celebrated for their anti-inflammatory benefits and can serve as excellent alternatives to highly processed or simple carbohydrate-heavy options:

Leafy greens: Vegetables like spinach and kale are packed with vitamins, minerals and antioxidants that help reduce inflammation. Add them to salads, smoothies or stir-fries for a nutritious boost.

Berries: Blueberries, strawberries and raspberries are rich in flavonoids – antioxidants that combat inflammation. Enjoy them as a snack or mix them into your breakfast or desserts.

Nuts and seeds: Almonds, walnuts, chia seeds and flaxseeds contain healthy fats and antioxidants that help reduce inflammation. They're great for snacks or as additions to salads and yoghurts.

Fatty fish: Fish like salmon, mackerel and sardines are high in omega-3 fatty acids, known for their anti-inflammatory benefits. Regularly eating fatty fish can support heart health and reduce inflammation.

Olive oil: Extra-virgin olive oil is rich in oleocanthal, a compound with anti-inflammatory effects. Use it for cooking or in salad dressings as a healthy fat option.

Bright red, yellow and orange vegetables: Incorporating colourful vegetables into your diet is a fantastic way to combat inflammation. Vegetables such as carrots and beetroot are rich in antioxidants, vitamins and minerals that help neutralise harmful free radicals and reduce inflammation. The vibrant pigments in these vegetables, such as beta-carotene and anthocyanins, provide a range of health benefits, including supporting immune function and reducing oxidative stress.

Turmeric: Turmeric is an excellent spice for fighting inflammation. It contains curcumin, a compound that can help reduce inflammation and support joint health. However, curcumin on its own has low bioavailability, meaning it's not easily absorbed by your body. To boost absorption, choose turmeric supplements that include piperine (black pepper), which enhances curcumin's effectiveness.

Ginger: Ginger is well-known for its pain-relieving and immune-supporting properties. It's a great addition to your diet for overall inflammation reduction.

An anti-inflammatory diet should be straightforward to implement. Aim to fill your plate with a variety of colourful fruits and vegetables, whole grains, lean proteins and healthy fats. Cutting back on processed foods, sugary snacks and unhealthy fats will help keep inflammation in check. If you have any underlying health issues, it's best to consult a medical professional before making changes to your diet.

EMBRACING THE MEDITERRANEAN DIET

The Mediterranean diet has time and again been validated by academics and social scientists for its extraordinary benefits for longevity. The research by Dan Buettner on the Blue Zones is of course the most high-profile study of the Mediterranean diet, pointing to the five zones in the world where people live the longest: Okinawa in Japan, Ikaria in Greece, Sardinia in Italy, Nicoya in Costa Rica and Loma Linda in California, each home to the world's largest populations of centenarians.[55]

The Blue Zones research points to these places as the home of the oldest, healthiest and happiest people on earth. And there are only a couple of things they all have in common. They each eat a Mediterranean-style diet rich in seasonal healthy fruits and vegetables, olive oil, whole grains and beans, and limited quantities of lean meats. They obtain their produce locally and enjoy their food in the company of their family and community. And they incorporate movement and incidental exercise into their everyday activities, participating in food production and other community activities until the very end of their lives.

The Mediterranean diet has been hailed for decreasing the risks of chronic age-related disease and lengthening lives. Its principles are not dissimilar to those of anti-inflammatory eating detailed earlier.

Here are eight ways to put the Mediterranean diet principles into practice.

1. **Fresh is best**: Load up on fresh fruits and veggies. Think vibrant salads, juicy tomatoes, and crunchy greens. The more colour on your plate, the better. It's a simple way to boost your nutrient intake, increase your filling quantities of healthy fibre, and keep things tasty.
2. **Olive oil over everything**: Swap out that butter and margarine for extra-virgin olive oil. It's your go-to for cooking, drizzling and dressing. Rich in healthy fats, olive oil is a cornerstone of the Mediterranean diet and perfect for heart health.
3. **Whole grains are gold**: Embrace whole grains like brown rice, quinoa and whole-wheat bread. They're packed with fibre and nutrients that keep you feeling full and satisfied, and they add a hearty, wholesome touch to any meal. And remember, as complex carbohydrates, they are good for maintaining stable blood sugar, which is also important for inflammation management.
4. **Fish a few times a week**: Include fish in your diet a couple of times a week. Rich in omega-3 fatty acids, fish such as salmon, mackerel and sardines are fantastic for your heart and brain. Plus, they add a delicious and nutritious twist to your meals.
5. **Nuts and seeds galore**: Snack on nuts and seeds like almonds, walnuts and chia seeds. They're packed with healthy fats,

protein and fibre, making them perfect for a quick and satisfying snack or a crunchy topping for your salads.
6. **Lean protein, please**: When it comes to meat, think lean and in moderation. Chicken and turkey are great choices, but don't forget to mix things up with plant-based proteins like legumes and tofu. They're good for your gut health too.
7. **Lunch like the Greeks**: Make lunch your main meal of the day. In Mediterranean cultures, lunch is often the biggest and most social meal. Enjoy it with family or friends, and fill your plate with a balanced mix of whole grains, lean protein and plenty of veggies. This approach helps keep your energy levels steady and supports better digestion.
8. **Wine's fine but drink it wisely**: If you enjoy a glass of wine, make it red. The Mediterraneans agree that a small glass with dinner can be a nice way to enhance your meal, but remember, moderation is key to reaping the benefits without the downsides.

CONTEMPLATING YOUR PROTEIN

As we hit our 50s, keeping our muscles strong and functional becomes increasingly important. That's where protein comes in. It's not just a building block for muscles; it's also essential for repairing tissues, supporting metabolism and maintaining overall health. Here's what you need to know about protein in this stage of life.

How much protein do you need?

For adults aged 50 and older, protein needs can vary slightly based on activity levels and overall health. However, general guidelines suggest aiming for around 1–1.2 grams of protein per kilogram of body weight per day. Here's a breakdown based on different body weights:
- **For a 60-kilogram person**: Aim for about 60–72 grams of protein daily.
- **For a 70-kilogram person**: Aim for about 70–84 grams of protein daily.

- **For an 80-kilogram person**: Aim for about 80–96 grams of protein daily.
- **For a 90-kilogram person**: Aim for about 90–108 grams of protein daily.

For those who are more active or aiming to build muscle, the protein needs might be slightly higher. If you're focusing on muscle strength or endurance, consider aiming for the higher end of the range or even up to 1.5 grams per kilogram.

How do you get your protein?

Not all proteins are created equal, so focusing on quality sources can make a big difference. Here's how you can meet your protein needs effectively:

Lean meats: Chicken, turkey and lean cuts of beef and pork are excellent sources of high-quality protein. Aim for grilled, baked or steamed options to keep things heart-healthy.

Fish and seafood: Fish such as salmon, trout and sardines not only provide protein but also offer those beneficial omega-3 fatty acids. Try to include fish in your diet at least twice a week.

Dairy products: Greek yoghurt, cottage cheese and low-fat milk are great sources of protein. They also provide calcium, which is important for bone health.

Eggs: Versatile and nutrient-packed, eggs are a fantastic source of protein. They're also rich in vitamins and minerals that support overall health.

Legumes and beans: Lentils, chickpeas, black beans and other legumes are excellent plant-based protein sources. They're also high in fibre and can help keep you full.

Nuts and seeds: Almonds, chia seeds and hemp seeds are not only good protein sources but also provide healthy fats and fibre.

Tofu and tempeh: As plant-based options, tofu and tempeh are rich in protein and can be a great addition to your diet, especially if you're reducing your meat consumption.

Protein supplements

Protein supplements, including powders and shakes, can be a practical solution if you're struggling to meet your daily protein needs through food alone. They offer a convenient way to boost your protein intake, especially if you have a busy lifestyle, dietary restrictions, or increased protein requirements due to health goals or conditions. But, not all protein supplements are created equal. Seek advice from your GP or a nutritionist if you have any underlying health issues.

I choose high-quality protein powders with minimal additives. Look for options that list protein as the primary ingredient and avoid those with excessive fillers, artificial sweeteners or added sugars. Also keep in mind that different protein powders are derived from various sources, such as whey, casein, soy, pea or hemp. Each type has its benefits, so choose one that aligns with your dietary preferences and needs. For example, whey protein is quickly absorbed and supports muscle recovery, while plant-based proteins are suitable for those who follow a vegetarian or vegan diet.

Supermarket protein powders can sometimes be filled with unnecessary additives, artificial flavours and sweeteners. Always check the ingredient list and nutritional information to ensure you're getting a product that's both effective and free from unwanted extras. It also pays to seek out natural brands that can be ordered online – in my experience, these provide the cleanest, most reasonably priced protein powders.

Overall, protein supplements can be a useful tool to enhance your diet, but focusing on whole food sources of protein should really be a priority for a balanced and nutrient-rich diet.

Bonus lesson
Health insurance – the things no-one tells you

As you transition into the second half of life and your kids leave home, you might start questioning whether to keep paying for health insurance – because it costs so much! It's a common dilemma, and the decision can feel like a tricky one, especially when balancing the costs with your changing health needs.

One thing that isn't talked about enough, though, is how your health needs evolve as you age, because in midlife we can sometimes still feel invincible. So I'm going to be blunt: you're likely to need more healthcare services, not less, for every year that passes. While you might be in good shape now, the reality is that issues like joint replacements, cataract surgery and heart procedures can sneak up on you. These are expensive to have without private health cover, and public waitlists can be lengthy if the procedure isn't an emergency.

It's wise to consider your insurance needs in your midlife and lock in a commitment, if you can afford to. This is something the government is really trying to encourage with its lifetime health cover (LHC) initiative, which encourages you to purchase and maintain private patient hospital cover earlier in life. If you have not taken out and maintained private patient hospital cover from the year you turn 31 and then you decide to take it out later in life, you will pay a 2 per cent LHC loading on top of your premium for every year you are aged over 30. So if you were a late starter, or if you drop your cover and decide to take it up again later, you could face this loading. After 10 years, the loading is removed, but until then it can really add up, making health insurance pricier when you might need it most.

Also, consider insuring yourself for extras cover, which is important for services that aren't always covered by basic health insurance. Look for policies that include dental care, physiotherapy and optical services like glasses and contact lenses. Hearing aids and podiatry services are also valuable, as hearing and foot health become more significant with age. Psychological services for managing stress and mental health are important too.

Think, too, about the peace of mind that comes with knowing you can access timely care. It's easy to take good health for granted, but having the right cover can make all the difference when something unexpected happens.

Health funds are now required to label their Gold, Silver, Bronze and Basic – policies consistently, based on standard clinical categories. Each tier must include a minimum level of cover, so when you're comparing your options, you're genuinely comparing apples with apples – not just clever marketing.

Gold policies cover all 38 clinical categories (including things like joint replacements, pregnancy and psychiatric care), while Silver and Bronze offer less – though some funds add extra benefits to these mid-tier policies. Basic policies offer very limited cover and are often used just to avoid the Lifetime Health Cover loading or Medicare Levy Surcharge.

When you're having a good look at what your cover includes, it's worth checking off the things you might need in the second half of your life that differ from the first half. Regarding your hospital cover, make sure your policy covers the major procedures that become more common with age, like hip, knee and other joint replacements; heart surgeries; hearing implants; and cataract surgery. You'll usually need 'gold' cover for these, which might be one level up from what you needed if you had children. Also ensure you have comprehensive cover for cancer treatments, so you can seek care without worrying about the costs.

It's worthwhile considering how your fund covers rehabilitation. Having cover for rehabilitation can help you recover more quickly from surgeries or chronic conditions, making it easier to regain your independence and wellbeing – something that everyone wants.

Of course, the Australian health system can be very good in an emergency situation. And we have great, government-supported rehabilitation services too. But if your need is not an emergency, it can be very difficult to get the treatment you need, so weigh up the idea of insurance very carefully.

If you decide it's time to check the pricing and offerings of health insurers, the best place to get an independent view is the Australian Government–run comparison website PrivateHealth.gov.au. It offers an impartial and comprehensive comparison of private health insurance policies. Be cautious of commercial platforms, where only insurers who pay for leads are featured; these sites are often biased by commissions.

And that's health insurance, another thing for you to consider the merits of in midlife. Add it to the pile of choices to make.

HOW MUCH DOES INSURANCE COST?

The typical healthy 50-year-old can expect to pay the following approximate average costs per year for 'gold' hospital and extras:
- Single: ~$3,060–$3,800 (estimated cost after rebate)
- Couple: ~$6,040–$7,600 (estimated cost after rebate).

You should expect your policy to rise in price by at least 10 per cent as you head toward 60 years of age.[56] These costs do not factor in the government private health rebate of up to 24.608 per cent, which you may be eligible for depending on your income. If your income is below a certain threshold, you may receive the full rebate; if it's above the threshold, the rebate amount may be reduced or phased out entirely.

The private health insurance rebate is available to retirees, including those who are eligible for the age pension.

Part 5
FAMILY AND COMMUNITY

As we head into the second half of life, the roles we play in our families start to shift. We naturally become the keepers of family stories, the caretakers of traditions and the guides for the next generation – whether we set out to or not. Known as the 'sandwich generation', we really are quite often the meat in the sandwich of life. It's a challenging spot to be in, but one that we can use to propel ourselves forward and prioritise what's really important.

Think about what truly matters in your family and consider whether it's time to reshape the narratives as teens turn into adults and adults into ageing parents. The relationship you've had with your kids as teens doesn't have to stay the same as they move into adulthood, and your relationship with your parents can evolve too. You have the chance to offer each relationship something new, something that reflects where you are now and what you want both for them and for yourself.

So what are your family goals for this next chapter? What do you want this phase to look like? How can you nurture closer bonds as everyone's needs and priorities shift? Midlife is your chance to create the family connections that feel right for this stage of life, bringing your loved ones closer in a way that works for everyone.

Setting family goals isn't about formal plans; it's about being intentional. Think about how you want your family to feel when it comes to connection, support and independence. These intentions can guide you as you support ageing parents, help grown kids find their footing, and nurture the relationship at the core of it all – your partnership.

There are heaps of family issues to navigate in midlife, and I don't have the space or knowledge to touch on half of them. So I've focused the lessons in this section on the three biggest issues that I think affect almost everyone in midlife – things which, when pointed out, make great sense to prioritise, at least in my world:

1. Prioritising your primary loving relationship
2. Revelling in your gradually emptying nest before it refills with grandchildren.
3. Giving your parents a good last leg.

Lesson 19
Prioritise your primary loving relationship

WE ALL KNOW THAT RELATIONSHIPS TAKE WORK, BUT WHAT MIGHT SURPRISE YOU IS how much they impact your health and happiness, especially as you age. I refer again to the Harvard Study of Adult Development, the longest ever study of human happiness which ran for over 80 years, that tells us that the quality of our relationships is the single most important factor in predicting happiness, health and even longevity.[57] The study followed 724 men initially and later their families, from two very different backgrounds: a cohort of Harvard students, and a cohort of disadvantaged men from inner-city Boston. As the men aged and lived through the many transitions of their life, the study clearly showed that while a certain amount of wealth and social status is helpful in life, it is not the key to happiness. True longstanding happiness comes from how deeply connected you are with those closest to you, especially your partner.

The most recent curator of the study, Robert Waldinger, has repeatedly revealed his favourite finding from the study: that those who were most satisfied in their relationships at age 50 were the healthiest at age 80.[58] He says that strong, supportive relationships, not wealth or fame, are key predictors of long-term physical and mental health.

According to the study, close, positive relationships not only protect your mental health but also your physical wellbeing. Couples who feel emotionally connected experience lower levels of chronic stress, and this has a direct impact on the cortisol levels in your body. Cortisol, the stress hormone, when chronically elevated, has been linked to a host of health issues, including heart disease, high blood pressure, inflammation and even cognitive decline.[59]

Interestingly, research shows that it's not just about avoiding loneliness but the quality of your connections that truly matters. A study published in the *Journal of Social and Personal Relationships* found that people in toxic or ambivalent relationships (those that swing between affection and conflict) are at a higher risk of both mental and physical health problems than those who are single.[60] So it's not just about being in any relationship. It's about fostering a healthy, supportive partnership that you can genuinely enjoy over the course of your life.

Sounds ideal, doesn't it? Yet so many people find themselves feeling lethargic or lost in their relationships during midlife, somewhat or fully disconnected from their partner as they go about the routines of life with relative independence: meeting to tackle chores, manage logistics and handle finances, and sitting side by side on the couch in silence at other times. Between the demands of work, maintaining a household, raising nearly-adult kids and caring for ageing parents, couples can often feel isolated from each other even if they lie in bed beside each other at night. The reality is that many couples in midlife experience 'relationship drift', a gradual distancing as attention shifts toward external responsibilities and away from a nurturing of the partnership. But midlife also presents an opportunity for renewal, as life begins to change again, freeing up time to dedicate to each other again – if you choose to. This is another of those choices you get in midlife, this time to get your relationship back on track and higher on your priority list.

If this drift sounds familiar, I want to suggest five priorities for you to focus on to help it thrive. After all, thriving relationships are something we all need to live longer, healthier and happier lives.

1. UNDERSTAND WHERE YOU ARE AT AND ACKNOWLEDGE WHAT'S AFFECTING YOU BOTH

Midlife is often marked by significant transitions: kids leaving home, career changes, even a sense of personal reinvention. While these transitions are natural, they can create strain in relationships. A common issue in this phase is the 'empty nest syndrome', where couples who have been focused on parenting suddenly find themselves with more time, but less sense of shared purpose. Without the daily routines of raising children, some couples struggle to re-establish their connection, unsure of how to relate without the buffer of kids or work.

Another challenge is the midlife identity shift. Many people undergo a period of reflection in midlife, questioning their purpose, goals and priorities. This shift can go in one of two directions. Some may feel disengaged or lost, while others may experience a burst of personal growth that can leave their partner feeling left behind or like they don't recognise the other person – particularly if one person is pursuing new interests, friendships or career paths while the other is less engaged in change. This can cause a rift, as one partner feels neglected or unsure of how to reconnect with the 'new' version of their spouse.

If you're feeling this type of transition or disconnection, it helps to identify it, talk about your feelings, and be open about your intention to find that connection again.

2. RECOGNISE COMMUNICATIONS CHALLENGES AND MAKE AN EFFORT TO RESET

Then there are communication styles to consider. Some communication patterns can become deeply ingrained in long-term relationships, and not all of them are healthy. By midlife, some couples may have developed a passive style, where they avoid conflict and important conversations, thinking it's easier than confronting the issues head-on. This is particularly common when both partners are fatigued by the pressures of life and feel like it's too late to change.

Other couples might experience more frequent arguments as they adjust to the boiling troubles of life, with stressors triggering defensive communication patterns. For instance, some might feel blamed or judged by their partner's frustrations, leading to defensiveness or an emotional shutting down. Research by Dr John Gottman, one of the world leaders in marital relationships, shows that these types of communication breakdowns, if left unchecked, can create a cycle of emotional distance and resentment.[61]

Gottman identified four communication styles that can destroy a relationship, which he called the 'Four Horsemen': criticism, defensiveness, contempt and stonewalling. His research, spanning decades, reveals that couples who avoid these destructive patterns and instead practise what he calls 'repair attempts', or who make a conscious effort to de-escalate tension during conflict, are far more likely to stay together and stay happy. This could be as simple as injecting humour, expressing affection or offering an apology, even in the heat of the moment. Gottman says it's about signalling to your partner that you value the relationship more than the argument itself.

Recognising these communications patterns and behaviours really is the first step, and the good news is that Gottman's research shows that couples can successfully break these negative patterns.

Of course, everything in a relationship can be improved with more active listening, which means focusing on your partner's perspective without planning a rebuttal. It helps to rebuild a real emotional connection. Gottman's research found that couples who regularly practise kindness, repair, active listening and the connection that comes with each, not only reduce conflict but also strengthen their bond, and that creates a more supportive, nurturing relationship over time.

3. TAKE INTIMACY SERIOUSLY

Rebuilding or simply reconnecting in midlife often means rediscovering both emotional and physical intimacy. Let's face it: emotional intimacy might've taken a back seat during the chaos of family and work demands, and physically, things are changing in midlife that no-one really talks about. But it's worth tackling these things head-on because both are key to keeping those long-term bonds strong and driving your happiness.

The best way to reconnect emotionally, according to research in the *Journal of Social and Personal Relationships*, is by taking active steps like spending quality time together, revisiting old interests, and having real conversations about every part of your lives.[62] It sounds simple, but in midlife, it takes real time and energy to rebuild and maintain that connection.

Gottman's research shows that staying emotionally connected is all about how couples respond to each other's bids for connection, those little moments when your partner seeks attention, affection or even just a chat.[63] Whether it's asking how their day went, sharing a joke or reaching for their hand, acknowledging these bids strengthens emotional intimacy over time.

The National Marriage Project at the University of Virginia found that couples who carve out quality time together at least once a week, whether it's a casual date night or a shared activity, are three times more likely to say they're 'very happy' in their relationship. It doesn't have to be fancy, just consistent.[64]

And here's something interesting: another study in the *Journal of Personality and Social Psychology* shows that trying new and exciting things together can give your relationship a boost.[65] This is a big one in midlife, when routines can feel stale. Doing something fresh –a trip, a hobby, a new adventure or a project together – can reignite that spark and create new memories to share.

And then there's physical intimacy. It can really become a source of strain in midlife relationships, even if you've been together forever. Between hormonal changes, health issues, changes in body shape and stress, both men and women can experience shifts that reduce sexual desire and create discomfort. The key here is to talk openly about what's going on, rather than brushing it under the rug. Facing it together can take a lot of the pressure off.

Sometimes it's about making simple lifestyle changes – getting more sleep, managing stress, staying active – that can give both of you a bit more energy and desire. If needed, there's also medical support like hormone therapy or addressing specific health concerns that might help you feel more comfortable and confident. And don't underestimate the value of counselling if you're struggling to communicate your needs or want to reignite that connection.

Remember that sexual health and physical affection are still really important, even as things shift with age. It doesn't always have to be about sex, either. Holding hands, hugging or just being close physically can go a long way. The goal is to keep that connection alive and growing, even as life changes.

4. REDISCOVER A SHARED PURPOSE AND GOALS

In midlife, many couples often find they need to rebuild a shared sense of purpose. After years of focusing on kids, careers and other responsibilities, it's time to refocus on each other. Research shows that couples who engage in shared activities tend to feel more emotionally connected.[66] Doing things together creates a renewed sense of partnership, offering fresh ways to bond and actually enjoy each other's company again.

Now is also the perfect time to revisit and redefine your future goals as a couple. Start thinking about what the years ahead might look like. What will your Prime Time look and feel like? How do you want to spend your time? What new adventures are on the horizon, and what do you want to share? What will your house and the lifestyle you live look like as the kids gradually become independent, and how can you share in building the next phase of your life together a little more?

Setting goals together not only gives you both a sense of direction, it can also reignite palpable excitement for the future.

5. EMBRACE THE CHANGES

Finally, reconnecting in midlife is about embracing the natural changes that come with this stage of life.

Midlife is a time for growth, reflection and often reinvention – and your relationship is part of that. Instead of seeing the challenges that come with midlife as a threat, look at them as an opportunity to build something even stronger. Research on relationship resilience shows that couples who tackle these challenges together, and see them as opportunities to grow, come out the other side more connected and solid than ever before.[67]

LOOKING FOR SOME IDEAS TO HELP RE-ESTABLISH YOUR LOVE CONNECTION?

Reignite shared interests: If you feel like you've drifted apart, reigniting shared interests can help. Whether it's a hobby, sport or creative pursuit, spending time together doing something you both enjoy is key to rebuilding emotional intimacy.

Create new rituals: It could be weekly date nights, morning coffee together, or even a short walk at the end of the day. Regardless, new, enjoyable rituals help bring consistency to your time together and strengthen your bond. It shows each of you that the other one values time spent together.

Schedule regular 'dream sessions': Take time to sit down together, maybe once a month, to chat about your future. No pressure, just a chance to throw around ideas about what you both want and what makes you excited for the next phase.

Plan a getaway: It doesn't have to be an expensive trip. A weekend away or a local adventure can give you both time to relax, enjoy each other's company, and talk about what's next.

Show appreciation every day: Simple acts of gratitude and appreciation go a long way, such as saying thanks and being genuinely grateful for the effort your partner puts in. Studies show that partners who regularly express appreciation for one another experience deeper satisfaction and connection.

Support each other's health goals: Whether it's joining your partner in a workout, eating healthily alongside them as peer support, or helping them manage stress, being a healthy ally for each other has a lot of lasting benefits for your relationship and your feeling of wellbeing.

Don't be afraid to get some counselling: If the issues seem too big to handle alone, couples counselling can be incredibly helpful – if both partners are open to it. A trained relationship counsellor can provide the tools to help break negative communication cycles, resolve past conflicts and create a more positive relationship dynamic. Look for someone with specific experience tackling the age and stage of life you're at.

Lesson 20
Revel in your gradually emptying nest

FOR MANY PARENTS, THE SO-CALLED EMPTY NEST CAN FEEL LIKE AN EMOTIONAL rollercoaster – I'm right in the thick of it myself. One minute they're home, then they're gone! Suddenly, they're back – but wait, now they've got other priorities. And just like that, they're off again.

After years of focusing on the kids, the house suddenly feels quieter, and life shifts in ways that can feel unfamiliar. It is quieter, but remember, there was a life before kids when we loved this stillness and time to do things that were all about us. Sure, the transition might bring moments of grief or even a sense of loss, but it's also packed with possibility – a chance to reframe, rediscover, and redefine what this new chapter can be. Of course, the empty nest isn't a clean break for most people. It's rarely a one-way ticket to freedom. Kids stay home for longer, then they bounce in and out, especially these days with those overseas trips, long university holidays, job changes and even boomerang moves back home. It's a constant dance of letting go, then welcoming them back, which sometimes feels like a loop that should've ended but might never do so. Many people's nests aren't emptying out quite as fast as they'd imagined.

So how do you find balance in this new reality?

This stage of life is more about building bridges back to your kids than fully cutting ties. Yes, they've left, but they're not gone, and relationships evolve. New family habits need to be set, creating space for their independence while maintaining a connection in a way that respects their adult life. What it's really about is finding those moments to reconnect as equals rather than as parent and child. This is where you start to see your relationship with your kids in a whole new light, more collaborative than directive and easier to enjoy.

Setting new expectations is so important. Sounds simple, right? But it's often easier said than done, especially as they transition from being financially dependent to … well, a bit less dependent – if you can manage it. Let's dive into how this shift might feel and explore what you can do as your nest empties, not just to cope but to truly embrace this new chapter, often long before your nest fills up with grandchildren.

RECOGNISE THE EMOTIONAL ROLLERCOASTER AND REFRAME

It can be a crazy time for parents. If the kids are gone, you feel like you constantly want them back; if they're there, you feel like you want them gone. When kids do leave home, it's completely normal for parents to feel all over the place emotionally. For some, it hits hard – a sense of grief and this weird loss of purpose creeps in. Psychologist Nancy Schlossberg, who knows a thing or two about life transitions, talks about how this shift can leave parents feeling a deep emptiness. You find yourself asking, 'What now?' or 'Who am I if I'm not a full-time parent?'[68]

Schlossberg's research shows that how parents deal with this transition is all over the map. Some dive deep into loneliness or even depression, while others feel a strange relief, excited to have more freedom but also hesitant about what to do with it.[69] It's natural to grieve one chapter while not knowing what to do with the next. That emotional tug-of-war of 'an ending' is real. The trick is to remember that it's perfectly okay to feel a mix of everything: sadness for the chapter that's closing, and excitement for what comes next. Remember the lessons in the 'Work, purpose and happiness' section of this book (Part 3) on transitions; it's not dissimilar here.

And remember that after all 'endings' there is a chance for self-discovery or a 'middle zone', and then the green shoots of personal growth. It's about reframing. Instead of focusing on what you've lost, ask yourself, 'What opportunities does this new phase offer?' This isn't about forgetting your role as a parent but embracing a new chapter where you get to rediscover yourself and your passions. The empty nest can become your gateway to finding new purpose and joy. It's about shifting your mindset from 'What have I lost?' to 'What can I explore now?'

SET UP NEW FAMILY HABITS

Let's talk about the practical stuff, because even when the kids have grown up and moved out of the house, they're not out of your life. Setting up new family habits as they transition into adulthood is vital. The dynamic has changed, and that means the way you interact needs to shift too.

At first they might still be under your roof, but they're asserting their independence, maybe coming and going on their own terms while still being part of the day-to-day life of the household. Later, they may not live with you full-time anymore, but you still want them to be a big part of your life. This is where you can start creating new rituals. Maybe it's family dinners once a week, a phone call every Sunday, a yearly trip together, or just texting each other throughout the day. You need to let go of control and allow the relationship to evolve. It's time to ask, 'What kind of relationship do we want now?', and then listen to what your children need as adults. This is not always easy, but it's crucial for building lasting, healthy connections as your kids grow and change.

When they're living at home as adults, set boundaries that work for both of you. What are the house rules now? What's expected of the children? How do you maintain your own space and independence, particularly if they're only temporarily back home on a boomerang move? And how will you both work to build more financial independence?

When they've left the nest, it's time to set rhythms that feel natural to both of you. Find ways to stay connected and keep that warmth alive without falling into old habits of trying to manage their lives.

EMERGING ADULTS NEED LOW-PRESSURE RITUALS

Psychologist Jeffrey Arnett coined the term 'emerging adulthood' to describe the period from ages 18 to 29 when young adults are figuring out their identity, independence and life direction.[70] During this time, the relationship with parents typically shifts from a hierarchical dynamic to one based more on mutual respect. Arnett's research shows that young adults still value their relationships with parents but want space to figure things out on their own. This explains why regular, low-pressure rituals like family dinners or check-in calls are helpful, as they allow for connection without overstepping the mark into managing their lives.

FINANCIAL INDEPENDENCE AND SETTING UP FOR THE NEXT PHASE OF YOUR LIFE

Financial independence for your kids can be a sticking point. It's natural to want to help your kids, but at the same time it's important to make sure you're setting yourself up for the future too. Let's face it: you need a financial ending so you can have a fresh beginning and they need a financial beginning to learn financial literacy slowly and carefully. You have to admit, it's hard to fully transition into the set-up phase of your Prime Time when you're still carrying some (or all) of your children's financial weight. While most of us parents are happy to help, there comes a time when your own financial independence has to take centre stage. This is about drawing a line between supporting your kids and making sure you're setting yourself up for the Prime Time of your life. The two most difficult expenses to separate are bearing their motor vehicle expenses and private health insurance costs. Make sure you notice these as you bid them farewell.

As hard as it is, helping your kids transition financially, whether it's through saving plans, teaching them about budgeting, or even charging them rent if they move back into the home, sets both of you up for success. You're giving them the tools to stand on their own two feet while also making sure your own future is protected. That's not selfish, it's practical.

Speaking of which, here are some practical steps to get you there.

HAVE THE MONEY TALK

Be open and honest about where things stand. Explain that while you're happy to help with money, it's time for them to take more responsibility for their finances. If they're moving back home temporarily, set clear expectations about how they'll contribute, whether it's financially or by helping with household tasks.

SET A BUDGET TOGETHER

Help them create a realistic budget if they don't already have one. Walk them through their income, expenses and saving goals. Apps like Pocketbook and Frollo are great tools to help them track spending and build good financial habits.

ENCOURAGE THEIR SAVING GOALS

Guide them in setting up a dedicated savings plan, whether it's for a house deposit, emergency fund or long-term financial goals. Matching or supporting their savings contributions can be a motivating way to encourage them to take saving more seriously.

CHARGE RENT IF YOU NEED TO

If they're living at home, consider charging them rent. It helps prepare them for future financial responsibilities and gives you a little relief. You could even stash some of this money away for them, creating a savings cushion they can use when they eventually move out to rent or buy a home.

REVISIT YOUR OWN FINANCIAL GOALS

Now is the time to focus on your own finances. What does your retirement look like? Are there adventures or projects you've been putting off because your kids were your main focus? Take a deep dive into your savings, investments and superannuation. This is the chance to make sure your own plans for Prime Time are on track. You might want to talk to a financial adviser to help fine-tune your strategy.

REKINDLING YOUR RELATIONSHIP WITH YOUR PARTNER

And let's not forget about your partner in all this. Once the kids leave, you're left with more time together – sometimes a lot more. And you're likely nowhere near retirement yet! It can feel strange, even awkward at first, to be back to just the two of you after years of focusing on family life. And, in my experience, many are afraid of what it will be like.

It helps to see it as an opportunity to rediscover each other, to reset the way you do things at home. Find some ways to have fun together and enjoy being together again, without the distractions and interruptions of others around you.

A study from the *Journal of Marriage and Family* shows that couples often experience a resurgence in their relationship once the kids are gone.[71] Without the day-to-day stress of parenting, there's real space to reconnect. We've just learned about that in the last section.

PRIORITISE YOURSELF AGAIN

Remember the catchcry of the Prime Timer, the line I use on my podcast to explain what your Prime Time is: 'When your kids have got their P-plates and the mortgage is almost paid off, it's time to put *you* back in the picture.' And so it is!

With the nest empty (or mostly empty), it's time to turn back to yourself. That might feel really foreign. In fact, you might have completely forgotten what it feels like to be selfish. But take a minute and remember being a 20-something and living life to the fullest with only you as the priority. This can be yours again now – with new perspective.

So think about it. What have you been putting off? This is your time to reinvest in your sense of purpose, health and emotional wellbeing. It's time to do stuff just because you want to, again. Maybe it's time to explore a new hobby, pick up a class, do something creative, organise a book club, go out with the girls. Whatever it is, remember that staying mentally and socially engaged has been shown to boost both cognitive and emotional health.

Don't let the quiet house make you feel like you've slowed down. Use this time to speed up in the areas that matter most to you.

Lesson 21
Give your parents a good last leg

AT THE BEGINNING OF THIS BOOK, WE TALKED ABOUT TWO LIFE STAGES WE FACE — ageing and frailty. But now, as your closest relatives get to this point, things get very real – sometimes fast!

Our parents looked after us our whole lives, so when it comes to their later years, if our relationship with them is strong, it feels right to try to give them the best 'last leg' we can. That doesn't mean you need to become a full-time carer or even bring them into your own home. It's about making sure they feel secure, respected and loved. It's about understanding their needs as they age and, as best we can, doing what we can to meet them.

Many of us haven't needed to navigate this part of life before, and when our parents reach that stage, it can catch us off guard. There's no user manual for this. In fact, I'm told by many that it can be an incredible privilege and a heavy burden at the same time. My parents are still in their 70s, not yet traversing the ageing phase fully. But I've gathered some of the best lessons from people who have already walked this road – insights they wish they'd known from the start.

Here's how to manage it without losing your balance.

GET CURIOUS – FIND OUT WHAT A GOOD LAST LEG MEANS TO YOUR PARENTS

Growing older means something different for everyone, and different families do it differently. So the first thing you need to understand is what your parents hope for in their ageing years. It's a worthwhile conversation to have when they're still healthy enough but can see their friends ageing around them. For some, there's an incredible desire to remain independent, within their community. For others, there's a hunger to be near their family and feel supported, loved and included.

If they're a couple, there's a natural fear of losing a partner, a home and friends, and what life will look like if one of them is gone. Remember this, and look out for it along the way. Change is hard, and it's even harder when we're old.

The one thing no-one wants is to die alone in an institution surrounded by strangers. If you and your family can support your parents to age with the love, attention and care of their loved ones around them, you're doing something truly special.

UNDERSTAND THE SIGNS OF AGEING

Spotting the early signs of ageing in your parents can be tricky, especially when it's up to you to address it and they don't see (or don't want to see) an issue. It's a tough but important role, as these small changes we notice early on can often be signs of what's ahead. Whether it's hearing loss, balance issues, memory lapses or more obvious declines in health, catching these sooner rather than later can make all the difference in setting up support that can help them stay safe, maintain their independence and quality of life.

Jessie's story is a good example. Living in Melbourne, she only visited her parents on the Gold Coast a few times a year. One Christmas, Jessie noticed her mum was struggling: repeating stories in a loop, and even getting lost once on a quick trip to the shops, then calling later from a completely different suburb. Concerned, Jessie suggested her mum see their family doctor, but these events were brushed off as typical forgetfulness. Reassured, Jessie went back to her life and work.

A few months later, Jessie returned to the Gold Coast to find her mum still looping, but now more noticeably. She tried raising her concerns privately with her dad, who again dismissed them, saying he didn't see any problems 'day to day'. But by the following Christmas, Jessie's mum's symptoms were clear as she really struggled with small details and increasingly seemed confused. This time, Jessie knew something needed to be done.

Moments like these can feel daunting, especially when you're the one seeing the change and your parents are resisting the idea that they might need extra help – sometimes even working together to deny ageing. But noticing these signs is often a call to step in, observe patterns and gently raise options for support.

Once Jessie leaned in more firmly, her father opened up, admitting it had been tough for him – that he'd been reluctant to worry her and her brother and he didn't want it to become real. From there, it became easier for Jessie and her dad to work together and talk to her mum, addressing both her mum's medical needs and finding the right support for her dad too.

Having that open, compassionate conversation can make all the difference. It allows you to break through fears of ageing and concerns about losing independence, and it opens the door to discussing ways to help your parents stay safe, respected and supported through their journey. There are many ways to help them live their last leg in comfort and dignity. The first is with open two-way conversations.

TIDY UP THE PAPERWORK EARLY

Paperwork is boring, often untidy and out of date, but things can get much more stressful if it's not in order later in life. One of the best ways to avoid future stress is to get all the paperwork for ageing parents in order early on – or to encourage them to do this and share it as part of a proactive approach to ageing well. This includes knowing where important documents such as wills, powers of attorney, health directives, superannuation statements and insurance policies are kept. If possible, create a digital back-up or at least a checklist of what exists, where to find it, and who their advisers are. As your parents' needs grow, having everything organised will make it far easier for them to manage their affairs and for you or a sibling to step in when needed. Plus, it can give you and them peace of mind knowing that nothing important will be overlooked later on.

HAVE A HARD TALK ABOUT HOUSING

One of the trickiest things to manage later in life is housing. Inappropriate or unmanageable homes can be a huge factor in a crisis, sometimes even leading to the last-minute move of a parent into your home. The best advice I can give? Start the conversation about housing much earlier in their ageing process.

The reality is that the easier their home is to get around – think fewer stairs, safer bathrooms and easy access – the longer they're likely to stay there. And for most people, that's a big deal.

If they live far away but want more connection, encourage them to think about moving closer to you. Being nearby can be helpful for everyone, especially if support needs increase over time.

If they're considering a retirement community, remember that the ideal time to make that move is when they're healthy enough to enjoy the social side of it, not just the care.

And if they're a couple, get them talking about where they'd want to live if one day only one of them remains, and making those decisions together now. It's an opportunity to leave the big home and memories behind and to build new connections together, so one of them doesn't have to do it all alone while grieving.

Don't shy away from talking about their real housing needs now and in the future. It can make all the difference for a smoother, more independent life later on.

KNOW THAT EVEN THE SMARTEST PEOPLE LOSE FINANCIAL LITERACY

Talking about money with our parents is something we often avoid, but it's a crucial conversation to have. Many older people are on a fixed income, and aged care, health support and even simple in-home modifications can be costly and frightening. Working together to understand their financial situation, including any pensions, super and savings, is a smart move.

Know that as they age, even the most financially savvy parents might experience a dip in financial literacy. It's not about intelligence or losing their edge, just a natural part of cognitive ageing that can affect how quickly and how accurately they handle complex decisions. Studies by the Center for Retirement Research at Boston College show that financial decision-making ability tends to decline by around 1 per cent per year after 60.[72] Understanding complex financial statements, grasping unfamiliar concepts and making tricky calculations can all start to feel a bit harder. Your parents' foundational knowledge can stay solid, but adapting to new financial complexities can become challenging, potentially leading to costly mistakes or even vulnerability to scams. Keep in mind, too, that while cognitive changes happen, many older people retain a high level of confidence in their financial skills – refusing to relinquish control, making it challenging for you to help.

Here's how you can help if your mum, dad or both are ageing yet still confidently handling their finances:

- **Start conversations early**: Gently suggest involving a trusted family member, advocate or adviser to add a layer of support.
- **Encourage financial check-ins**: Sit down periodically to review finances, go over statements and discuss any concerns.
- **Discuss power of attorney options**: Early conversations about a financial power of attorney can make future transitions smoother.
- **Stay informed and observant**: Watch for signs like missed payments or difficulty managing investments, which may indicate a need for more support.

- **Discuss how you'll support the surviving parent**: When one parent passes, especially if it's the father who may have traditionally handled the finances, there can be a lot of worry. It can help to discuss and build a strategy to support the surviving parent upfront.

Don't forget to protect your own financial future. Supporting ageing parents is important, but avoid jeopardising your own retirement plans. Balance helping them with maintaining your own stability.

MAKE SURE THEY KNOW THEY MIGHT NEED SOME SUPPORT

As our parents age, their needs change, and the support they require often progresses in stages. Knowing what to expect – and when – can make a huge difference in ensuring they remain comfortable, independent and safe for as long as possible. This gradual approach also helps us, as carers and loved ones, adapt to increasing responsibilities over time without feeling overwhelmed.

Care needs usually start with light assistance with daily tasks or support to recover from surgery. The first type of help people usually access is simple stuff like getting assistance with the shopping, having meals delivered so they don't have to cook, arranging medication delivery in pre-prepared packaging for easy monitoring, and being transported to doctor's appointments. Being involved in this is typically the easiest way to be supportive and keep your parents independent in most areas – but you can also pay home help service providers to assist from this early stage.

At this point, most people also begin looking into government assessments for care services through the My Aged Care portal. There can be long wait times for assessment, and accessing government-supported care services can be tricky, but persevere. Tackling your parents' needs early on makes it easier to move through the system as their needs progress.

The next step is usually to support them with cleaning, gardening and home maintenance, making sure they're able to stay in their home as long as possible. From there, the need for in-home assistance can often increase gradually, with a personal carer to help with bathing and dressing, a nurse for medical tasks, and more support with mobility. As health and mobility decline, more regular and increased clinical care services might be needed to help them each day.

If managing alone becomes too difficult or unsafe, it may be time to explore more comprehensive options, like full-time in-home care or moving into assisted living. This level of care covers all daily needs while keeping them as comfortable and independent as possible.

For those needing 24-hour care, options like residential aged care facilities offer intensive support, which is especially helpful when mobility or medical needs become complex. This stage includes constant assistance with personal care, health monitoring and opportunities for social engagement.

SET SOME BOUNDARIES ON YOUR CAREGIVING

This is one that often gets lost. Your parents' last leg is important, but so are your prime time years. Caregivers can sometimes find themselves in an all-or-nothing tug-of-war in caring for a parent, but that's just not sensible. Set some boundaries, and if you have siblings, engage them in the process. If your siblings or other loved ones who want to help are far away (or less helpful), lean on them for respite or other support. Put the right balance of professional care in place – daily, weekly or respite services – because people often live longer than doctors predict. Also, carers aren't always fun to be around if they're not getting out for some proper social contact. Remember this, and look out for other carers around you too.

As a carer, you need to live your own life, so keep up your friendships and relationships and even your work – and, for goodness' sake, exercise! At your age, you need to maintain your own health, financial security and career progress. Being a martyr by your parents' side could severely limit your ability to stay professionally relevant, healthy and able to care for the other people in your life – like your partner and children, who are your ongoing priorities.

FIND SOME SHARED THINGS YOU CAN DO TOGETHER

The last leg isn't just about caregiving, finances and powers of attorney. It's also about sharing, enjoying your parents' company and spending quality time together. This is a wonderful time to dive into their memories and photo albums, listening to the stories of their life and giving them the chance to relive those moments.

Some of the best memories Prime Timers have of this stage with their parents are the simple things: watching TV or movies together, chatting about current affairs stories in the newspaper, and reflecting on the past, comparing it to today. It's these shared moments that create the lasting connections and memories you'll cherish.

REMEMBER: MANY PEOPLE BECOME SINGLE LATER IN LIFE – OFTEN FOR YEARS

At some point in the second half of life, many people face the reality of becoming single – whether through the loss of a partner or a late-in-life divorce. It's a major life transition, often bringing a mix of emotional, social and financial challenges. Being prepared to support your parents through this stage both practically and emotionally can make all the difference.

When someone becomes single later in life, it's not just their emotional world that shifts. Financial realities often change too, and these two aspects are deeply intertwined. For widowed parents, this might mean navigating their partner's estate, adjusting superannuation drawdowns, or learning to manage their finances alone for the first time. For divorced parents, the process of dividing assets or rethinking their retirement plans can be equally daunting.

This is where your role becomes pivotal. Beyond being there emotionally to listen, to support, to help them rebuild, you can also help them feel secure and able to navigate it. Practical steps such as reviewing their financial position or ensuring they're accessing the right entitlements (such as the age pension or other benefits) can alleviate stress. But remember, the focus isn't on solving everything for them, it's about helping them feel equipped and empowered to navigate these changes themselves.

At the same time, this is an opportunity to strengthen your relationship. For a parent who's widowed, this might involve guiding them through the grieving process while encouraging them to re-engage with the world. For divorced parents, it's about helping them find their footing again socially, emotionally and financially, and reminding them that it's never too late to create a new chapter.

Practical preparedness can help smooth the road. This could mean helping your parents review their wills, update powers of attorney, or organise their superannuation accounts, knowing their financial situation is important too – for both people in a couple, not just one. It's not about overwhelming them with responsibilities and details but making sure the knowledge and practicalities are in place so they can focus on what matters most: rediscovering purpose, staying connected, and building a life they love, even in the face of big changes.

And remember, loneliness is a huge risk for older people, particularly those adjusting to life on their own. You can help by introducing them to community groups, hobby clubs or even online tools to stay socially connected. Small actions, like regular check-ins or shared meals, go a long way in making them feel supported and seen. For those ready, exploring things like dating apps or social activities for older singles might even be part of their new journey.

KNOW THAT AGEING CAN SOMETIMES CAUSE ANGER

Ageing isn't just about physical changes. It's also about facing a loss of control over your own life as it bears down on you, and that can come out as anger. My grandmother made life hell for my father in her final year. She despised the carers, complained about the food he had delivered, and nitpicked over everything – even the way her bed was made by the lady who came to clean. She was frustrated, and she made sure he knew it. Her whole world felt out of her hands, and she took it out on the one person doing the most for her. She even told everyone she could that it was my dad's fault, that he'd somehow chosen the wrong carers and cleaners, and that he just didn't understand what she needed.

When I came to visit, though, I was an angel in her eyes. She showered me with her good vibes. He got grumpy grandma and I got grateful grandma.

When our loved ones lose their grip on the everyday things that once defined their independence, it can be incredibly upsetting for them. Imagine knowing exactly how you want things done but no longer having the power to make it happen. It's not just frustrating but also frightening. This feeling can lead them to direct anger toward those closest to them, often the very people trying their hardest to help. For many, the hardest part of ageing is knowing they could do things better, but realising they can't anymore.

When an ageing parent's anger surfaces, especially when they direct it at you, it's important to keep it in perspective. Remind yourself that their frustration isn't really about you. It's rooted in their struggle with losing independence. They're dealing with feelings of fear, helplessness and sometimes even grief over the life they once controlled.

Instead, acknowledge their feelings, redirect the conversation, and look for small wins together that will offer some semblance of control to them. Stay compassionate and keep doing your best. And whatever you do, don't let their anger divide you and your siblings. Working together as a family is how you'll weather this storm.

REMEMBER WHAT REALLY MATTERS

Despite the heartache of watching your parents age, there are only three things any older person truly wants, and it's worth keeping these close:

1. To know their family loves them dearly
2. To know they played a special role in making you who you are today, and that you value them for that in their later years
3. To not be alone, sad or lonely at the end.

Remembering this can help you stay grounded and give meaning to the hard moments.

Part 6
TRAVEL AND ADVENTURE

When you're working, especially in midlife, you need adventure as much as you need travel. In fact, the two often go hand in hand, yet they serve very different purposes. We Australians, as some of the most curious and adventurous travellers in the Western world, have a particular hunger to see, experience and enjoy the richness that other cultures have to offer. But in midlife it's not just about hopping on a plane for a holiday. It's about weaving travel and adventure into our lives, finding ways to make both part of the way we live, and using our health and physical and mental capability well, while they are in good form.

As we head into midlife in this new generation, many of us having saved our superannuation for decades, we often have a bit more time and opportunity for travel than we might have previously imagined – and a little more money to do it with, if we're lucky or have planned well. And we've got lots of options for how we can go about this.

I could write endlessly on travel because I love doing it and I love inspiring people to do more of it! But alas, there just isn't enough space. So I've focused this travel section on the five biggest lessons I think we all want to understand in midlife:

1. Embrace challenge, adventure and active travel: understand your options
2. Seek out sabbaticals – several times in your life
3. Learn the tricks of the travel trade and get better value
4. Don't be afraid to go solo.
5. Understand travel money and insurance, and know what to watch out for.

Lesson 22
Embrace challenge, adventure and active travel: understand your options

As we hit midlife, it seems a bit silly to wait for full retirement before we start truly experiencing life. The potential we have right now is enormous, and travel and adventure are essential ingredients for a fulfilling Prime Time. But here's the thing – the kinds of trips that make sense at this stage of life often differ from what you might envision for your later, full retirement years.

In your Prime Time, you're still balancing work and squeezing in travel and adventure whenever you can. But there's a shift that happens when you become more aware that time isn't endless. You start to realise just how important it is to make the most of the time and health you have, to do the things you've always dreamed of, and to spend that time with the people you love.

For me, travel and adventure aren't just about the big, once-a-year family holidays. They're about separating the two – travel and adventure – and making sure both have a place in your life, whether it's a quick weekend getaway or an ambitious adventure you've always had on your bucket list.

Think about it: travel is when you plan, pack your bags and set off on a journey. You leave home, explore new places and take time away from your regular routine. It's exciting, immersive and often deeply fulfilling.

Adventure, on the other hand, doesn't always mean hopping on a plane. Adventure can be woven into your everyday life: exploring a new part of town on a weekend, trying something different after work or diving into a passion project. It's the spirit of discovery, whether it's far-flung or right around the corner.

I think we deserve both travel and adventure in our Prime Time. But the catch is that, for many of us, it takes a bit of a mindset shift. We need to recognise that if we want more out of life, we have to be more proactive.

If there's one priority I'd urge you to focus on, it's tackling the toughest trips first: the challenges, the gap years, the active adventure travel and the bucket list trips you've always wanted to take. Because there's no escaping this truth: while we're all told we might live longer than we expect, there's also a very real possibility that we won't, or that our health will limit us.

So how do you make sure you're not leaving your biggest adventures until it's too late? It's pretty simple – you start now. And you keep reminding yourself to do it while you can!

Don't put off the trips that are physically challenging or that require a bit more endurance. In your Prime Time, you've still got the health and energy to take them on. So make a list of those dream trips, especially the ones that will be harder to do later, and prioritise them.

At the same time, weave in those smaller, everyday adventures. They don't require long flights or big budgets, but they bring just as much joy and fulfilment. Whether it's a weekend road trip, a group expedition aligned with a new hobby or exploring a local rail or walking trail, these little adventures keep your sense of curiosity alive and remind you that life is for living, right now, in the moments between the big milestones.

Now we're going to look at the many wonderful ways in which you can do that, so you don't feel lost for inspiration.

THE TYPES OF TRAVEL TO CONTEMPLATE

As we enter Prime Time, we're not necessarily looking to give up work entirely, but most of us seek more flexibility to fit travel and adventure into our lives – and our travel goals are different to those we've had in our peak family years.

I like to break prime time travel into 10 key areas. Each of them has a place in midlife, in my opinion. Different types of travel can be combined, or you can choose the hardest types of travel first. Again, it's a real choose-your-own adventure.

1. PRIME TIME CHALLENGES

Prime Time challenges get me excited, and I'm increasingly seeing 50-somethings embrace them. I think this part of the travel market is set to skyrocket. This type of travel pushes you out of your comfort zone and gives you a sense of physical and mental achievement. It might involve hiking the Overland Track or the Three Capes Track in Tasmania, doing the Rottnest Channel Swim in Western Australia, walking the Camino de Santiago in north-western Spain or doing the Annapurna Base Camp Trek in Nepal, cycle-touring the Italian Alps or running the New York Marathon.

Clever travel operators are making these types of challenges more accessible, building multi-day hikes, sporting challenges and extreme expeditions, many of which are aimed at Prime Timers. They are the kinds of experiences that are physically and mentally challenging but incredibly rewarding.

Why now? In their 40s, 50s and 60s, most people still have the energy and health to take on really adventurous trips, and these challenges provide a sense of purpose and growth. They give you something to train for, and a sense of reward when you complete them.

> ## SOME REAL-LIFE CHALLENGES
>
> Janelle completed the coast-to-coast Astungkara Way across Bali: 'A hundred and forty kilometres over 10 days. The scenery was stunning, the food was exceptional, and I learned so much about the culture, regenerative farming and the impact of commercial tourism. It was an inspiring and unforgettable trip.'
>
> Sandy joined a ladies' walking group in her 50s to push herself to do more: 'I've hiked the Cinque Terre in Italy and done a hiking adventure in Vietnam. Back home, we've tackled the Sapphire Coast, explored around Bowral, and even hiked while houseboating down the Murray in South Australia. Friends from the group have hiked the UK coast to coast and visited Africa, among many other adventures. Getting older doesn't stop the adventure!'
>
> Col completed an epic trek in Nepal from Kathmandu to the Gokyo Lakes and Everest Base Camp with two prime time mates. Over 16 days, they hiked through unseasonal snow, the first September snowfall at the base camp in 15 years: 'Somehow, we made it to EBC and back. Three Prime Timers, one 53 and two 59, and looking back about 35 per cent of it was fitness and preparation, and the other 65 per cent was pure belief and determination. There's no such thing as too old.'

2. ADVENTURE TRAVEL AND TOURING

Unlike the more physically demanding 'challenges', adventure travel is about exploration, discovery and enjoying new experiences. It's the kind of travel many people embrace in midlife as they seek to make the most of their health, wealth and agility, and get a dopamine hit as they do so. While these trips may not be about conquering big challenges, they are filled with enriching and exciting adventures that leave lasting memories.

Many people seek out tours and cruises that will maximise their adventure experiences, whether it's going on safari in Africa, cycling through the villages of Vietnam or cruising the Ganges River in India. Choosing the right touring company, one with deep cultural experience and a track record of serving 'people like you', is the key.

Adventure travel comes in so many different forms, but typically the common thread is an active experience. It could be touring Tuscany or Machu Picchu in Peru, exploring Norway's fjords, or cycling through the Loire Valley in France. It could be a culinary tour of the Mediterranean, diving in the Galapagos Islands, or a cycle, hike and sail trip in Croatia. It's about creating lasting memories by immersing yourself in the culture, action and activity, while enjoying the journey and the freedom that comes with it.

Why now? You're probably at the peak of your curiosity, your experience in life and your cultural appreciation. You've got fewer responsibilities than you've had in years, meaning you can take off on a holiday for a few weeks. And you can use a guided touring company to access their expertise, to make sure you see and do things that are spectacular.

THE KEY TO SUCCESSFUL ADVENTURE TRAVEL AND TOURING HOLIDAYS

The secret to travelling in groups is to find an operator who is highly experienced in the type of active adventures you enjoy and in the destinations you want to travel to. Decide if you're a traveller who prefers a small-group journey or someone who's happy to travel in a larger group, and always choose a company whose signature style is aligned with your own. Check their track record, ask around for reviews, and consider choosing a themed adventure that fits with your interests. That could be a culinary tour, walking expeditions, a golfing tour, a history jaunt – the list goes on.

> Ultimately, what's important is that you travel with like-minded people in a style of travel that suits you. It might take you a few goes to find an operator who offers the right types of experiences at the right price point for you. Look carefully – there's something for everyone in travel.

Adventure experiences closer to home

Adventures are experiences that add excitement to our lives. They break the monotony of daily routines and offer opportunities to explore, learn and grow. And they don't have to be costly or time-consuming. In fact, some of the most enriching experiences are right on our doorstep and can be enjoyed inexpensively.

> **PLEDGE TO PUT MORE ADVENTURE INTO YOUR LIFE**
>
> Set yourself the midlife adventure goal of adding one local adventure a month, getting out and about and finding things you haven't done before or haven't done in a while. It might be the nudge you need to see the city and region around you and bring more joy and purpose into your life.

Road trips close to home

Taking a road trip in your local area gets you out of the house and allows you to discover hidden gems in your own region. It might be a quaint village, a historic landmark, a scenic lookout or a country bakery. There's always something new to explore, and you can do it without straying too far from home.

City breaks

Short trips to a nearby city can offer a refreshing change of pace. Dive into a new urban atmosphere by visiting museums, art galleries, parks and local markets, or schedule your trip around a sporting game or event you want to go to.

Camping trips

Camping is a fantastic way to reconnect with nature and unwind from the digital world. And if you already have equipment, it can be really cost-effective. I keep a list of camping locations to try, so when I'm feeling inspired I can simply book something new.

Weekenders at the beach or in the country

A weekend getaway to the beach or countryside provides a quick escape from urban life. Sometimes we fall into the habit of only going to one beach spot, but adventure means variety. So switch things up occasionally to refresh your approach.

Foodie activities

Exploring food cultures is a real adventure for the senses. Whether you're a seasoned cook or just love to eat, you can consider food courses, food festivals or simply heading to food-growing regions for a farm-door roadtrip, each of which is a great way to make food or wine an adventure.

Festivals and concerts

Music festivals, art fairs and cultural celebrations are packed with midlifers looking to life-it-up, and the tours of many ageing musicians, artists and entertainers have become very successful as a result. In recent years we've found a couple of friends with similar interests, and we each keep a watch on the ticketing websites and suggest upcoming events we could go to together.

Hikes, bushwalks, cycling journeys

Heading into the great outdoors for a hike, bushwalk or cycling journey is not only healthy but also deeply rejuvenating. Walking lets you immerse yourself in natural landscapes, observe wildlife, and savour the peace and quiet of being away from it all. Whether you're strolling a local trail or tackling a multi-day trek, there's something special about discovering new scenery on foot. Start by choosing trails that match your fitness level and interests, build up your hiking kit, and set out to explore nature's beauty.

Cycling, on the other hand, adds a sense of adventure and freedom. With rail trails and dedicated cycle paths popping up all over, it's easier than ever to plan a multi-day ride that blends exploration, fitness and fun.

3. SLOW TRAVEL

Slow travel is the mindset of taking your travel more slowly than usual and immersing yourself in what a town or city or region has to offer. Instead of rushing from place to place, slow travel encourages you to stay in one location for an extended period of time so you can build more meaningful connections with the place and the people around you.

Slow travel looks different for everyone. Some might plan a six-week holiday, choosing to spend a week in each new location and explore it thoroughly before moving on to the next one. Others might book an eight-week trip to a single destination and sink deeply into the local scene, getting to know the neighbourhood and the locals.

One of the greatest advantages of slow travel is that it allows you to 'live like the locals'. Instead of staying in hotels, slow travellers often choose apartments or holiday lets. This tends to be more affordable and gives you access to a kitchen.

Contrary to what you might think, slow travel can be surprisingly affordable. The longer stays often come with discounted rates on accommodation. Booking during the shoulder seasons – the months just before or after the peak tourist times – makes it even more budget-friendly. Destinations are less crowded, accommodation is cheaper, and you can still enjoy pleasant weather without the chaos of peak season.

Why now? Slow travel is an ideal option for midlifers who want to take a break from the fast pace of their regular lives and enjoy a more mindful travel experience. After decades of working, raising families and perhaps travelling in more traditional, fast-paced ways, midlife is the perfect time to shift into a slower, more intentional approach to exploration. You've earned the time to linger, reflect and really get to know a place.

4. WORK AND TRAVEL (DIGITAL NOMAD STYLE)

In your Prime Time, you might not want to retire fully, but that doesn't mean you're tied to a nine-to-five routine or fixed to one location. With remote working on the rise, many capable professionals are choosing to combine work with travel, living in different cities or countries while continuing to work, and often using the tools of digital nomads to make it possible. This gives them the flexibility to explore on their weekends and spare time, and it allows the costs of their travel to be a little easier to manage as they are supported by work.

Why now? You really can enjoy the best of both worlds – working and earning your salary (on your own terms) – while exploring new places. It's ideal for those who want to keep working but crave flexibility and a change of scenery.

5. BLEISURE TRAVEL

Bleisure travel combines business and leisure, and it's something we're already familiar with – taking a work trip and tacking on a holiday before or after. You might be attending a conference and then take a week or two afterward to have a holiday, go on a tour or head off on an adventure. Or you might be on a work sales or operational trip and ask your partner to meet you afterward for a leisure holiday.

The great thing about bleisure holidays is their cost-effectiveness. The company is likely paying for your airline ticket and some accommodation, so if you tack on a tour or cruise, it's not as prohibitive financially. They may not mind if your partner tags along and spends the evenings with you on the work days of your trip if it's not costing them anything and your obligations are light in the evenings.

Why now? If you're in the type of career that allows you to travel, bleisure holidays can be a very cost-effective way to enjoy subsidised travel in your Prime Time. If you can afford the side trips, why not!

6. WELLNESS AND MEDITATION RETREATS

Ever felt the need to take time out just for you? To escape the pressures of daily life, learn how to meditate, or focus on your physical, mental and spiritual health? Whether it's a yoga retreat in Bali, a mindfulness course in Thailand, a spa getaway in Europe, or a meditation retreat in the middle of nowhere, these trips are designed to offer deep rejuvenation and self-care. At a time when many people feel an 'inner death', often mistaking burnout, career exhaustion and a lack of self-care for a desire to retire early, wellness retreats offer a much-needed reset.

Taking a wellness or meditation retreat is something you do purely for yourself. It's about prioritising your most important asset – your health and wellbeing – and finding some inner peace, reconnecting with yourself on a deeper level, and for many it can be a profound, life-changing experience.

Why now? As you juggle work, home life and the urge to travel, a wellness retreat offers the perfect space to recharge and recalibrate. It's an opportunity to stay healthy and focused, allowing you to continue pursuing your goals with renewed energy in this phase of life. It could be a reset to help you adjust your eating habits, sleeping behaviours and mindfulness practices, or it could be a learning experience where you grow your skills in a type of therapy or practice that interests you.

JANE TARA'S JOURNEY WITH MEDITATION

In her 50s, Jane finally found the meditation practice that truly worked for her. After years of exploring different styles, she realised that meditation didn't have to be rigid or gruelling to be effective.

Jane had tried Vipassana, known for its 10-day silent retreats with strict rules: no speaking, no eye contact and hours of meditation each day. She recalled how, after five days of mental struggle, she had a brief but powerful moment of clarity – fully present, connected to nature, free from the constant chatter of her mind. But despite the benefits, the practice always felt like a massive effort, and she never truly looked forward to it.

As she approached 50, Jane turned to science and neuroplasticity, realising that her brain's wiring could be changed. This led her to Dr Joe Dispenza's retreats, which were a revelation. There were no strict rules, just a mix of intense meditation, joy and community. The experience was completely different from Vipassana, and Jane embraced the variety and vibrancy. Evenings were spent sharing stories with others over a glass of wine – her kind of enlightenment.

Now, Jane is a firm believer in the cognitive and psychological benefits of meditation. It's where she became aware of her deep-seated beliefs and habits, and learned how to change them. 'It took time, but finding the right practice has been life-changing,' she says. Jane encourages others to explore until they find their own path.

Jane Tara is the author of bestselling novel Tilda is Visible, *about women, midlife and being seen.*

7. CELEBRATION HOLIDAYS AND MULTI-GENERATIONAL FAMILY TRIPS

Creating life-fulfilling memories with our beloved family members is one of the greatest gifts we can offer them, and our Prime Time is the perfect time to do it. Time is precious, and celebration travel is all about bringing together the people you love to share in the big moments, perhaps a special birthday or a milestone wedding anniversary. And what's unique about the present day is that as our average life span increases, for the first time in history, the travel industry is at times experiencing up to five generations of the same family travelling together.

These are called multi-generational holidays, and they offer a unique opportunity to strengthen family bonds while exploring new destinations. Some families build a culture of taking trips together regularly, while others do it as a very rare and special event. Think about what you want for your family and start something, if your family has no organised holiday framework.

Why now? There are greater opportunities for these trips for today's Prime Timers than there were for previous generations because our parents are living longer, and they're healthier until later in life too. Even so, your early Prime Time might be one of your last chances to bring your parents and children together for unforgettable multi-generational trips that create lasting memories.

8. FLOP-AND-DROP HOLIDAYS

I look at flop-and-drop holidays as not so much 'nice to have' but actually 'need to have', especially if you're still working full-time. Flop-and-drop holidays are all about pure relaxation, where you simply switch off and enjoy the peace. Whether it's lounging on a beach on the Gold Coast or in Fiji, staying at a beach apartment or a luxury resort or taking a leisurely cruise, these trips offer complete rejuvenation and no responsibility.

Why now? After years of juggling work, family and responsibilities, a flop-and-drop holiday provides you with the perfect opportunity to rest and recharge. Many people report that scheduling a week of relaxation somewhere not too far from home is an essential annual investment in their health, and this kind of travel should not break the bank if well planned.

9. CARAVANNING AROUND AUSTRALIA

Caravanning around Australia is something that more than 40 per cent of pre-retirees want to do, either before or after retirement. Most people take the iconic anti-clockwise circuit of Australia on their biggest trip, heading north in April or May as the end of the wet season arrives. They drive up the east coast to Cairns before taking the Savannah Way to the Northern Territory, and then it's on to the Kimberley and Broome. Then they travel down the continent's west coast, looking to time their trip back across the Nullarbor Plain with the winter trade winds pushing them along from June to October. Then it's back home for a grease and oil change and a clothing swap before heading south for the summer.

Why now? This is one of those trips that you need to do while you can. Many people I meet talk about how fantastic it was to drive a caravan around Australia. They also tell me that it can be a lot of work, and requires you to be in good health. You also need to think about the fact that you'll want to hike, climb and enjoy yourself physically in a lot of the destinations you visit. So bear that in mind and plan for it in your best years.

10. CRUISING

Cruising is magical. You wheel your suitcase on board the ship and only unpack once. From that moment, you get to enjoy days or weeks of relaxation and adventure, usually in great comfort and with nightly entertainment. There are four main types of cruises: expedition cruises, river cruises, ocean cruises and luxury small-ship cruises. And within each category there's an extraordinary depth of different operators, each with unique approaches to cruising.

Expedition cruises offer access to some of the world's most remote locations, with purpose-built ships equipped to tackle the more challenging environments. Examples include the polar regions, the Northwest Passage and the Galapagos Islands.

River cruising offers all the benefits of a floating boutique hotel, and is great for those who prefer enclosed waters, meeting new like-minded people, and travel in smaller groups, usually with about 150 people on board.

Ocean cruises come in all shapes and sizes, from very large ships that are like mini cities, catering to up to 5000 guests with every facility or entertainment you can imagine, to exclusive and immersive small-ship experiences. Regardless, as a general rule of thumb, the larger the ship, the lower the price. The cost typically covers accommodation, food and activities, but be aware of what you do actually need to pay for onboard.

Luxury small-ship cruising is a growing trend, especially among Prime Timers and Epic Retirees who enjoy a high degree of comfort. Sometimes called 'yachting', these voyages might be done on intimate vessels carrying 100–200 guests, or larger ships accommodating up to 500 people. They focus on delivering incredibly scenic trips through breathtaking regions such as the Greek Islands, the Mediterranean and the Kimberley.

Why now? There's a reason why cruising is the fastest-growing segment of the travel industry, offering you an exceptional holiday experience that cuts across many travel categories, from expedition to multi-generational and celebration, to adventure and beyond. You can see whole regions of the world in a few weeks, or choose an expedition-style cruise to explore more remote locations. Your Prime Time is made for this.

Lesson 23
Seek out sabbaticals or 'golden gap years' – several times in your life

MANY OF US HAVE WORKED ALMOST NON-STOP FOR 30 OR 40 YEARS. EXHAUSTION sets in and we lose clarity on what excites us and, worse, on what direction we should head in next. The grind can leave us feeling stuck, running on autopilot, with no clear passion or purpose.

Unsurprisingly, many people in their late 40s and 50s reach out to me feeling completely exhausted. They tell me they want to retire, but the reality is often more nuanced. It's not necessarily retirement they're seeking but a break. They need space to recover from the burnout, refocus, and find that *spark* again.

When I bring up the idea of a sabbatical, something shifts in them. For most, the thought of taking a proper break – a sabbatical to pause, breathe and reassess their path – has never even crossed their mind. And yet, when we were younger, during our early career transitions, gap years or sabbaticals were completely normal. We gave ourselves permission to step away, explore and find new direction. Why not do the same thing now in midlife?

Sabbaticals offer you a chance to hit the pause button, whether it's for a few months or a year, and give yourself the space to recharge and rediscover what lights you up.

Some people do sabbaticals in midlife instead of retiring early, taking one or more periods of long release from work. Others use them to try retirement on. They are often negotiated as extended leave without pay, or created by combining long service leave and holiday leave. Many people also take a sabbatical at the end of a long role, as a break.

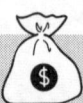

SMART MONEY AND SABBATICALS

If you're fortunate enough to have accrued long service leave, consider using it to take a sabbatical before your official retirement date rather than getting paid out for it. There are some smart financial reasons to do this:

- During the long service leave period, you continue receiving a normal salary, and you also receive superannuation contributions on that salary, effectively increasing your overall retirement savings. If the leave were paid out as a lump sum, the superannuation component might not be included.
- You can enjoy a break while building your savings – your nest egg – and staying insured. Additionally, you may remain insured for total and permanent disability and keep receiving income protection if your company provides these benefits during your leave period.
- During your long service leave, you may continue to accrue annual leave and sick leave which would not have been paid out. Annual leave can be paid out when you finally retire, adding another boost to your savings.

Here are a half-dozen big types of sabbaticals or golden gap years.

SLOW TRAVEL SABBATICALS

If you've ever dreamed of immersing yourself in another culture, beyond what a typical holiday allows, then a slow travel sabbatical might be perfect for you. This type of sabbatical involves setting up a temporary home in a foreign place, living more like a local than a tourist. Or you travel slowly through a series of destinations, staying more than a week in each so you can see it through the lens of the locals. Whether you're renting a villa in Tuscany, living in a coastal town in Portugal, driving your way around Scotland and Ireland, hopping your way around the Greek Islands or spending time in the beachside streets of Kata in Thailand, slow travel sabbaticals offer a mix of adventure and rest. They are perfect for people who are reconsidering their priorities, or looking to rediscover themselves and find inspiration by getting out of their daily routine.

SKILL-BUILDING SABBATICALS

If you've hit midlife and still crave growth and learning, skill-building sabbaticals could be for you. They are all about intentional learning, where you purposefully take time off work to dive into an education or development program that excites you or benefits the next phase of your career. It's a way to step out of your everyday routine, more deeply immerse yourself in a learning process, and come back with fresh perspectives, new skills and maybe even an entirely different direction in life.

The possibilities for skill-building sabbaticals are endless. Maybe you've always wanted to take a pastry-making course in France, or perhaps a leadership program at Harvard in the United States has been on your radar. If you're more creatively inclined, you could focus on art or photography, looking for programs that excite you in places you've always wanted to go.

Skill-building sabbaticals aren't just for career advancement. They're also about exploring passions that may have taken a backseat to other things, but now you're able to give yourself permission to pursue them.

EXPLORATORY SABBATICALS

Midlife can be a time of existential questioning: what's next? Am I doing what I want? Should I switch paths? An exploratory sabbatical is all about taking time off to experiment with what your future could look like. You could spend time working with a non-profit, start a creative project, or test the waters of a new industry you've been curious about. You don't even have to leave home to do this type of sabbatical, but if your kids have flown the nest and you're interested in seeing what's out there, then why not?

> **WANT TO HEAR REAL PRIME TIME SABBATICAL STORIES? TUNE IN TO THE PRIME TIME PODCAST**
>
> We've talked to some truly inspiring Prime Timers who've taken sabbaticals across Europe, Thailand and beyond. Their stories are full of adventure, personal insights, and lessons learned along the way. It's the perfect way to get a fresh perspective on what a sabbatical could mean for you.
>
> Catch their journeys and experiences by searching Prime Time with Bec Wilson wherever you get your podcasts. Don't miss out – your next adventure might just start here.

RESTING SABBATICALS

Let's face it: midlife is tiring. After decades of balancing career, family and personal obligations, many people simply need to pause and rest. A rest and reflection sabbatical allows you to focus on self-care, mindfulness and reconnecting with yourself. It might see you live by a beach in Thailand, Spain or Greece for several months, or it might simply mean you unplug from work and regular life for a while to recharge mentally and physically at a nearby seaside town. A resting sabbatical is about replenishing your energy reserves so you can return to life with renewed clarity and purpose.

ADVENTURE SABBATICALS

Adventure sabbaticals are for those who want to combine their time off with excitement and exploration. This could involve trekking through the Himalayas, cycling through Vietnam or Italy or exploring the jungles of Costa Rica. Adventure sabbaticals push you out of your comfort zone, physically and mentally, giving you a sense of accomplishment and a dopamine hit as you embrace new challenges. While they can be demanding, these sabbaticals often leave you feeling rejuvenated, inspired and more connected to the world around you. They're perfect for midlifers who are looking to remind themselves of their strength and resilience.

A SABBATICAL THAT LOOKS MORE LIKE A RELOCATION

Then there's the sabbatical with no planned 'ending'. These are for when you want to pack up the house and head off into the sunset to try something completely different. This type of sabbatical appeals to those who are less interested in a fixed timeline and more excited about a complete life refresh. You might be ready for something different, but you don't want to limit yourself with a return date. A relocation sabbatical allows you to truly live somewhere new, rather than just visit. It's a great way to explore not just new countries, but new lifestyles, career possibilities and ways of being.

SCHENGEN VISA RULES

For Australian, British and US citizens taking a sabbatical in countries within the Schengen Area, which contains 29 European countries, it's important to be aware of the Schengen visa rules. Australians can stay in Schengen countries for up to 90 days within a 180-day period. This applies across the entire Schengen zone cumulatively, so time spent in any and all countries in the zone count toward your total. Planning your stay within this timeframe, or extending your travels beyond the Schengen Area, is key for Australians looking to take longer sabbaticals in Europe. Many do their 90 days in Europe and then spend 90 days in non-Schengen countries like the UK.

The Schengen zone countries are Austria, Belgium, Bulgaria, Croatia, Czech Republic, Denmark, Estonia, Finland, France, Germany, Greece, Hungary, Iceland, Ireland, Italy, Latvia, Liechtenstein, Lithuania, Luxembourg, Malta, Netherlands, Norway, Poland, Portugal, Slovakia, Slovenia, Spain, Sweden and Switzerland.

Lesson 24
Get better value when you travel

WHEN YOU SHIFT FROM TRAVELLING AS A FAMILY TO TRAVELLING AS A COUPLE OR A single person, which most people do in their midlife, your opportunities to save improve dramatically. As someone who ran a travel company for six years and became immersed in the industry's ways, I'm going to take you through my best tips for anyone shifting gears to a more travel-centric lifestyle in their midlife. These are tips that will keep helping you all through your retirement years too.

DECIDE WHICH TYPE OF TRAVELLER YOU ARE FOR EACH TRIP

Know that the type of traveller you are will change, depending on the trip. You're either a strategic traveller or an opportunistic traveller, but very rarely can you be both.

Strategic travellers generally are constrained by time and date, either due to what's happening while they are away, or what's happening back at home. They might be travelling with their family in peak season because they need to work around school holidays, or they could be celebrating an event like a 50th wedding anniversary, or a wedding somewhere overseas. When you are limited to specific dates, or want to travel in peak season, you need to make bookings a long time in advance and do detailed planning. Some destinations will be extremely busy during the time you are there (think Italy in the summer, or skiing in Japan in January), and certain trips like cruises can sell out a long time before they begin or offer the best prices when bookings commence. Ideally, you would map these out in your 'strategic travel plan' 3–5 years ahead of when you want to do them, if you can.

Outside peak season, travel companies still have to fill the same capacity, even though demand might be lower. So they price it lower to move it. This creates possibilities for those who want a great deal and can travel often at very short notice: the opportunistic traveller. Opportunistic holidays are where you can get a great deal if you're flexible on the place you want to go or the dates you'll travel on. They can be a great thing to slot in in-between strategic holidays.

As some people head toward retirement, with less pressure on their time, they become very opportunistic, choosing to pick up great deals that work for them as they come up. It certainly makes their money go further. More holidays for the same budget – something that makes everyone happy.

MAKE YOUR STRATEGIC VERSUS OPPORTUNISTIC HOLIDAYS LIST

Let's get practical and make two lists for your prime time and early retirement years: one for strategic holidays and one for opportunistic holidays. Brainstorm them first, then number the trips according to how you prioritise them.

Strategic	Opportunistic
1	1
2	2
3	3
4	4
5	5
6	6
7	7
8	8

RECOGNISE THE ROLE A GOOD TRAVEL ADVISER CAN PLAY

If you've built a travel bucket list for the years ahead – with both strategic and non-strategic holidays – it might be worth building a relationship with a travel adviser so they can bring you great opportunities when they pop up, and plan your more strategic and challenging holidays for you. A good travel adviser will get to know you as a long-term client and will want to know your travel goals, travel preferences and target destinations. They'll also want to know your likes and dislikes, what's important to you, and what kind of financial investment you want to make in travel, and then help you use them most effectively.

A word of advice here: there is a difference between a travel agent and travel adviser. A travel agent is working to sell their preferred partner products for a commission, often discounting to get the deal over the line. A professional travel adviser has many years of experience and access to a black book of contacts all over the world. Of course, they still have access to the same, if not more, travel content from around the world, but they'll sit on the same side of the desk as you (figuratively of course) and work in your best interests to curate bespoke experiences. You may well (and you should!) pay a small advisory fee in addition to your trip costs for access to this expertise, but the value and benefits a travel adviser can bring will be worth every cent. The critical point to remember is that within your budget, both product quality and service are essential to successful travel experiences.

CONSIDER TRAVELLING OFF-PEAK OR EVEN LAST MINUTE

If you are willing to travel off-peak, in what's called the shoulder season or, if you dare, in the low season, you'll usually get much better prices. Destinations will be less crowded, and the people who live and work in the tourism sector will be keen to encourage travellers during these months to spread their bookings across a broader period of time. As a result, the price difference between peak and shoulder seasons can be quite substantial, sometimes up to 25 per cent less. Timing your travel to happen outside of peak season is therefore one of the best ways to secure a better deal.

If you're a spontaneous type who loves seizing the moment, last-minute travel deals can offer both excitement and value. Here's a helpful tip that not everyone knows. As tours and cruises approach their departure dates – typically within two to three months – operators often have a few unsold seats or cabins. Once they've covered their basic costs for the wider departure, they're keen to fill these remaining spots to maximise their income. Rather than depart with empty spaces that earn nothing, they offer these spots at discounted rates. But they usually only offer them discreetly, not wanting to sabotage demand for their full-priced holidays or disillusion existing customers. The best way to find these deals is to sign up for email lists and newsletters from tour companies and cruise lines directly, or join the different 'discount holiday providers'. Being flexible and ready to act quickly will be crucial.

So keep an eye out, and you might just find yourself on an unexpected adventure at a fraction of the cost.

UNDERSTAND AIRLINE BOOKING ALGORITHMS

Airline ticket prices often seem unpredictable, changing from day to day or even hour to hour. This is because airlines and travel websites use complex algorithms to adjust prices based on various factors. By understanding the basics of how these systems work, you can find better deals on international flights.

There are four main reasons why flight prices change:
1. **Supply and demand**: When a flight is popular and seats are selling quickly, prices go up. If there are many empty seats, airlines may lower prices to attract more passengers.
2. **Timing**: Airlines often offer the best prices several months before the departure date. Last-minute bookings can be

expensive because airlines know some travellers are willing to pay more to get a seat.
3. **Competition**: Airlines monitor each other's prices. If one airline lowers fares on a route, others might do the same to stay competitive.
4. **Seasonality and events**: Prices increase during peak travel seasons, holidays and major events. Travelling during off-peak times can result in lower fares.

Knowing this, how do you get better prices? I have eight suggestions for you to employ:
1. **Be flexible with your dates and times**: Flying on weekdays, early mornings or late at night can be cheaper than peak times. Sometimes it's worth considering leaving at 2 am for a better price.
2. **Book in advance**: Try to purchase tickets two to three months before your trip for better deals. Very popular international flights are usually launched 11 months before departure and the day they drop can be when they're at their cheapest.
3. **Use multiple websites**: Compare prices on different travel sites and check airline websites directly. Some discount sites have special deals to clear seats at low prices. Always check the terms and conditions.
4. **Set fare alerts**: Many airlines have tools to notify you when prices drop for your desired route. Give them a try.
5. **Consider alternative airports**: Flying into or out of secondary airports might save you money.
6. **Clear your browser cookies or use private browsing**: There's a lot of evidence that airline prices can increase based on your search history, so always search using incognito modes.
7. **Join loyalty programs and newsletters**: Airlines and major hotel groups frequently offer special deals to their subscribers and frequent flyers.
8. **Avoid peak seasons**: If you can, travel during less busy times of the year if price is an important driver for you.

CONSIDER ALTERNATIVES TO BUSINESS CLASS TRAVEL

Many people want to travel business or premium economy because of the comfort they offer. But the costs can be prohibitive. It's worth considering the alternatives, especially if your body doesn't enjoy flying long-haul.

For Australians, around-the-world travel is broken up into two main zones: Europe and America. For each, you can consider these:

Going to Europe: Choose from stopovers in Singapore, Doha, Dubai or Hong Kong.

Going to America: Choose from Auckland, Santiago, Vancouver, Honolulu or Nadi.

Many airlines will offer you a very low-cost stopover in one of the major centres on your way to Europe or America if you choose to stay a full day or more, allowing you to break up your flight, have a little adventure and arrive feeling refreshed, and at a much lower cost than flying business class.

Even if you don't have time for a full 24-hour stopover, some of the world's great airports now sell transit hotel rooms by the hour, inside the terminal, without you needing to exit through immigration. In Singapore and Dubai, for example, you can book a room for eight hours to sleep even if you have just a 12-hour wait for your next flight. In doing so, you'll arrive at your final destination refreshed and ready to go.

UNDERSTAND THE BEST WAY TO USE YOUR AIRLINE CURRENCIES

People build up frequent flyer points in one of two ways: by spending on credit cards or by travelling consistently with one airline. They usually gather them with the goal of using them to subsidise big holidays, securing long-haul flights for excellent prices.

But there are other really effective ways to use them as well. In fact, many don't realise they'll get much better bang for their buck with most frequent flyer programs if they use their points to travel domestically, and to bid on upgrades in the days before departure for larger trips or to book fares by sector rather than as a multi-stop ticket.

You may also find that from time to time, airlines release some extra special deals that are only available to their frequent fliers, to exclusive destinations. Keep your eye out for these. Now, let's have a closer look at the ways in which you can leverage those points most effectively:

LONG-HAUL AND BUSINESS-CLASS FLIGHTS

The reality is that getting 'classic' reward seats (the best-value rewards) in peak season for flights from Australia to places like Europe and America is really, really hard in business class. And it's getting tough to get economy seats too. Asian destinations aren't too bad, and there are plenty of seats domestically. But for those valuable international seats, it's only possible if you know how airline travel is booked and work with the system.

If you're looking for business class or other popular international frequent flier tickets, you might want to consider breaking your trip up into sectors and booking each one separately.

DOMESTIC ECONOMY FARES

These fares represent one of the best value ways to use your frequent flyer miles. There's usually plenty of classic rewards seats between capital cities, so long as you are not looking to travel at the same time as a major event is on.

For more tourism-centric destinations, it's worth watching the airlines' emails for extra-value fares for frequent flyer members. Airlines regularly get offered subsidies by state and regional governments to stimulate travel to tourist areas like Cairns, the Gold Coast, the Northern Territory and the Whitsundays. These subsidies are usually offered to large airlines to underwrite fare discounting that brings tourists in when organic bookings are low.

Most airlines release their discount emails at 4 pm on a Thursday in Australia, and each week there are different offers. It's a great way to be an opportunistic traveller in your own backyard!

A GREAT FLIGHT DEAL FOR LOYAL CUSTOMERS

One of the best and most unique Qantas routes for frequent flyer deals is the one from Sydney to Lord Howe Island. It's available from time to time for just 8000 points and $88 in taxes each way, when it would normally cost up to $700. You do need to keep an eye out for them, but they represent fantastic value. What a deal!

UNDERSTAND STATUS CREDITS

An airline's status is used to offer you a range of exclusive benefits within its frequent flyer program. The most coveted benefit is usually exclusive access to airline lounges all over the world. These lounges offer a comfortable and relaxing environment in which to enjoy complimentary food and beverages, wi-fi and showering facilities before your flight.

Access is extended through airline alliances such as Star Alliance, Oneworld and SkyTeam. This means that earning status with one airline can grant you lounge access and other privileges across a network of partner airlines worldwide.

Status credits are typically earned by flying regularly with the airline or its partners. The number of status credits you earn depends on several factors:

- **The distance you fly**: Longer flights generally earn more status credits
- **The class of fare**: Premium cabins like business or first class earn more status credits than economy class
- **The booking class**: Even within economy, different fare types can earn different amounts of status credits
- **Flights with partner airlines**: Flights with partner airlines may also earn status credits, sometimes at different rates.

Some airlines also offer status credits through credit card spending or promotional offers, allowing you to accumulate credits without flying.

> ### ACCESSING AIRLINE LOUNGES
>
> If you don't have elite status, there are still ways to enjoy the airline lounges:
> **Purchase a day pass**: Some airlines offer one-time access to their lounges for a fee
> **Use your credit card benefits**: Certain premium credit cards include lounge access as a perk
> **Buy an annual lounge membership**: Buy an annual membership to an airline's lounge program or independent networks like Priority Pass
> **Fly in premium cabins**: Business and first-class tickets usually include lounge access for the trip.

BOOK DOMESTIC FLIGHTS EARLY AND TRAVEL OFF-PEAK

There's a smart but simple strategy for booking domestic flights that you'll do well to adhere to if you want to get better pricing. Where you can, book your interstate flights more than two weeks before your departure date and avoid peak travel hours, which are typically 6–9 am and 4–7 pm.

Monday mornings and Friday afternoons are often the busiest times for domestic flights, which are filled with people travelling to and from major cities for work. To keep their planes operational throughout the day, airlines aim to fill seats during midweek periods when demand is lower by offering lower prices. Ticket prices usually stay relatively stable until about two weeks before departure, at which point demand from business travellers can cause prices to rise.

UNDERSTAND CRUISING BETTER

Cruise companies have a whole different way of doing things that, if you plan on cruising at all, you'll need to learn. Most of the cruise ships come into the South Pacific during what's called 'wave season', from November to May, which is when waves roll through the oceans of the Northern Hemisphere. This is also the time when most of the cruise ship deals are released for future years. The longer the cruise you are seeking to go on, the more in advance you have to book it. But you will see a lot of deals released as we head into the Australian summer for a full year ahead, and only last-minute deals for the year we're in.

If you haven't cruised much, you will find it beneficial to book using a travel adviser, so your expectations and standards are aligned with the operator, and you won't be disappointed. Otherwise, keep in mind that every cruise company has a different strategy for how they sell their rooms, and there are a few things to compare to get good value for money.

MEAL AND DRINKS PACKAGES

Some cruise lines bundle meal and drink packages into the initial booking price, while others sell them separately. In some cases, once you're on board, you won't need to reach for your credit card at all, or only for a limited number of extras. However, other lines sell you just the room upfront, and once you're on board, you'll be paying full price for everything from coffee to meals and drinks. While the lower initial cost of a cruise might be appealing, it's essential to understand exactly what's included so you're not caught out.

ONBOARD CREDIT

Some companies will use an onboard credit to lure you in, which is essentially free spending money provided by the cruise line to use during your voyage. This credit is used to pay for costs you might otherwise have paid out of your own pocket.

The credit can typically be used for expenses such as specialty dining, beverages, spa services, shore excursions, internet access and shopping. While it doesn't lower the upfront cost of the cruise, it adds value by reducing your onboard expenses. This can make a higher-priced cruise more attractive if you plan to take advantage of these amenities.

So look out for onboard credit deals when you're booking. Travel advisers are offered extra onboard credits by some brands to pass on to their clients to stimulate cruise sales. More often, cruise companies use big onboard credit promotions to drive people to book directly with them. Understand what you expect to spend on board, then explore any restrictions, as some onboard credits may have limitations on where or how they can be used; for example, they might exclude casino spending or gratuities. And check if you can combine onboard credit offers with other promotions, like your loyalty program benefits or group discounts.

SHORE EXCURSIONS

Shore excursions are a big part of the cruise experience, and how they are priced varies significantly between cruise lines. Some companies offer a range of included activities, while others charge for every excursion you take off the ship. To avoid unexpected costs, make sure you understand which excursions, if any, are included in your fare. If excursions aren't included, research the costs of these beforehand to budget appropriately. Also, don't forget to check whether you'll need specific visas or travel documents to participate in the excursions at each destination.

UNDERSTAND HOW DISCOUNT HOLIDAY PROVIDERS WORK AND LEVERAGE THEM

In Australia, several discount package holiday providers have evolved their approach since COVID-19 and offer fantastic deals – if you know how to navigate their promotions. Companies like Trip a Deal (now owned by Qantas), My Cruises and Luxury Escapes provide a diverse range of holidays, but each deal is available for only a short window – usually a week or two – so you have to act quickly; in the case of cruises and tours, these are only available on certain departure dates. Unlike in the past, these companies aren't just about last-minute offers. Instead, they work by securing bulk room nights in hotels, cabins on cruises and seats on tours from major operators. During the 1–2 week promotional period, they offer these at discounted prices to help operators fill their forward bookings; once the promotion ends, the deal is no longer available.

This model means the travel dates could be far in the future, but the sale itself is time-limited, making it more of a short-dated sale rather than a last-minute deal. It's a brilliant way to score a well-priced tour or cruise that you can build an entire holiday around. But you can't linger on the decision. Recognising a great deal when it comes through and acting fast is the key.

Lesson 25
Don't be afraid to travel solo

I COULD NOT BE A BIGGER SUPPORTER OF SOLO TRAVEL. IT'S A GROWING SPACE: growing in the number of people who are travelling solo, and growing in the number of options you have if you want to travel solo.

Before I dive in here, I want to point out that solo travel sometimes means single people travelling, but more than ever, married people are travelling solo too, particularly if one person in a couple doesn't enjoy travelling or is suffering health issues that limit their ability to travel. Whatever your situation, the desire to embrace travel is limited only by your courage and your finances.

The biggest challenge many solo travellers face is how the travel industry prices accommodation and tours. Typically, prices are based on double occupancy, meaning the cost of a room or tour is calculated with the expectation that two people will share it. When only one person stays in the room, they are often required to pay nearly the same rate as two people would, effectively increasing the cost for solo travellers to almost double what those travelling as a couple would pay per person. This additional charge is known as the single supplement. And this is not something that's going to change.

So, you have two choices. You can get angry about single supplements and let them scare or frustrate you, or you can get smart and adopt strategies that can help you minimise or avoid the additional costs that come from travelling solo. Here are some ways to make solo travel more affordable:

Choose solo-friendly operators for tours and cruises: Some tour companies and cruise lines specialise in providing good accommodation for solo travellers. They may offer trips without a single supplement or have programs to match you with a roommate of the same gender, so you can share costs without sacrificing comfort.

Travel during off-peak seasons: Off-peak periods often see travel companies offering lower prices with more flexibility. Hotels and tour operators may be more willing to waive or reduce the single supplement during periods of lower demand to fill their rooms and bookings.

Look for single rooms: Seek out hotels and cruises that offer single rooms designed specifically for one person. These rooms are usually smaller and less expensive than standard double rooms, providing a lower-cost option without the extra charges. Yet they may still be in the best locations and in the most high-end hotel and cruise chains. They are increasingly being developed in response to the surging demand from solo passengers, but you'll still usually have to book early to secure them.

Negotiate directly with hotels and guesthouses: Contact hotels, guesthouses or bed and breakfasts directly. Independent operators may have more flexibility to negotiate rates, and they might offer discounts to solo travellers to secure your booking without having to pay hefty fees to online platforms.

Use apartment rental and homestay websites: Consider staying in hostels or homestays, or renting a room through online apartment rental platforms to bring your costs down and open your options up. These often cater to solo travellers and can provide a more personal and cost-effective experience.

Join group tours for solo travellers: There are travel groups and companies that organise tours exclusively for solo travellers. These groups often have no single supplement or include it in a way that is more cost-effective because they have access to group rates.

Be open to sharing a room: If you're comfortable with it, sharing a room with another solo traveller can eliminate the single supplement. Many tour operators offer a matching service to pair you with a roommate of the same gender and similar age. Remember, though, that the risks of ending up with a snorer or a chronic chatterer are on you.

Leverage loyalty programs and memberships for better prices: Join hotel loyalty programs or travel clubs that offer perks to members. These benefits can include discounted rates, free upgrades or waived single supplements, which can make your solo travels more affordable. Sticking with one hotel group when you find one you like can allow you to build points and get freebies too.

Monitor for special solo traveller deals: Keep an eye out for deals targeted at solo travellers. Quite a few companies offer deals where the single supplement is reduced or completely waived, especially during special events or celebrations. Why not build a list of operators you want to track, and keep an eye out for them.

Plan and book your trip early: Early planners often reap the rewards of lower prices and get access to the very scarce solo rooms that might be available. By booking well in advance, you might be able to pick up early-bird discounts too.

Consider shorter trips: If international solo travel seems too costly, explore destinations closer to home. Shorter trips or local tours can satisfy your travel itch without the added expense of long-haul flights and high single supplements.

Use travel advisers that specialise in solo travel: A travel adviser with expertise in solo travel can help you find the best deals and navigate the complexities of single supplements. They often have access to exclusive offers not advertised to the general public too.

Lesson 26
Understand travel money and insurance – and know what to watch out for

WHEN YOU'RE TRAVELLING, TWO ESSENTIAL THINGS TO GET RIGHT ARE YOUR TRAVEL money and insurance, as these can often trip people up. The reality is that many travellers don't fully understand how these systems work or the potential pitfalls that come with them. And they don't learn the easy way, either. They make mistakes and learn the hard way. Like blowing hundreds of dollars on unnecessary credit card fees that could've been avoided simply by thinking out their money options well before they travelled. Or by buying insurance that didn't actually cover the risks they were taking, and then, when a health issue or a cancellation hit unexpectedly, they were stuck paying the costs out of pocket, simply because they didn't read the fine print or chose the wrong policy.

Understanding insurance and travel money options up-front can save you a lot of financial stress later, trust me!

UNDERSTANDING TRAVEL INSURANCE

Travel insurance covers a wide range of risks, many of which you might not fully appreciate until you're exposed to a real disaster. As you enter what could be the most travelled years of your life, it's essential to understand how travel insurance works and the crucial role it plays in your holiday planning.

Good travel insurance should be taken out as soon as you book your trip, not just before you head to the airport. Why? Travel insurance covers cancellation due to unforeseen circumstances, such as illness, injury or a sudden change in travel conditions at your destination. For example, if you're diagnosed with an illness or sustain an injury before departure, your policy can provide a refund for your trip, including non-refundable tickets. And once you're on your trip, it covers a range of other potential problems, such as accidents, delayed or missed connections, lost luggage, and making an emergency return home for family reasons.

When you purchase travel insurance, there are a few things you should be aware of.

PRE-EXISTING CONDITIONS WILL COST YOU MORE

Insurance companies assess risk, so if you have a pre-existing medical condition, expect to pay more. Many policies will allow you to exclude coverage for specific conditions to reduce costs, but this shifts the risk back to you. For example, someone with a manageable thyroid condition might opt to exclude it from coverage, effectively self-insuring against complications from the thyroid issue while still being covered for everything else, whereas someone with a heart issue might not want to exclude it knowing it could cost hundreds of thousands of dollars if they require surgery, ICU and support in a foreign country.

ALCOHOL CONSUMPTION LIMITS

Be mindful of alcohol limits. Most travel insurance policies include a clause voiding coverage if your blood alcohol level exceeds a certain limit (often 0.05 per cent) at the time of an incident. This can apply in a car accident even if you're not driving, voiding your insurance and leading to significant expenses.

UNDERSTAND YOUR APPROACH TO AGEING PARENTS

Keep in mind that most travel insurance policies exclude coverage for people over 80. If you're counting on your insurance to cover the costs of getting home or cancelling in the event that one of your elderly parents falls ill or takes a turn for the worse, you might be in for an unpleasant surprise. Always read the fine print carefully and have a back-up plan for emergencies involving ageing parents while you're away.

ANNUAL POLICIES

Annual travel policies are great for frequent travellers, but pay attention to clauses around trip duration. Some policies only cover trips up to 30 days at a time. If you regularly take extended trips, look for policies with longer coverage periods.

AGE

I have not yet come across a type of travel insurance that doesn't go up in price as you age. Travel insurers recognise that as we get older, we have more health issues, and we're more at risk of falls, heart attacks and strokes, among other things. Since they are in the business of minimising their own risk, as you get older, the price of your insurance goes up. Once you reach the age of 80, you might find your options are severely limited and quite expensive – it's worthwhile being aware of this and getting the bulk of your international travel dreams achieved before that point.

IS CREDIT CARD TRAVEL INSURANCE ENOUGH?

This is a question I'm asked all the time. Not all credit card insurance is the same. Do your research to fully understand your own credit card insurance and draw a conclusion you can live with. Most of these policies activate insurance when you pay for your holiday using your credit card. This will cost you about 1.3–1.5 per cent of your holiday for most cards, which *can* add up to the price of a more comprehensive policy!

In my experience, some credit card policies are not comprehensive enough for families with pre-existing conditions or those who love active travel. They tend to come with long exclusion lists and limited coverage options. However, some Australian banks offer more comprehensive policies through their credit cards. For example, Commonwealth Bank's Platinum Mastercard includes travel insurance underwritten by Covermore, which allows you to add additional paid coverage for cruises, skiing and other activities, and properly account for pre-existing conditions. This policy can provide a solid alternative to standalone travel insurance, and it's one of the reasons I keep my Platinum Mastercard despite the annual fee.

TRAVEL MONEY

Travel credit, debit and money cards have quietly evolved over the past few years as global banking has become more digital and interconnected. If you're keen to avoid being hit with hefty fees for international transactions, there are a few smart options that will help you keep costs down while you explore the world.

CREDIT CARDS WITHOUT INTERNATIONAL FEES

Several credit cards in Australia offer fee-free international transactions to attract frequent travellers. When looking for credit cards without international transaction fees, there are a few standout options that cater to different needs and budgets. AMEX is renowned for offering robust travel perks, but it typically comes with hefty annual fees, so you'll want to consider whether the benefits justify the cost. On the other hand, the Bankwest Zero Platinum Mastercard is a favourite among frequent travellers because it offers no annual fee and no foreign transaction fees, plus it comes with the added bonus of complimentary travel insurance underwritten by Covermore.

For those looking to earn rewards while travelling, the Coles Rewards Mastercard stands out by not only waiving international transaction fees but also allowing you to collect Flybuys points, which can add extra value to your overseas spending. If you're a digital nomad or someone who travels for extended periods, the 28 Degrees

Mastercard could be worth a look as it offers no foreign transaction fees and no annual fee, although be cautious of the immediate interest applied to cash advances. Finally, for those seeking more luxury travel benefits, the Macquarie Black Card offers perks like complimentary lounge access and travel insurance, but again, with a higher annual fee, making it better suited to those who travel often and appreciate premium benefits.

TRAVEL MONEY CARDS

Travel money cards are a form of debit card onto which you can load money in your home currency, then select the currency you want to transact in, and the card holds it. They've traditionally been issued by banks and Australia Post. They're convenient, but for most, the downside is the rates are usually quite unfavourable, allowing the bank to make its margin this way. The cards are convenient, but frankly, not the most secure way to carry money, as if you lose one (and we've lost a couple over the years), it can't be replaced easily as they are not attached to your identity.

But there are new players in the travel money industry over the last couple of years that we have to talk about. In fact, there are three companies changing the game, becoming the industry standard for travel money in the new world – Wise, Revolut and Monzo.

Wise, Revolut and Monzo are three standout travel money cards and services for international travellers looking to avoid the hefty fees and poor exchange rates often associated with traditional banking. And they're taking international money management to a whole new dimension.

> **Disclaimer:** The products mentioned here are examples of popular travel money options available at the time of writing. I'm not affiliated with Wise, Revolut, Monzo, CBA or any other providers mentioned. This is general information only and not financial advice. Fees, features, and availability may change over time, so please check with the provider directly and consider whether the product suits your personal needs before signing up.

Wise

Wise, formerly TransferWise, initially specialised in low-cost, transparent international money transfers and currency exchange – you might have seen them in international airports. Then came the Wise card, an internationally available travel debit card that has gained popularity among travellers and expats. Its innovative card now allows users to hold and manage over 50 currencies in a single account, accessible via both virtual and physical cards. The card offers mid-market exchange rates with no hidden mark-ups, and any fees for currency conversion are clearly disclosed. Additionally, the card's connection to your identity ensures that funds remain secure, even in the event of loss, with easy replacement options.

Revolut

Revolut has built a reputation as a versatile travel money card with additional features beyond basic currency management. It's also known for low currency conversion fees and offers mid-market exchange rates (with certain limits based on the plan you choose). Revolut supports spending in over 30 currencies and also includes a range of extras such as budgeting tools, cryptocurrency trading and saving vaults. While Wise is excellent for straightforward travel money management, Revolut offers a broader scope of financial tools.

Monzo

Monzo is a digital bank that is particularly popular in the UK and offers travel-friendly features similar to Wise and Revolut. While Monzo operates primarily as a bank, it provides fee-free international spending and easy-to-manage accounts through its mobile app. Monzo's prepaid card allows users to spend overseas without incurring any fees (up to a certain limit), and like Wise and Revolut, it uses near-mid-market rates for currency conversions. Monzo is a great option for those looking for a banking service that integrates travel money management with a full range of personal banking features.

Part 7
TAKING ACTION

READING ABOUT HOW TO HAVE AN AMAZING PRIME TIME IS ONE THING, MAKING IT happen is another. If you want to live long, live well and make your Prime Time count, it's time to turn ideas into action.

The second half of life isn't something that just falls into place, it's something you build, step by step. There's no set template, no easy formula. It's not about hitting a certain age and suddenly knowing exactly what's next. The people who thrive in this stage of life aren't necessarily the wealthiest or the luckiest. They're the ones who take deliberate steps toward the life *they* want, rather than waiting for the 'right time'. The changes they make to their lives happen in small, incremental steps – choosing to focus on health today, setting up financial security and financial confidence piece by piece, or carving out time for the people and experiences that matter. Each small decision adds up, shaping your future in ways that don't seem obvious at first but make an enormous amount of difference over time.

So don't wait for the perfect plan or the perfect moment. Just start.

WHY ACTION MATTERS MORE THAN KNOWLEDGE

A lot of people put off making changes in midlife – not because they don't care, but because it feels too big, too complicated or too uncomfortable. Waiting for the perfect plan, though? That's a trap.

Most people say they'll get around to it later, whether it's improving their health, sorting out their finances, understanding their super or figuring out what's next for their work and their sense of purpose. But the longer you wait, the harder it gets.

The people who make the most of their Prime Time don't just drift into it, they shape it, test things out, and adjust as they go. They don't wait until they have everything perfectly figured out. They just start, knowing that modest, consistent steps matter more than big, dramatic plans that never get off the ground.

- If you want to be fit, strong and healthy later in life, start moving today.
- If you want financial confidence, work on your budget, understand your super and start building a financial plan that works for you.
- If you want more adventure, excitement or connection, go looking for it.
- And if you want a deeper sense of purpose, start exploring what truly brings you joy and meaning.

Frankly, the second half of life is too important to leave to chance. If you want to love the life you're living in the decades ahead, don't just think about it, build it.

NOW LET'S TURN INSPIRATION INTO ACTION

The lesson in this section is all about making your Prime Time count and preparing for an Epic Retirement. I'll show you how to roll up your sleeves and start making a plan – not just a wish list, but a real, practical roadmap for the next stage of your life.

Lesson 27

Make your Prime Time count and prepare for an Epic Retirement

CONGRATULATIONS! YOU'VE REACHED THE FINAL LESSON OF *PRIME TIME*, BUT IN many ways, this is where your practical journey really begins. This last lesson isn't just about closing a book, it's about opening a door to a new, exciting phase of life, full of possibilities. Here, you have both a big responsibility and a big opportunity ahead of you: to make your Prime Time count in ways that are meaningful, fulfilling and uniquely yours.

I want you to look within and consider what you truly want from this next phase of life, then set some meaningful goals. Don't wait until retirement to start living fully; make your Prime Time count. These extra years in your healthiest, most capable stage are a gift, an opportunity to design a life filled with purpose, joy and fulfilment right now.

I want you to put your head down early and do the financial work: budgeting and investing well earlier in life, paying off your debts, taking advantage of the tax breaks available to grow your wealth, and mastering superannuation and compound investing so the rest of your life can be lived with true financial confidence.

I want you to look after your body like there's no more important priority in your life. Embrace exercise and nutrition, stay proactive in monitoring your health, and pay attention to any early signs of potential issues. Make health and wellness a foundation for everything else you do, so you can fully enjoy all the wonderful years ahead.

I want you to find happiness, joy and a sense of purpose in your life, blending work you enjoy with activities you're passionate about. As you do, focus on building a supportive, vibrant community around you, a circle of people who enrich your life and share in your journey.

I want you to embrace the changes in your family and build new bridges that connect everyone as you and they get older. Rediscover your passion for life with your partner, be there for your kids, and help your parents as they age, knowing family is at the heart of a good midlife.

And I want you to travel, and have a great time doing it.

This phase of life is not one to passively coast through or hide from. It's about making active choices that will shape your wellbeing, financial security and overall happiness for many years to come. So lean into it. Stay open and curious, explore the unknowns, and let each experience guide you toward a clearer vision of what you want your Prime Time and, later, your Epic Retirement to look like.

As you step into this new chapter, remember that this is just the beginning. Your choices today are paving the way for a future that's entirely within your grasp. Take it one step at a time, stay committed, and make each day of your Prime Time as intentional as it is inspiring. Here's to making your Prime Time count, and to the Epic Retirement waiting on the other side.

TELL ME ABOUT YOUR PRIME TIME JOURNEY

As you head off to make your Prime Time count, I want you to know you're not alone. I'll be sitting here watching and waiting to hear your stories of success, triumph and the challenges in-between.

In a year or two, when you've got stories to share, send me an email at bec@primetimers.net. Tell me how your prime time journey is going, what you've discovered about yourself, money and the meaning of midlife. Share with me the transitions you've grappled with and the investments you've made that built your confidence. Tell me about how your views on work have changed, and what you're doing now for fulfilment. Share your healthy living lessons and tell me about your family and your travels – all the wonderful adventures you've had and the ones you have planned.

I'll read the emails aloud on my podcast Prime Time, if you tell me I can. Otherwise I'll read them to my husband Brett, and we'll smile with pride in you together.

Action and reflection plan

To help you check off all the things you've learned and take action, I've compiled a little action and reflection plan for you, walking you lesson by lesson through the actions I hope you'll take as you start to explore how you'll tackle your Prime Time.

Remember, some of these lessons are here to help you think differently about your life, while others are all about inspiring you to take action. But through each step, keep this in mind: *this is your Prime Time*. It's not a final destination. It's an amazing phase of life where you can take intentional, fulfilling steps, each decision contributing to a richer, more meaningful life.

Good luck on the journey. And remember, I'm with you every step of the way.

UNDERSTAND YOUR POWER TO MAKE CHOICES

1. **Recognise that the shape of life has changed**
   The templates of what a good life is have changed, so stop now and reconsider your vision and expectations of life.
   You've got a new phase of life, your Prime Time, to enjoy – a phase of life that is well-suited to working, lifestyling and part-timing. And you get to choose how you do them.
   Reflection: Think about your assumptions around how work, lifestyle and retirement come together, then reconsider them. Build a big-picture vision of what the next 20+ years might look like.

2. **Consider that retirement isn't the ultimate goal**
   It's time to get practical and set some goals for the prime time years of your life, the next 15–20 healthy years – seriously! You've read the book, soaked up the lessons, now head back to this section of the book and write the big goals down.
   Action: Write down your goals. Work through the questions on page 24. Make a vision board if that's your thing, or a list will do just fine.

3. **Learn to make active choices**
   It's time to put yourself back at the centre of your picture, making choices that are right for *you*.
   Reflection: Commit to re-prioritising important things in your life, and start to look for ways in which you can put yourself first.

PUT AN ACTION PLAN IN PLACE FOR YOUR FINANCES

4. **Stop taking shortcuts**
   Recognise that quick and dirty efforts won't get you anywhere nearly as far as doing the hard work on your finances will.
   Reflection: Identify the shortcuts you've been taking and stop taking them. Think about the ways you can instead be getting more strategic with your money and using it to build your Prime Time.

5. **Understand the foundations of financial confidence and put them in place**
   Each of the financial foundations is important, and by midlife, it's worth taking them seriously. There's a long list of actions you should take from the learnings in this section.
   Actions:
   - Organise your intentional dinner with your partner or friend (or by yourself) and have your first conversation about your midlife money expectations.

- Create a detailed household budget, built off what you spend today.
- Put together your current big financial picture. Use the Excel template provided at Becwilson.net.
- Understand how much you might need to live in comfort. Also understand the benchmarks and acknowledge whether these feel high or low to you.
- Read about compounding and make sure you grasp how your investments are growing through it.
- Think about the tax concessions available to you. Are there any obvious ones you can better take advantage of? Make a list and start.
- Reconsider your home, mortgage and housing needs in the future, and build a strategy and timeline for when you can pay off your mortgage or how to get your mortgage into good shape so you can enjoy your prime time years.
- Contemplate when or if there might be a good time to downsize or right-size your home.
- Review your superannuation – consider your fund's performance, fees and the services they offer in the next phase of life. Think about how you can increase your super contributions, and leverage the tax concessions available to you.
- If you have investments, of any kind, stop and consider whether they are the best investments for you at this time of your life.
- Understand your age pension eligibility – it's handy to know whether you'll be eligible for it later in your life, so you can be conscious of the rules around assets and housing if you think you will be.

6. **Learn the new lessons of midlife money management – about time, income and spending**
It's time to really think about what will change, about how different things will be, as you move into a phase of life when

some income is active and some is passive – and you'll want to understand both so you can make great choices.

Actions:
- Work out your life expectancy – set yourself a goal 'number' you can plan to.
- Map out the number of years you'd like to spend in each phase of life. Really think about it and fill out the table provided on page 202.
- Consider what your income layers might look like in the next stage of life. Write them down – identify the different layers and consciously map these into stages of your life – pointing out to yourself when different layers might drop away or kick in.
- Build your future budget, leaning on the current-day budget you produced above to help you. Plan a budget you will look forward to living on right through the next phase of life, if you possibly can.

7. **Review your big financial picture and plan your budget**

    This is a hands-on and practical lesson where you make action plans and build your own budget for the future. It comes as two big parts.

    Actions:

    Think about the lessons laid out in lesson 7 and how you want to apply them in your life. Make some practical plans on how you will:
    - Demolish your debts
    - Assess your age pension eligibility
    - Optimise income-generating assets
    - Evaluate your home's suitability
    - Ensure accessible funds outside super
    - Review your super investments.

    Then, develop a forward-looking budget to manage your income and expenses confidently. Break it down into:

1. **Cost-of-living and lifestyle budget**: Cover essential expenses and discretionary activities like travel and leisure.
2. **One-off expenditure budget**: Plan for large, irregular costs like home maintenance, a new car, or future care needs.
3. **Lifestyle lump sums and epic experiences**: Allocate funds for milestones like sabbaticals, caravans or big celebrations.

8. **Work out how much is 'enough'**
   This is the step where you bring it all together and work through all the inputs, to prepare yourself for proper financial planning.
   Action: Work through the activities starting on page 197, completing the tables with your answers to give you perspective on what 'enough' looks like for you.

9. **Get appropriate advice for your situation**
   Take the time to think about the types of financial advice available to you, and what advice you need to get yourself on track.
   Action: Seek advice from the right type of financial adviser for you, setting yourself on track for your Prime Time and Epic Retirement with a plan you properly understand.

10. **Take a modern, proactive approach to your legacy**
    Do some thinking about what legacy really means to you, and how you want to provide both financial and non-financial legacies.
    Reflection: Consciously consider what you want to do for or with your loved ones while you are alive, and the relationships and financial legacy you want to leave.
    Actions:
    - Make sure you have in place the following-end-of life documents, and that they are all up to date:
      - Binding death nomination with your super fund
      - Your will

- Enduring power of attorney
- Advance care directive.
- Have the end-of-life talk with your family.
- Understand if you'll need to take action to avoid the Superannuation Death Benefits Tax long before you turn 75 – ask your super fund advice team or a financial adviser for help.
- Reconsider your life, total and permanent disablement, income protection and trauma insurances.

EXPLORE THE NEXT PHASE OF YOUR WORK, PURPOSE AND HAPPINESS

11. Recognise the outdated models of work and retirement: understand your true options

Redefine your options for what life could look like in Prime Time, examining where you'd like to spend your time and how you want to contribute or create value.

Action: Reflect on what draws your curiosity, what gives you purpose, and how you want your next chapter to unfold.

12. Design your path out of the workforce

Think through how long you want to work, and consider possible career changes, part-time options and gradual retirement paths.

Action: Set a timeline for when and how you'll reduce work hours or shift to different kinds of fulfilling roles.

13. Rediscover what brings you joy and fulfilment

This section has a long list of actions, designed to help you think about what brings you joy and go looking for things that offer you fulfilment.

Actions:
- Think back to moments or activities that once made you feel energised and content. Write down what you enjoyed about them.

- Make a list of past hobbies, passions and experiences that brought you happiness. Circle a few you'd like to revisit or explore further.
- Clarify your personal values to understand what truly matters to you and aligns with a fulfilling life. Write down your top five values (for example, creativity, community, health, adventure, innovation) and think of ways to incorporate them more fully into your day-to-day.
- Schedule some 'joy breaks' – regularly set aside the time for activities that bring you happiness, even if it's just 15 minutes a day.
- Develop your self-awareness by practising mindfulness, which helps you connect with what brings you true contentment. Try a daily mindfulness exercise, like journaling or meditation, to check in with yourself and identify what's fulfilling.
- Visualise what a joyful and fulfilling life looks like for you by crafting a vision board with images, words and symbols that resonate with you.
- Set a monthly or quarterly check-in with yourself to reflect on whether you're making time for joy and fulfilment. Each month, ask yourself: 'What brought me joy this month? What could I do differently to bring in more fulfilment?'

14. **Look beyond work to hobbies, pursuits and communities**
    Always remember that when you're lying on your deathbed, you'll never say 'I wish I worked more'. But what will you wish you'd done more of? It's an important question to stop and think about now.
    Actions:
    - Build a list of pursuits you'd like to invest yourself in becoming better at, or activities you'd like to explore as pursuits.
    - Experiment on these pursuits to see if they fit you. Try out some new pursuits, volunteer roles or creative activities to

discover fresh sources of joy. Choose one new activity to explore each month, whether it's learning an instrument, hiking, joining a club or taking a class.
- Seek out like-minded people through activities you enjoy and interests you have. Forge connections with others who share your interests and values. Join a local group or online community where you can connect with people who have similar passions and discuss what makes life meaningful.

15. **Recognise transitions and embrace the journey they offer**
Reflect on recent changes or milestones in your life to see how they've shaped you.
Actions:
- List three challenging transitions you've successfully navigated in the past. Think about how you overcame them and what helped you through.
- Each week, take a moment to check in on how you're feeling about recent changes. Write down any self-kindness statements, like 'I'm adapting at my own pace, and that's okay'.

16. **Remind yourself that curiosity, learning and flexibility are crucial**
Ultimately, the world is evolving, and so must we – inside and outside the workplace.
Actions:
- Consider what you would like to learn in the next phase of your life. Explore your own interest in formal education, courses and personal development and prime time pursuits. Make a list of things to act on.
- Think of topics that pique your curiosity and start small in exploring them, then go deeper. Embrace the ones that you become more drawn to.

- Consciously look for ways to act with greater courage. Try something you might previously have stood back from, such as speaking up in a meeting.
- Complete the five purposeful activities on page 310.

PUT YOUR HEALTH HIGHEST ON YOUR PRIORITY LIST

17. **Make your health your top priority**
    You can live a fulfilling life without a lot of money, but you absolutely cannot live a fulfilling life without your body and mind being in good shape.
    Reflection: Reflect on whether your health is your top priority, and if not, what you can do to ensure it is. Take your own health into your hands by learning more about your biometrics, and taking your prevention testing seriously.
    Actions:
    - Identify a list of biometrics that you want to monitor and improve. Set yourself specific goals.
    - Work through the list of prevention tests that you should be having at your age, and check them off as you have them done.
    - Review your health insurance – make sure it's ready to support you through the next stage with the right inclusions.

18. **Learn how to age better according to science**
    Understand the science of modern ageing and how you can use some of its principles to improve your health, lengthen your healthspan and make your quality of life better over the long haul.
    Reflection: Consider the ways in which you can put more of the practical lessons from the science of modern ageing into practice.

Action: Make some solid commitments to exercise, to improve nutrition and healthy living, and check in with yourself about these quarterly.

EMBRACE THIS NEW PHASE OF FAMILY LIFE

19. **Prioritise your primary loving relationship**
    Embrace your relationship – literally – and take active steps to improve your connection. Bear in mind the quote by Robert Waldinger that 'those who were most satisfied in their relationships at age 50 were the healthiest at age 80'.
    Action: Reignite the fire in your relationship, making a good effort using the many ways I explore in this section. Work on your connection, your intimacy and your shared sense of purpose and goals.

20. **Revel in your gradually emptying nest before it fills up with grandchildren**
    Think about how you can morph your relationship with your children into a healthy adult one, setting new expectations of each other and building new bridges to connect.
    Reflection: Think about the new family habits and rituals you can put into practice to help your adult and gradually more independent children connect with you.

21. **Give your parents a good last leg**
    Reflect on what it means to you to be there for your parents as they age. Decide how you want to help them.
    Actions:
    - Have a conversation with your ageing parents about what ageing well means to them. Listen!
    - Work with your parents to ensure there is tidy paperwork in place. Wills, power of attorney documents, health directives, superannuation statements and other material

should all be brought together and organised so either parent can interact with the documents when needed.
- Have a hard talk about housing, including whether their home is a suitable place to age in – really!
- Prepare yourself for the fact that your parents will lose some of their financial literacy.
- Know your options for care services and exercise them early. Waitlists can be long!
- Find some things you can do with your parents. Have fun!

TRAVEL – AS MUCH AND AS FAR AS YOU CAN

22. Embrace challenge, adventure and active travel: understand your options

For me, this isn't just about the big, once-a-year family holiday. It's about separating travel and adventure and making sure both have a place in your life.

Actions:
- Make a bucket list of travel you want to do in your prime time years – sabbaticals, holidays, active adventures – then put them in priority order!
- Think about how you can get more incremental adventures into your life.

23. Seek out sabbaticals or 'golden gap years' – several times in your life

Really think about the difference a sabbatical might make in your life in allowing you time and space to step off the treadmill, gain clarity and explore.

Reflection: Contemplate the opportunities in your years ahead, when you might be able to do a sabbatical, and explore what types of sabbatical interest you.

24. Get better value when you travel

Having run a travel company for six years, I love to teach people how they can get better value when they travel, especially knowing what a huge role travel plays in most Prime Timers' happiness goals.

Actions:

- Consider your bucket list holidays, and break them into a strategic and opportunistic holidays list, considering all the holidays you want to take in your Prime Time.
- Reflect on how you'll use the tricks of the travel trade to get yourself better value when you travel.

25. Don't be afraid to go solo

Many people feel a bit hesitant about solo travel in their Prime Time, but there's no reason not to give it a go.

Reflection: Think about how you could embrace solo travel. Consider destinations, activities and the freedom solo travel offers. Take the first step by making some plans.

26. Understand travel money and insurance – and know what to watch out for

Explore the benefits of emerging travel money cards and make sure you're fully across your travel insurance before you buy it.

Actions:

- Review your travel insurance policy to confirm it covers not only your planned activities but also the entire length of your stay and any alcohol consumption. Understand exactly what you're covered for and where the gaps are.
- Look into travel money cards that offer convenience and savings, helping you manage your finances on the go more easily and affordably.

27. **Make your Prime Time count, and then have an Epic Retirement**

And finally, remember that this journey is yours to shape. Every choice, every goal and every step forward is about creating a life that feels authentically *you*. Embrace the possibilities, stay intentional with your time and resources, and invest in the people, experiences and values that truly matter. And seriously, get onto compound investing as early as you can. It's one of the best ways to build your future.

This is your Prime Time, so make it count. Then, when the time is right, and you finally do give up work forever, make sure you're ready for an Epic Retirement!

KEEP IN TOUCH

The Prime Time newsletter goes out weekly at primetimers.net.

You can listen to the *Prime Time* podcast by searching for 'Prime Time with Bec Wilson' wherever you get your podcasts.

My website has heaps of resources – and it will only get better. Visit becwilson.net and sign up for the resources, newsletters and tools on offer.

And you can always email me at bec@primetimers.net

Acknowledgements

WHEN I WROTE MY FIRST BOOK, *How to Have an Epic Retirement*, I WORKED quietly, with my dad and a couple of deeply trusted financial experts as my greatest helpers.

This time, my dad was still there, plugging away with me (thank you, Dad!), but it felt as though the collective light of Australia's finance sector was shining all around me, guiding the way. So many incredible people have helped me bring the insights in *Prime Time* to life – sharing their perspectives, listening to mine and helping to shape a conversation for a new generation of pre-retirees navigating a stage of life no one has truly prepared them for.

Being 50-ish in a post-superannuation world is unlike any midlife we've experienced before. It's a whole new stage of life, and one that deserves its own roadmap.

First, I owe a huge thank you to Sophie Hamley, my publisher and biggest supporter, along with the brilliant team at Hachette Australia who surround her. The concept for *Prime Time* grew from observing younger pre-retirees – those not quite ready for an Epic Retirement – seeking help and guidance in the same envelope. Over the past two years, through countless conversations about what people need to know, how life is evolving and how we can offer support, you've helped shape and hone this vision. Sophie, your belief in me means more than I can express.

To Luke, the cover designer, wow! You've outdone yourself again. What a cover! And to Jacquie Brown, the editor of this book, thank you for your skill and care in polishing my words. You managed to refine the manuscript beautifully without cutting too many of the (far more than contracted) words I handed over.

To everyone who has contributed to this journey, thank you for shining your light on this project. Your support has helped make *Prime Time* come to life.

This book tackles complex financial topics and trend analysis, subjects that no one should develop an opinion on in isolation. It would be unwise to do so when I have access to incredible subject matter experts who have spent decades working in the finance industry on behavioural data and policy. Their insights, guidance and willingness to review the material have been invaluable and I am deeply grateful for their support.

A special thanks goes to Aaron Minney at Challenger Financial Services for his profound insights into spending behaviours and longevity trends and for helping to tie the lessons of midlife into a coherent and practical framework. I'm also incredibly grateful to Mark Lapedus and Tim Hegarty at Allianz Retire+ for his expertise on longevity and for compiling data that demystifies life expectancy, making it both technically accurate and easy to digest. To Ian Fryer from Chant West – thank you for the sense-checking and shaping of our superannuation criteria for the Epic Retirement Tick. To Neville Azzopardi and Jen Harding – thanks for reviewing and guiding me on the constantly changing shape of the advice sector. And to Jason Hunt, Patrick Clarke, Jim Hennington, David Orford and Ben Hillier for sharing their insights into longevity solutions and the superannuation industry alongside many others who really know the underpinnings of the industry. Apologies if I've accidentally forgotten some of the many wonderful direct and indirect expert contributors along the way – please don't feel left out.

My heartfelt gratitude goes to David Lane from Ord Minnett. As an exceptionally experienced financial adviser and investment expert, he has been instrumental in refining the investing section of this book. His careful reviews have been invaluable, and he was the planner beside me, nudging them into real-feeling shape, calculating and checking the numbers behind the mock financial examples that are available for download with this book.

This book also delves into the travel sector, exploring how to travel well in ways that only industry insiders truly understand. For this, I've drawn not just on my own experiences but on the incredible knowledge of Fiona Dalton, a 30-plus year veteran of the travel industry who has more expertise in her little finger than I could ever hope to have.

Thank you, Fiona, for sharing your invaluable insights, lessons and stories as you navigate your own Prime Time. Your wisdom has added depth and richness to this book, and I'm so grateful for your generosity.

To Barry Bloch, one of my longest-standing mentors and a truly remarkable leader in championing third act careers and finding joy in your job, thank you. Your insights on the lattice have been invaluable and your encouragement to dive deeper into explaining it has truly enriched this work.

To the experts who've joined me on the *Prime Time with Bec Wilson* podcast over the past 18 months, thank you. You may not realise just how much your expertise has shaped the ideas and insights that have found their way into this book.

From Dr Ginni Mansberg on menopause, Carly Barlow on metabolic health, and Jonathan Freeman on exercise, diet and protein, to Dr Dan Blackmore on cognitive health and exercise, Brian Herd on legacy and Dr Nahum Kozak on relationships, and many, many more – your conversations have been invaluable. To all of you, thank you for leaning in, sharing your wisdom on the show and helping ensure that the voice of *Prime Time* is grounded in the best possible advice and insights.

Then there are the stories and storytellers. To Jane Tara and Tim Burrowes, thank you for sharing your unique perspectives, shaped by your own insights and journeys.

And to everyone who contributed or told me their stories (whether you realised it or not!), the many real-life Prime Timers in my world and my online community who have inspired this book simply by living meaningful and purposeful lives, thank you. I feel so lucky to know people like you who are redefining what the new midlife looks like, giving me the privilege of telling your stories. To Stuart, Sue-En, Therese, Fiona, Jillian, David, Barry, Sharon, Geoff, Annie, Jill, Carolyn, Susan, Greg, Wendy, Gary, and so many others ... thanks for being part of the story.

To the team at 9Podcasts – who brought the *Prime Time* podcast to life, knowing the conversations about midlife are changing, thanks! To my producers Genevieve Rule and Emilia Fuller, thanks for shaping it and me into the wonderful world of podcasting. To Mia and Sam and all the people at Nine who produce, sell and make the show, thanks for getting behind it and making it happen. And to the wonderful sponsors that support the show – a huge thank you.

To my editor at *The Age* and the *Sydney Morning Herald*, Dominic Powell, thanks for supporting my will to shape a conversation not just around retirement, but around this new generation of midlifers who want more and can actively strive for it financially.

And to the biggest contributors of all – the incredible community around me. We launched The Epic Retirement Newsletter in 2023 (Aussie and International editions now exist, can you believe), and both have grown at lightning speed. By early 2024, it inspired the creation of the *Prime Time* podcast, which is closing in on a million downloads as I write this, and The Epic Retirement Club on Facebook, a group that now includes hundreds of thousands of people worldwide, moderated by the most wonderful team of volunteers.

To the community: thank you for inspiring me to write this book.

To the moderators: an enormous thank you for everything you do. A special shoutout to David Halliday, who has taken on the role of chief moderator in ways I could never have imagined – it's more than I could have dreamed.

What struck me early on was that so many in this community, learning how to 'epic', aren't actually at retirement age. Instead, they're craving a Prime Time life, a phase of living that no one has really given them a language for.

So, this book is for you. For those who aren't ready for the 'R-word' but know there's more to life and want to embrace it fully. Thank you for being the heart of this journey.

Lastly, to my family and my best friends – my husband, Brett; my dad, Tony, and my three kids, Paris, Sienna and Reubs, as well as my wonderful extended family and friends cheer squad – Mum, Nanny, the Willos, Gaz and Jules, Sio and Simon and all my siblings. I couldn't do what I do without your constant support (okay, maybe I could, but let's face it – it wouldn't be nearly as much fun without knowing you're there to smile if it works and share in the stories). You are my rocks, my laughter and the reason this journey feels so worthwhile.

Thank you for embracing our adventure into Prime Time – with all its shifting goals, emptying nests, work dynamics, layered income streams, opportunities to travel and our shared hunger to be healthier and live life to the fullest. You inspire me every single day.

Endnotes

1 Life expectancies based on Australian Government Actuary, 'Australian Life Tables 2015–17', with 25-year mortality improvement factors.
2 Australian Institute of Health and Welfare (2023), *Australian Burden of Disease Study 2023*, AIHW.
3 Australian Government Actuary, 'Australian Life Tables 2015–17'.
4 DG Blanchflower and AJ Oswald, 'Is well-being U-shaped over the life cycle?' *Soc Sci Med*. 2008 Apr; 66(8): 1733–49. doi: 10.1016/j.socscimed.2008.01.030. Epub 2008 Mar 7. PMID: 18316146.
5 DG Blanchflower, 'Is happiness U-shaped everywhere? Age and subjective well-being in 145 countries', *J Popul Econ* 34, 575–624 (2021). doi.org/10.1007/s00148-020-00797-z
6 ET Berkman (2018), 'The neuroscience of goals and behavior change', *Consulting Psychology Journal*, 70(1):28–44.
7 Harvard Study of Adult Development. (n.d.). Retrieved from adultdevelopmentstudy.org.
8 McKinsey Health Institute (2023), 'Age is just a number: How older adults view healthy ageing', 22 May, mckinsey.com/mhi/our-insights/age-is-just-a-number-how-older-adults-view-healthy-aging#/ (viewed December 2024).
9 C Kidd and BY Hayden (2015), 'The psychology and neuroscience of curiosity', *Neuron*, 88(3): 449–60.
10 MC Schippers and N Ziegler (2019), 'Life crafting as a way to find purpose and meaning in life', *Frontiers in Psychology*, 10:2778.
11 LL Carstensen, (2011). *A Long Bright future: An action plan for a lifetime of happiness, health, and financial security*. PublicAffairs, New York.
12 Australian Bureau of Statistics (2022–23), Retirement and Retirement Intentions, Australia, ABS website, accessed 20 December 2024.
13 CareSuper (2024), 'Compare my spend', spiritsuper.com.au/Retirement/Compare-my-spend (viewed December 2024). The publicly available spending data used in this tool is provided by a major bank from the 2023 calendar year. All data used or represented is anonymised and aggregated before analysis. The spending data covers all digital transactions of de-identified bank

customers using the following payment methods: debit card, credit card, direct debit, BPAY transactions, ATM and POS cash withdrawals.
14 Association of Superannuation Funds of Australia (2024), 'The ASFA Retirement Standard', superannuation.asn.au/resources/retirement-standard (viewed December 2024).
15 Ibid.
16 T Lawless (2022), 'The long game … 30 years of housing values', CoreLogic, 29 August, corelogic.com.au/news-research/news/2022/the-long-game-30-years-of-housing-values (viewed December 2024).
17 Australian Bureau of Statistics (2022), 'Housing Occupancy and Costs', 25 May, abs.gov.au/statistics/people/housing/housing-occupancy-and-costs/latest-release (viewed December 2024).
18 Chant West (2023/24), 'Retirement ratings'.
19 Australian Government Actuary, 'Australian Life Tables 2015–17'.
20 Figures provided by Optimum Pensions. The table uses the latest Australian Life Tables (ALT2020-22) and the 25-year improvement rates. The figures reflect the full Australian population including all health states, lifestyles and socio-economic groups. The 25-year improvement rates are generally more conservative in the context of financial planning. Ages have been rounded up.
21 F Modigliani and R Brumberg (1954), 'Utility analysis and the consumption function: An interpretation of cross-section data', in KK Kurihara (ed.), *Post-Keynesian Economics*, Rutgers University Press, New York.
22 A Minney, *Adding Direction to the Consumption Rate in Retirement*, The Journal of Retirement, Vol. 5, No. 1 (2017), pp. 106–116. Available at: https://www.pm-research.com/content/iijretire/5/1/106
23 Figures were provided by Optimum Pensions. The table uses the latest Australian Life Tables (ALT2020-22) and the 25-year improvement rates. The figures reflect the full Australian population including all health states, lifestyles and socio-economic groups. The 25-year improvement rates are generally more conservative in the context of financial planning. Ages have been rounded up.
24 DG Blanchflower and AJ Oswald, 'Is well-being U-shaped over the life cycle?' Soc Sci Med. 2008 Apr; 66(8): 1733–49. doi: 10.1016/j.socscimed.2008.01.030. Epub 2008 Mar 7. PMID: 18316146.
25 LL Carstensen, DM Isaacowitz and ST Charles (1999), 'Taking time seriously: A theory of socioemotional selectivity', *American Psychologist*, 54(3): 165–81.
26 P Moen (2016), *Encore Adulthood: Boomers on the edge of risk, renewal and purpose*, Oxford University Press, Oxford, p. 29.
27 M Goldberg et al. (2007), 'Cohort profile: The GAZEL Cohort Study', *International Journal of Epidemiology*, 36(1): 32–9.

28 HS Friedman and LR Martin (2011), *The Longevity Project: Surprising discoveries for health and long life from the landmark eight-decade study*, Hudson Street Press/Penguin Group USA.
29 A Colby et al, (2017), Purpose in the encore years: Shaping lives of meaning and contribution', Encore.org, cogenerate.org/wp-content/uploads/2022/09/PEP-Full-Report.pdf (viewed December 2024).
30 MEP Seligman (2011), *Flourish: A visionary new understanding of happiness and well-being*, Atria Books; M Csikszentmihalyi (1990), *Flow: The psychology of optimal experience*, Harper & Row.
31 RJ Waldinger and MS Schulz (2016), *The Good Life: Lessons from the longest study on happiness*, Harvard University Press.
32 D Buettner (2008), *The Blue Zones: Lessons for living longer from the people who've lived the longest*, National Geographic Books.
33 W Bridges (2004), *Transitions: Making sense of life's changes*, Da Capo Press.
34 BS McEwen, In pursuit of resilience: stress, epigenetics, and brain plasticity', *Ann N Y Acad Sci*. 2016 Jun;1373(1):56-64. doi: 10.1111/nyas.13020. Epub 2016 Feb 25. PMID: 26919273.
35 WJ Kraemer and NA Ratamess (2005), 'Hormonal responses and adaptations to resistance exercise and training', *Sports Medicine*, 35(4): 339–61.
36 *Journal of the International Society of Sports Nutrition*. (n.d.). Effects of protein intake on testosterone levels. Retrieved 20 December 2024, from medshun.com/article/does-protein-effect-testosterone-levels
37 Stephan, Blossom CM et al (2024), 'Population attributable fractions of modifiable risk factors for dementia: a systematic review and meta-analysis', *The Lancet Healthy Longevity*, Volume 5, Issue 6, e406–e421.
38 The Lancet Commission on Dementia Prevention, Intervention, and Care. Dementia prevention, intervention, and care: 2020 report. *The Lancet*, 2020; 396(10248): 413-446. DOI: 10.1016/S0140-6736(20)30367-6.
39 DA Sinclair and MD LaPlante (2019), *Lifespan: Why we age – and why we don't have to*, Atria Books.
40 C López-Otín, MA Blasco, L Partridge, M Serrano, G Kroemer, ' The hallmarks of aging', *Cell*. 2013;153(6):1194-1217. DOI: 10.1016/j.cell.2013.05.039.
41 J Campisi, P Kapahi, GJ Lithgow, S Melov, JC Newman, E Verdin, 'From discoveries in ageing research to therapeutics for healthy ageing', *Nature*. 2019;571(7764): 183–192. DOI: 10.1038/s41586-019-1365-2.
42 DA Sinclair and MD LaPlante (2019), *Lifespan: Why We Age – and Why We Don't Have To*. Atria Books, New York.
43 VD Longo (2018), *The Longevity Diet: Slow Aging, Fight Disease, Optimize Weight*, Avery, New York.

44 JA Mattison et al (2017), 'Caloric restriction improves health and survival of rhesus monkeys', *Nature Communications*, 8(1): 14063.
45 L Fontana, L Partridge and VD Longo (2010), 'Extending Healthy Life Span: From yeast to humans', *Science*, 328(5976): 321–26.
46 VD Longo and MP Mattson (2014), 'Fasting: Molecular mechanisms and clinical applications', *Cell Metabolism*, 19(2): 181–92.
47 MP Mattson et al (2017), 'Impact of intermittent fasting on health and disease processes', *Ageing Research Reviews*, 39: 46–58.
48 S Imai and DA Sinclair (2016), 'NAD+ and sirtuins in aging and disease', *Trends in Cell Biology*, 26(8): 583–95.
49 E Verdin (2015), 'NAD+ in aging, metabolism, and neurodegeneration', *Science*, 350(6265): 1208–13.
50 DG Blackmore et al (2024), 'Long-term improvement in hippocampal-dependent learning ability in healthy, aged individuals following high intensity interval training', *Aging and Disease*.
51 DA Hood et al (2019), 'Maintenance of skeletal muscle mitochondrial function in health, exercise, and aging', *Annual Review of Physiology*, 81: 19–41.
52 LM McMorris and MS Howard (2017), 'Aerobic exercise and neuroplasticity: A review of the evidence', *Neuroscience & Biobehavioral Reviews*, 83: 1–15.
53 Blackmore et al (2024), 'Long-term improvement in hippocampal-dependent learning ability'.
54 MG Benedetti et al (2018), 'The effectiveness of physical exercise on bone density in osteoporotic patients', *BioMed Research International*.
55 Buettner, *The Blue Zones*.
56 A Duncan (2024), 'How much does private health insurance cost', Canstar, 30 July, canstar.com.au/health-insurance/what-does-health-insurance-cost (viewed December 2024).
57 R Waldinger et al (2017), 'The Harvard Study of Adult Development: Lessons from the longest study on happiness and human flourishing', *Harvard Gazette*.
58 R Waldinger (2015), 'What makes a good life? Lessons from the longest study on happiness', TED, November, ted.com/talks/robert_waldinger_what_makes_a_good_life_lessons_from_the_longest_study_on_happiness?subtitle=en (viewed December 2024).
59 A Sic, K Cvetkovic, E Manchanda and NN Knezevic, 'Neurobiological Implications of Chronic Stress and Metabolic Dysregulation in Inflammatory Bowel Diseases', *Diseases* 2024, 12, 220. doi.org/10.3390/diseases12090220
60 G MacDonald, KD Locke, SS Spielmann and S Joel (2012), 'Insecure attachment predicts ambivalent social threat and reward perceptions in romantic relationships', *Journal of Social and Personal Relationships, 30*(5), 647–661. doi.org/10.1177/0265407512465221.

61 J Gottman and N Silver (1999), *The Seven Principles for Making Marriage Work*, Harmony Books; J Gottman and J DeClaire (2011), *The Science of Trust: Emotional attunement for couples*, W.W. Norton & Company, New York.

62 CA Sanderson and FC Dickson (1996), 'Maintenance of romantic relationships: An analysis of individual and dyadic strategies', *Journal of Social and Personal Relationships*, 13(4): 489–506.

63 Gottman and Silver, *The Seven Principles for Making Marriage Work*.

64 WB Wilcox and J Dew (2012), *The Date Night Opportunity: What does couple time tell us about the quality of relationships?*, The National Marriage Project.

65 A Aron (2000), 'Couples' shared participation in novel and arousing activities and experienced relationship quality', *Journal of Personality and Social Psychology*, 78(2): 273–84.

66 Aron, Arthur & Norman, Christina & Aron, Elaine & McKenna, Colin & Heyman, Richard. (2000). 'Couples' shared participation in novel and arousing activities and experienced relationship quality,' *Journal of personality and social psychology*, 78. 273-84. 10.1037//0022-3514.78.2.273.

67 J Gottman and J DeClaire (2002), *The Relationship Cure: A 5 step guide to strengthening your marriage, family, and friendships*, Three Rivers Press, New York.

68 NK Schlossberg (2009), *Revitalizing Retirement: Reshaping your identity, relationships, and purpose*, American Psychological Association.

69 NK Schlossberg (1989), *Overwhelmed: Coping with life's ups and downs*, Lexington Books, Maryland.

70 JJ Arnett (2004), *Emerging Adulthood: The winding road from the late teens through the twenties*, Oxford University Press, Oxford.

71 SM Gorchoff, JM Pasupathi and LL Carstensen (2008), 'Dyadic adjustment and changes in life satisfaction during the empty nest transition: A longitudinal study', *Journal of Marriage and Family*, 70(2): 373–82.

72 KJ Gamble et al (2015), 'How does ageing affect financial decision making?', no. 15-1, Center for Retirement Research, Boston College, USA.